Medical Microbiology *Volume 4*

Medical Microbiology *Volume 4*

edited by

C. S. F. EASMON
Department of Medical Microbiology
Wright Fleming Institute
St Mary's Hospital Medical School
London, UK

J. JELJASZEWICZ
National Institute of Hygiene
Warsaw, Poland

ACADEMIC PRESS · 1984

(Harcourt Brace Jovanovich, Publishers)

London · Orlando · San Diego · New York
Toronto · Montreal · Sydney · Tokyo

ACADEMIC PRESS INC. (LONDON) LTD.
24-28 Oval Road,
London NW1 7DX

United States Edition published by
ACADEMIC PRESS, INC.
Orlando, Florida 32887

British Library Cataloguing in Publication Data

Medical microbiology.—Vol. 4
    1. Medical microbiology
    616.01'05   QR46

ISBN 0−12−228004−0

LCCCN 83-71539

PRINTED IN THE UNITED STATES OF AMERICA

84 85 86 87   9 8 7 6 5 4 3 2 1

Contributors

D. Armstrong
Infectious Disease Service
Memorial Sloan-Kettering Cancer
Center
New York, New York 10021, USA
and Cornell University Medical
College
New York, New York 10021, USA

D. P. Bonner
The Squibb Institute for Medical
Research
Princeton, New Jersey 08540, USA

P. J. Chesney
Department of Pediatrics
Clinical Science Center
University of Wisconsin Center for
Health Sciences
Madison, Wisconsin 53792, USA

G. W. Csonka
St Stephen's Hospital
Chelsea, London SW10 9TH, UK

J. P. Davis
Acute and Communicable Disease
Epidemiology Section
Department of Health and Social
Services
Division of Health, State of
Wisconsin
Madison, Wisconsin 53701, USA

C. S. F. Easmon
Department of Medical Microbiology
Wright Fleming Institute
St Mary's Hospital Medical School
London W2 1PG, UK

C. G. Gemmell
Department of Bacteriology
University of Glasgow
Royal Infirmary
Glasgow G4 0SF, Scotland, UK

S. Hafiz
Department of Medical Microbiology
The University of Sheffield Medical
School
Sheffield S10 2RX, UK

C. A. Ison
Department of Medical Microbiology
Wright Fleming Institute
St Mary's Hospital Medical School
London W2 1PG, UK

G. R. Kinghorn
Department of Genitourinary
Medicine
The Royal Hallamshire Hospital
Sheffield S10 2JF, UK

M. G. McEntegart
Department of Medical Microbiology
The University of Sheffield Medical
School
Sheffield S10 2RX, UK

M. B. Skirrow
Worcester Royal Infirmary
Worcester WRI 3AS, UK

S. L. Squires
Research Laboratories
May and Baker Ltd.
Dagenham, Essex, UK

R. B. Sykes
The Squibb Institute for Medical
Research
Princeton, New Jersey 08540, USA

T. J. Trust
Department of Biochemistry and
Microbiology
University of Victoria
Victoria, British Columbia V8W 2Y2,
Canada

A. S. Tyms
Department of Medical Microbiology
Division of Virology
Wright Fleming Institute
St Mary's Hospital Medical School
London W2 1PG, UK

D. van der Waaij
Laboratory for Medical Microbiology
University Hospital
9713 EZ Groningen, The Netherlands

J. M. Vergeront
Acute and Communicable Disease
Epidemiology Section
Department of Health and Social
Services
Division of Health, State of
Wisconsin
Madison, Wisconsin 53701, USA

T. Wadström
Department of Bacteriology and
Epizootology
College of Veterinary Medicine
Swedish University of Agricultural
Sciences
Biomedicum
S-751 23 Uppsala, Sweden

J. D. Williamson
Department of Medical Microbiology
Division of Virology
Wright Fleming Institute
St Mary's Hospital Medical School
London W2 1PG, UK

Preface

With Volume 4 the series returns to the multi-theme format. Toxic-shock syndrome is yet another "new" bacterial disease which has taught us a number of lessons in pathogenicity and epidemiology. A few years ago campylobacter infections were at a similar stage but they have perhaps now come of age. Four of the chapters deal with sexually transmitted or associated infections, including acquired immune deficiency syndrome, while a further four are concerned with antimicrobial agents, but from very different angles. The final chapter is a comprehensive review of bacterial surface lectins and their role in adherence and pathogenicity.

Charles Easmon   *Janusz Jeljaszewicz*
                                                        September 1984

Contents

Contents of Volume 1

Contents of Volume 2

Immunization Against Bacterial Disease

Contents of Volume 3

Role of the Envelope in the Survival of Bacteria in Infection

1 Toxic-shock syndrome— epidemiology, pathogenesis, clinical findings and management

JEFFREY P. DAVIS, P. JOAN CHESNEY
and JAMES M. VERGERONT

I. INTRODUCTION

Toxic-shock syndrome (TSS) is a term ascribed to an acute illness characterized by rapid onset of fever, hypotension, headache, myalgia, vomiting and diarrhea, mucous membrane hyperemia, laboratory evidence of multiple organ system dysfunction, and an erythematous rash with subsequent desquamation particularly on the palms and soles (Todd *et al.*, 1978). The spectrum of severity for TSS is broad, and fatalities do occur. Currently, a confirmatory test for TSS is not available and the diagnosis must be based on the typical constellation of abnormal clinical and laboratory findings (Davis *et al.*, 1980; Shands *et al.*, 1980). A strong correlation exists between the occurrence of TSS and the presence of *Staphylococcus aureus* during the acute phase of illness (Davis *et al.*, 1980; Shands *et al.*, 1980; Todd *et al.*, 1978), particularly strains of *S. aureus* that produce a marker protein or toxin called staphylococcal enterotoxin F (SEF) and pyrogenic exotoxin C (PEC) (Bergdoll *et al.*, 1981; Schlievert *et al.*, 1981). Although TSS does occasionally occur in males and nonmenstruating females, it most frequently occurs in conjunction with active menstruation in previously healthy women who have been using tampons (Davis *et al.*, 1980; Shands *et al.*, 1980).

II. HISTORY

Illnesses resembling TSS have been sporadically reported in the medical literature as far back as 1927 (Stevens, 1927). Todd *et al.* (1978) first used the term

Medical Microbiology, 4
ISBN 0-12-228004-0

toxic-shock syndrome to describe 3 males and 4 females aged 8 to 17 years who presented with acute onset of fever, headache, sore throat, erythroderma, diarrhea, refractory hypotension, confusion and laboratory evidence of acute renal failure and hepatic dysfunction. Six of the patients had desquamation of the palms and soles during convalescence; the seventh patient died during the acute illness. The illness in these patients was associated with strains of *S. aureus* of phage group I that produced a unique epidermal toxin.

Between July 1979 and January 1980, 7 patients with signs and symptoms similar to those reported by Todd were hospitalized in Madison, Wisconsin; 6 patients were menstruating at the time of onset of illness, and 1 was premenstrual (Davis *et al.*, 1980). In Minnesota, 5 patients with similar illnesses were hospitalized between December 1979 and January 1980; all 5 also had onset of illness during menstruation (Minnesota Department of Health, 1980; Schrock, 1980). State health officials reported these cases and the apparent association of illness with menses to the Centers for Disease Control (CDC) in January 1980 (Shands *et al.*, 1980). Over the succeeding months, both the public and the medical community interest in TSS began to grow. Requests for TSS case reports from physicians and newspaper publicity on TSS resulted in the reporting of cases by the public and physicians to state health departments (Davis and Vergeront, 1982).

In May 1980, the CDC reported on the case findings of 55 confirmed cases of TSS that had been reported nationally; this publication stimulated further nationwide reporting of TSS (Centers for Disease Control, 1980a). By June 1980, case-control studies completed by state health departments in Wisconsin (Davis *et al.*, 1980) and Utah (Kehrberg *et al.*, 1981) and by the CDC (Shands *et al.*, 1980) had statistically linked the onset of menstrual TSS with the use of tampons. In September 1980 the CDC reported that women using Rely® (Procter & Gamble Company) brand tampons were at a greater relative risk of developing TSS than those using other tampon brands, but that users of all brands had developed TSS (Centers for Disease Control, 1980b; Schlech *et al.*, 1982). Rely® was voluntarily withdrawn from the market by its manufacturer in September 1980. Subsequently, a case-control study involving collaborators in Minnesota, Wisconsin and Iowa, known as the Tri-State TSS Study, showed that the relative risk of developing TSS increases with increasing tampon absorbency, and that Rely® tampons were associated with a risk greater than that predicted by absorbency alone (Osterholm *et al.*, 1982a). Recommendations and health warnings that have incorporated the findings of these studies have been widely publicized (Institute of Medicine, 1982). Although there has been a decrease in the nationally reported incidence of TSS noted since November 1980, cases continue to occur in men and women in a variety of clinical settings (Centers for Disease Control, 1982a).

During the time these epidemiologic studies were being conducted, laboratory-based studies were under way to identify the etiologic agent of TSS. Pursuant to the original suggestion of Todd *et al.* (1978) that TSS was associated with *S. aureus* of phage group I that produced a unique epidermal toxin, bacterial studies established that a majority of patients with menstrual TSS had vaginal or cervical colonization with *S. aureus* (Davis *et al.*, 1980; Shands *et al.*, 1980). A study comparing patients with menstrual TSS to healthy menstruating women demonstrated a statistical correlation between illness onset and vaginal colonization with *S. aureus* (Shands *et al.*, 1980). Bergdoll *et al.* (1981) and Schlievert *et al.* (1981) isolated protein products from *S. aureus* strains that were obtained from TSS patients. Bergdoll described an enterotoxin-like protein called staphylococcal enterotoxin F (SEF) and noted that patients with acute TSS had low levels of antibody to SEF (anti-SEF) when compared to healthy and ill (non-TSS) controls. Schlievert *et al.* described a pyrogenic exotoxin labeled pyrogenic exotoxin C (PEC). SEF and PEC have been demonstrated to be antigenically identical (Melish *et al.*, 1982). Recent studies have demonstrated that SEF administered intravenously to female baboons will produce a majority of clinical manifestations of TSS seen in humans (Quimby *et al.*, 1984).

While no common name for these proteins has as yet been referenced in the literature, in all likelihood SEF and PEC will be renamed toxic-shock toxin. When the terms SEF and PEC are not used in this chapter, we have elected to use the term TSS toxin or toxin to refer to that staphylococcal protein produced by TSS-associated strains thought to be responsible for the clinical and laboratory manifestations of TSS.

III. EPIDEMIOLOGY

A. Surveillance and incidence

Statewide surveillances for TSS in the United States were first instituted in Wisconsin and Minnesota in January 1980 (Davis *et al.*, 1980; Osterholm and Forfang, 1982) and in Utah shortly thereafter (Kehrberg *et al.*, 1981). Passive surveillance activities in other states and in other countries began later, following the first national communications on TSS. In 1981, several states adopted TSS as an officially reportable disease, and by 1982, TSS was listed as a nationally reportable disease (Centers for Disease Control, 1982b).

For the purposes of surveillance and epidemiologic study, a case of TSS was considered to be confirmed if it met established diagnostic criteria (Davis *et al.*, 1980, 1982a; Reingold *et al.*, 1982c; Shands *et al.*, 1980) (Table I). A case was considered to be probable if it were one criterion short of meeting the definition for a confirmed case. Through March 26, 1983, a total of 2010 confirmed cases in the United States had been reported to the CDC. Of these cases, 1931 (96%)

Table 1 Toxic-shock syndrome case definition[a]

1. Fever—temperature ≥ 38.9°C (102°F)
2. Rash (diffuse macular erythroderma)
3. Desquamation, 1–2 weeks after onset of illness, particularly of palms and soles.
4. Hypotension (systolic blood pressure ≤ 90 mm Hg for adults or < 5th percentile by age for children < 16 years of age, or orthostatic syncope)
5. Involvement of three or more of the following organ systems:
   A. Gastrointestinal (vomiting or diarrhea at onset of illness)
   B. Muscular (severe myalgia or creatine phosphokinase level ≥2 × ULN[b])
   C. Mucous membrane (vaginal, oropharyngeal, or conjunctival hyperemia)
   D. Renal (BUN[c] or Cr[d] ≥ 2 × ULN or ≥ 5 white blood cells per high-power field—in the absence of a urinary-tract infection)
   E. Hepatic (total bilirubin, SGOT[e] or SGPT[f] ≥ 2 × ULN)
   F. Hematologic (platelets ≤ 100,000/mm³)
   G. Central nervous system (disorientation or alterations in consciousness without focal neurologic signs when fever and hypotension are absent)
6. Negative results on the following tests, if obtained:
   A. Blood, throat, or cerebrospinal fluid cultures
   B. Serologic tests for Rocky Mountain spotted fever, leptospirosis, or measles

---

[a] Original case definition. These criteria were modified in the summer of 1981 so that orthostatic dizziness is accepted as evidence of hypotension, and patients with *S. aureus* bacteremia are included as cases if they otherwise meet the case definition. A case is "confirmed" if it meets all the criteria, and "probable" if it is missing one of them. (Desquamation is unnecessary in fatal cases.) (Centers for Disease Control, 1980b.)
[b] Greater than or equal to twice the upper limits of normal for laboratory.
[c] Blood urea nitrogen level.
[d] Creatinine level.
[e] Serum glutamic oxaloacetic transaminase level.
[f] Serum glutamic pyruvic transaminase level.

had occurred in women. Of cases in women in which the menstrual history was known, 91% occurred during menstruation; and of these women in whom tampon use could be assessed, 99% were associated with tampon use. Of the total cases, 247 (12%) were definitely not associated with menstruation; 79 of the nonmenstrual cases occurred in men (A. L. Reingold, personal communication, May 9, 1983).

Prior to the report by Todd *et al.* (1978) few reports of TSS-like illness were made (Aranow and Wood, 1942; Dunnet and Schallibaum, 1960; Stevens, 1927). In Colorado, a review of medical records of patients 1 month to 30 years was made in two hospitals serving two separate communities (Wiesenthal *et al.*, 1982). Based on this review, the incidence of confirmed TSS in these two communities was equal in males and females and was at least 3 cases/100,000 population for each of the years 1970 to 1978. In one city, the male incidence increased to 7 cases/100,000 population in 1979, and the female incidence increased to 12 cases/100,000 population in 1980. Estimates of TSS incidence in 1980 in a variety of states and nationally ranged from 6 to 14 cases/100,000 menstruating women (Davis *et al.*, 1980; Kehrberg *et al.*, 1981; Osterholm and Forfang, 1982).

As depicted in Fig. 1, there was a rapid rise in 1980 and an ensuing rapid decline in the number of confirmed TSS cases reported nationally (Centers for Disease Control, 1982a). Numerous factors have been reported to have potentially affected the occurrence and reporting of TSS (Centers for Disease Control, 1981; Davis and Vergeront, 1982); these include (1) tampon-associated factors such as changes in the number of women using tampons and their wearing habits, the composition of tampons, and the withdrawal of Rely® brand tampons from the market, (2) surveillance-associated factors such as changes in the intensity and type of surveillance (i.e., active versus passive), media publicity regarding TSS, and the source of reports (i.e., patient or self-reported cases versus physician-reported cases), (3) public health–associated factors such as changes in the public and medical communities' awareness of TSS and earlier recognition and treatment of suspect cases of TSS leading to a reduction in the number of cases that fulfill the case definition, and (4) changes in the distribution of PEC- and

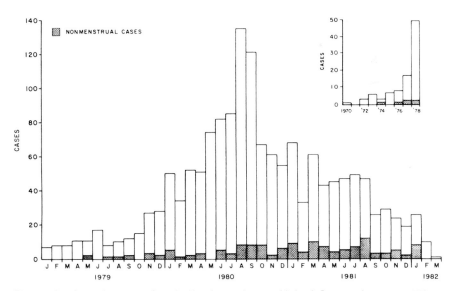

Fig. 1 Confirmed cases of toxic-shock syndrome, United States, January 1970 to March 1982 (reports received through April 9, 1982) (Centers for Disease Control, 1982a).

SEF-producing strains of *S. aureus* and in the general population's immunity against PEC and SEF.

During September and October 1980, there was considerable media publicity regarding TSS, in part because of the established association of TSS with menses and with tampon use. In Wisconsin, where surveillance was basically passive with a focal active component, one study demonstrated that intense publicity regarding TSS may have resulted in the increased number of reported TSS cases that occurred in August and September 1980 (Davis and Vergeront, 1982). During periods of peak publicity, a large number of patients self-reported their illness to the state health department. In Minnesota, where the degree of active surveillance was not changed during the 9 months prior to and the 9 months following the voluntary removal of Rely® brand tampons from the market in September 1980, no change was noted in the incidence of TSS (Osterholm and Forfang, 1982). Based on this active surveillance data, the incidence throughout this 18-month interval in Minnesota was roughly 8.9 cases/100,000 menstruating women.

While cases of TSS have been reported in every state of the United States, significant differences in the incidence of TSS are noted between states. Through April 9, 1982, five states—Wisconsin, Minnesota, Colorado, Utah and California—accounted for 44% of the total reported cases, although they represent only 16% of the United States population (Centers for Disease Control, 1982a). Intensified surveillance activities may be a factor contributing to these incidence differences, as the health departments and some of the universities in these states are very active in TSS investigation. In addition, regional differences in the degree of immunity against TSS toxin and in the distribution of toxin-producing organisms may be an important factor.

As of November 1981, more than 150 confirmed cases of TSS had been reported from other countries, including Australia, Canada, Denmark, Finland, France, Iceland, the Netherlands, New Zealand, Norway, Scotland, South Africa, Sweden, the United Kingdom, and West Germany (Institute of Medicine, 1982). When documented, the degree of menses association, tampon association, and the production of SEF or PEC by *S. aureus* strains obtained from these patients is comparable to that noted in the United States (Institute of Medicine, 1982). Active surveillance for TSS is not conducted in these countries, and their reported incidence rates are lower than those of the United States. However, the reported incidence of TSS through 1981 in Sweden approached that noted in the United States (Institute of Medicine, 1982). Surveillance factors affecting differences in the reported incidence of TSS in the United States are also operant in other countries. In addition, in contrast to the United States, where tampons account for 70% of the catamenial product usage, in most countries they represent less than 30% of the usage (Institute of Medicine, 1982).

B. Risk factors in menstrual TSS

Most confirmed cases of TSS occurred in healthy white menstruating women who were using tampons at the time of onset of illness. The combination of risk factors predisposing to this occurrence is complex.

1. Age

The age range of patients with menstrual TSS is 11–61 years, with a mean of 22.6 years (Reingold et al., 1982c); of the menstrual cases, 65% occurred in women less than 25 years old, and over one-third occurred in women 15–19 years old. The age-adjusted incidence of menstrual TSS in Wisconsin among menstruating white women who used tampons for 1980–1981 is depicted in Fig. 2. Patients with nonmenstrual TSS tend to be significantly older (mean 27 years) than patients with menstrual TSS (mean 22.6 years) (Reingold et al., 1982c).

2. Race

Since the early case series, it has been apparent that TSS occurs predominantly in whites; nationally, 97% of menstrual TSS cases have occurred in whites who comprise 83% of the U.S. population. However, this racial difference is not as marked for nonmenstrual TSS, where whites account for 87% of the cases (Reingold et al., 1982c). Disparity in the racial incidences of menstrual TSS may be due in part to age-specific differences in natural immunity or differences in menstrually related practices (Irwin and Millstein, 1982); reduced access to medical care and diagnostic difficulties are not likely to account for this racial disparity (Institute of Medicine, 1982). Similar racial differences are noted for cases of (menstrual) TSS occurring outside of the United States.

3. Menstruation and tampon use

Subsequent to the initial association of TSS with menstruation (Davis et al., 1980), all series have demonstrated that a high proportion of TSS cases have onset during menses (P. J. Chesney et al., 1981; Fisher et al., 1981; Helms et al., 1981; McKenna et al., 1980; Shands et al., 1980; Tofte and Williams, 1981a). All six of the case-control studies designed to assess risk factors in menstrual TSS have demonstrated that wearing tampons is associated with an increased risk of acquiring TSS (Davis et al., 1980; Helgerson and Foster, 1982; Kehrberg et al., 1981; Osterholm et al., 1982a; Schlech et al., 1982; Shands et al., 1980). In these studies at least 97% of the cases, as compared to 76–89% of matched controls, wore tampons during the period associated with illness onset. These studies used varying designs to select matched controls (best friend, neighborhood, clinic) and to match for menses. Although each study had different strengths, weaknesses and biases, the association of illness with tampon usage was found to be significant in each study. A comprehensive review of these case-

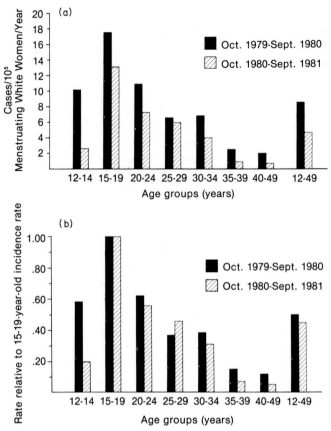

Fig. 2 (a) Age-specific incidence rates of toxic-shock syndrome in menstruating white women in Wisconsin during a 2-year period, October 1979–September 1981. (b) Relative age-specific incidence of toxic-shock syndrome. The relative rate among the highest incidence group, 15- to 19-year-old menstruating white women, was assigned as 1.0. Rates for each other age groups are expressed in relation to the relative rate for 15- to 19-year-old menstruating white women.

control studies concluded that the use of tampons is an adequate explanation for the excess risk of TSS in women over men, and that discontinuance of the use of tampons would be expected to reduce the incidence of TSS by 80–90% (Stallones, 1982).

The second CDC case-control study completed in September 1980 reported that the use of Rely® brand tampons was associated with a greater relative risk of developing menstrual TSS than the use of other brands, but that cases of TSS had occurred with the use of all brands (Schlech *et al.*, 1982). That study led to the voluntary withdrawal of Rely® tampons from the market by the manufacturer.

Subsequently, the Tri-State TSS Study demonstrated that the relative risk of developing menstrual TSS was 18-fold greater among women who used tampons versus those who did not use tampons, and that this risk varied between brands from 5.3 to 27.5 (Osterholm *et al.*, 1982a). In addition, the Tri-State TSS Study found that the best predictor for the risk of acquiring TSS was tampon absorbency: the greater the absorbency of the tampon, the greater the risk of acquiring TSS. In that study, the TSS risk associated with the use of Rely® brand tampons was significantly greater than that predicted by absorbency alone.

The precise mechanism by which tampons are associated with TSS is not known, nor is it clear why increased absorbency is significant. The Tri-State TSS Study was unable to separate the TSS risk associated with the chemical composition of tampons from the risk associated with absorbency. *In vitro* studies have demonstrated that specific tampon components may affect the ability of TSS-associated strains of *S. aureus* to produce and release SEF (Lee and Crass, 1983).

While the first CDC case-control study suggested that continuous use of tampons was associated with a greater risk of TSS than noncontinuous use (Shands *et al.*, 1980), the Tri-State TSS Study demonstrated that noncontinuous use was as significant as continuous use (Osterholm *et al.*, 1982a). No studies have demonstrated an association between TSS and the frequency of changing tampons. Cases of TSS have been associated with the use of sea sponges as catamenial devices; however, the risk of TSS developing in women who use sea sponges has not been evaluated in relation to the use of other tampons, napkins, or other catamenial products (Institute of Medicine, 1982; Smith *et al.*, 1982).

Diaphragms are used not only as contraceptive devices, but also to control menstrual flow. Sporadic reports of TSS associated with diaphragm use have appeared (Alcid *et al.*, 1982; Beahler *et al.*, 1982; DeYoung *et al.*, 1982). In these reports, diaphragms had been used for intervals ranging from 9 to 72 hours prior to onset of illness.

4. Other factors

Two early studies noted that fewer cases than controls practiced contraception (Davis *et al.*, 1980; Shands *et al.*, 1980). This difference in the overall use of contraceptive methods was not substantiated in the Tri-State TSS Study; however, this study did demonstrate that among those individuals using contraceptives, fewer cases (36%) than controls (61%) used oral contraceptives (Osterholm *et al.*, 1982a). This finding supported an earlier suggestion that oral contraceptive steroids may have an affect on vaginal *S. aureus* strains that produce a TSS-associated toxin (Davis *et al.*, 1980). Additional significant findings in the Tri-State TSS Study were: more cases than controls had a history of vaginitis in the year prior to onset of TSS; more cases than controls reported illness characterized by fever, diarrhea, dizziness, and vomiting during the menstrual period preceding the period associated with illness; and fewer cases than controls reported leisure-time exercise activities (Osterholm *et al.*, 1982a). Other factors such as sexual activities, douching, use of other vaginal products, types of clothing and various personal hygiene practices have not been shown to be significantly associated with TSS (Osterholm *et al.*, 1982a).

C. Nonmenstrual TSS and risk factors associated with nonmenstrual TSS

As of April 1982, 154 confirmed nonmenstrual cases of TSS had been reported to the CDC (Centers for Disease Control, 1982a). The age range of these patients was 1–75 years. Previously, the mean age for both males and females with nonmenstrual TSS was reported to be 26.8 years (Reingold *et al.*, 1982c). With the exception of recurrences, the clinical findings and complications in these patients were virtually identical to those patients with menstrual TSS. In 1981, the case fatality ratio in nonmenstrual TSS of roughly 6.0% was higher than the rate of 3.1% noted for menstrual TSS. The case fatility ratio has decreased over time for both entities. As the incidence of reported menstrual TSS has decreased, the relative proportion of nonmenstrual TSS reported to the CDC has increased (Centers for Disease Control, 1982a). Nonmenstrual TSS cases were associated with nonsurgical cutaneous and subcutaneous lesions (30%), childbirth or abortion (27%), surgical wound infections (18%), vaginal infections occurring at times other than during menstruation or the postpartum interval (5%), other sources of infection (6%) and unknown sources of infection (14%). The *S. aureus* strains obtained from infected sites in nonmenstrual TSS patients were similar to the strains obtained from menstrual TSS cases regarding antibiotic sensitivity, phage type and toxin production (Reingold *et al.*, 1982b).

Among 16 patients with postpartum TSS, none of 5 patients with onset early during the postpartum interval used tampons, but 10 of 11 patients with illness onset 2 or more weeks after delivery used tampons to control postpartum spotting or lochia flow (Reingold *et al.*, 1982b). Of the 17 cases of TSS associated with surgical wound infection, 10 occurred in women; 3 of these occurred postoperatively during menstruation, but were associated with wound cultures positive with *S. aureus* and vaginal cultures negative for *S. aureus*. To date, TSS has been reported after a wide variety of surgical procedures including spinal fusion, herniorrhaphy, reduction and augmentation mammoplasty, tubal ligation, arthroscopy, uterolithotomy, partial pleurectomy, nasal repair, joint repair, and cyst enucleation (Reingold *et al.*, 1982b). Nonmenstrual TSS has also been associated with a variety of deep-tissue staphylococcal infections including lymphadenitis, osteomyelitis, empyema, septic arthritis (Reingold *et al.*, 1982a,b), and pilonidal abscess (Cobb *et al.*, 1982); however, relatively few cases of TSS have been associated with deep-tissue infections. Typically, the surgical wounds associated with postoperative TSS have minimal or absent signs of inflammation but the lesions are colonized with strains of *S. aureus* that produce TSS-associated toxin. The interval from the specific operative or reference event to the onset of illness in nonmenstrual TSS is usually short, roughly 12–48 hours (Bartlett *et al.*, 1982; Reingold *et al.*, 1982a), but may be substantially longer.

IV. THE ORGANISM

The production of a characteristic extracellular protein, the heavy-metal susceptibility pattern, and lysogeny by one or more bacteriophage are the three features most consistently associated with *S. aureus* isolates from TSS patients compared to *S. aureus* isolates from non-TSS patients. Characteristic patterns of bacteriophage lysis, and the identification of other extracellular products and the biological activity of these organisms have also been described for TSS-associated strains of *S. aureus*.

A. Characteristic extracellular protein or toxin

The most striking difference between TSS and non-TSS strains of *S. aureus* is the production of a characteristic extracellular protein or exotoxin. This protein has a molecular weight of about 20,000–22,000 and an isoelectric point of 6.8–7.2. A standard nomenclature for this protein initially isolated by two laboratories and identified as staphylococcal enterotoxin F (SEF) (Bergdoll *et al.*, 1981) and pyrogenic exotoxin C (PEC) (Schlievert *et al.*, 1981) has not yet been agreed on, although both proteins are antigentically identical (Melish *et al.*, 1982) and it is likely that they are the same protein (Schlievert, 1983). A similar, probably identical protein has now been identified in other laboratories (Barbour, 1981; De Nooij *et al.*, 1982; Melish *et al.*, 1982; Notermans and Dufrenne, 1982).

1. Production of PEC and SEF

Quantitative differences in the production of PEC are related to individual strains and to culture conditions (Schlievert and Blomster, 1983). Although stationary-phase bacterial growth is the same, toxin production is significantly less at 30°C. Little or no bacterial growth or toxin production occurs at pH 5.0 and 9.0. Significant bacterial growth but no toxin production occurs at pH 6.0, and maximal cell growth and toxin production occur at pH 7.0 to 8.0. Toxin production is decreased 32-fold under anaerobic conditions, whereas bacterial growth is decreased only 2-fold (Schlievert and Blomster, 1983). Glucose concentrations of greater than 0.3% in artificial media inhibit both bacterial growth and toxin production, in contrast to control strains, which grew better in the presence of glucose.

Tampons can significantly alter the production of SEF *in vitro* (Lee and Crass, 1983), although they do not alter the growth of the organism (Lee and Crass, 1983; Broome *et al.*, 1982). The amount of toxin produced *in vitro* can vary from undetectable to 300 μg/ml, depending on the particular brand and style of tampon (Lee and Crass, 1983). Under the conditions of these experiments, toxin production did not vary at pH values as low as 4.5, although the growth of the organisms was retarded.

Thus, it is inferred that *in vivo,* PEC and SEF production may be maximal at 37°C in a well-oxygenated environment with a low glucose concentration and at pH 7.0–8.0, except in the presence of a tampon when pH may not be as critical.

2. Biological properties of PEC and SEF

Biological properties of PEC and SEF that have been studied in detail include altered immune function, pyrogenicity, lethality and enhanced endotoxin susceptibility.

(a)   Altered immune function

Although rabbits can make antibody to both SEF (Bergdoll *et al.*, 1981) and PEC (Schlievert, 1983), the response does not occur in all animals. Of 6 animals receiving a total of 6 subcutaneous injections of 50 μg PEC each over 105 days, only 3 developed anti-PEC antibody. However, all animals were capable of making antibodies to sheep erythrocytes, suggesting the presence of a specific unresponsiveness rather than a general immunodeficiency (Schlievert, 1983).

Although neither PEC nor endotoxin given alone suppresses the immune response of rabbits to sheep erythrocytes, when PEC was given i.v. and followed by endotoxin 4 hours later, the immune response was significantly suppressed 4 days later. In animals receiving a higher dose of endotoxin, the immune response remained suppressed for up to 12 days (Schlievert, 1983).

In vitro, PEC is a nonspecific T cell mitogen (Schlievert *et al.*, 1981). Nonspecific lymphocyte mitogenicity was evaluated using rabbit splenocytes and human peripheral T and B cell populations. There was a minimal response of the B cells to PEC, whereas PEC was an active mitogen for the T cell–enriched population.

Using the slide modification of the Jerne plaque assay, PEC has been shown to suppress IgM antibody synthesis of both murine and rabbit spleen cells to sheep erythrocytes (Schlievert *et al.*, 1981). PEC plus endotoxin further reduced the plaque-forming cell response compared to PEC alone (Schlievert, 1983).

Suppression of the clearance of colloidal carbon by the reticuloendothelial system (RES) was found to be unaffected by i.v. PEC (10 μg/kg). However, when PEC was given and followed by intravenous endotoxin 4 hours later, significant RES blockade occurred (Schlievert, 1983).

An additional biological activity of PEC is that of skin sensitization

(Schlievert, 1983). Rabbits given a subcutaneous injection of PEC every other week developed progressive increases in skin-test responsiveness to homologous toxin. Reaction diameters increased with progressive increases in the number of sensitizing doses and in progressive increases in the size of the challenge doses of PEC. In addition, rabbits previously sensitized only to PPD (heterologous antigen) demonstrated an enhanced skin-test reactivity when challenged with PPD plus PEC, as compared to challenge with PPD or PEC alone.

(b)   Pyrogenicity
In vivo, both purified PEC and an exoprotein antigenically identical to SEF have been demonstrated to be pyrogenic for rabbits (Schlievert *et al.,* 1981; Melish *et al.,* 1982). Antibody to PEV prevents the pyrogenic response (Schlievert, 1983).

   In vitro, culture supernatants of TSS-associated strains of *S. aureus* induce adherent human monocytes to release large quantities of leukocyte pyrogen and lymphocyte-activating factor (Ikejima *et al.,* 1983), identical molecules now know as interleukin I (IL-I) (Murphy *et al.,* 1980). Following gel filtration of the culture supernates, the IL-I inducing property, which was as potent as *Escherichia coli* endotoxin in terms of inducing IL-I production, was found in two peaks, a major peak of 20–25 kathodal duration and a minor peak of 9–10 kathodal duration. These findings suggest that some of the manifestations of TSS may be due to the massive release of IL-I.

(c)   Lethality and enhanced endotoxin susceptibility
The susceptibility of rabbits to PEC appears to depend on prior conditioning of the animals. Animals that were quarantined for 1 week prior to use, given tetracycline for visible signs of pulmonary infection, and restrained for 3 hours on a pyrogen test rack were relatively resistant to PEC. However, animals that were not conditioned were highly susceptible to PEC (Schlievert, 1983). Approximately 50% of these animals were killed by a single injection of either 10 or 30 µg PEC/kg, and 100% died after 3 doses of 10 µg/kg·day. Another exoprotein, antigenically identical to SEF, is lethal for rabbits at an LD_{50} of 60 µg/kg (Melish *et al.,* 1982). The lethality of PEC for rabbits is markedly enhanced following the administration of small doses of endotoxin (Schlievert, 1982), a phenomenon known as enhanced endotoxin susceptibility.

   In experiments demonstrating this enhanced endotoxin susceptibility, *S. typhimurium* endotoxin with an LD_{50} of 500 µg/kg was used (Schlievert, 1982). If rabbits were given an i.v. dose of 100 µg PEC/kg, followed by endotoxin at 4 hours, the LD_{50} dose of endotoxin was 0.01 µg/kg, a 50,000-fold enhanced susceptibility to endotoxin. Using a range of doses, a straight line was obtained when the log of the PEC pretreatment dose was plotted against the log LD_{50} of endotoxin. Death occurred in rabbits from 1–24 hours after challenge, depending on the dose used, and after an illness characterized by fever, hypothermia, diarrhea, and labored respirations. Other characteristics of this phenomenon included loss of the enhanced endotoxin susceptibility 12–24 hours after the endotoxin administration, and no enhanced endotoxin susceptibility using low doses of PEC unless 2 hours elapsed before repeated endotoxin administration.

In the rabbit model, when methylprednisolone or pooled human gamma globulin were given intravenously prior to the administration of PEC or endotoxin, mortality was significantly decreased. However, no single agent was protective after the administration of endotoxin, but the combined administration of methylprednisolone and gamma globulin decreased mortality. Ibuprofen was ineffective under all conditions (Peterson *et al.*, 1983).

3. Association of PEC and SEF with TSS
It has not yet been established that PEC or SEF cause TSS. *In vivo*, SEF has been identified in the breast milk of a woman with TSS (Vergeront *et al.*, 1982), and an antigenically identical protein has been identified in the serum urine and vaginal washings of patients (Melish *et al.*, 1982).

The most important animal model thus far examined is the baboon. Quimby *et al.* (1984) found that the intravenous administration of purified SEF into adult female baboons was associated with a marked decrease in blood pressure (60/45 mm Hg), orthostatic hypotension, ascites, hyperthermia, rash (abdomen and thighs), conjunctival hyperemia and thrombocytopenia, as well as chemical evidence for abnormalities involving muscle, liver, and kidney. Confirmation of this observation will be important.

B. Heavy-metal susceptibilities

TSS-associated *S. aureus* isolates are almost uniformly sensitive to mercury (Hg^S) and resistant to the effects of cadmium (Cd^R), arsenate (As^R) (Barbour, 1981; de Saxe *et al.*, 1982; Kreiswirth *et al.*, 1982) and penicillin (Pc^R) (Shands *et al.*, 1980). This resistance pattern of Cd^R, As^R, Pc^R, Hg^S, which is unrelated to bacteriophage type, has been found in 38–42% of non-TSS-related strains of *S. aureus* studied for epidemiologic purposes (Barbour, 1981). In *S. aureus*, as in other organisms, Pc^R is usually plasmid determined and Cd^R is always plasmid determined. As these TSS-associated isolates do not carry plasmids (Kreiswirth *et al.*, 1982), it is assumed that the resistance to Cd, As, and Pc is chromosomally mediated. In transduction experiments, Cd^R, As^R are always co-transferred, Pc^R is unlinked, and the chromosomally mediated determinant for PEC or SEF is not linked to either the Cd^R, As^R or Pc^R determinant. Thus, it has been concluded that the chromosomal determinant for PEC or SEF production is a heterologous insertion that is independent of two other well-defined insertions (Kreiswirth *et al.*, 1982). These findings suggest that there is a rather well-defined basic strain that is the nearly exclusive carrier of the chromosomal determinant for both PEC and SEF. A chromosomal fragment from *S. aureus* that expresses both SEF and PEC has been cloned in *E. coli* (Kreiswirth *et al.*, 1983). Periplasmic shockates of this clone contained most or all of the PEC or SEF as identified using specific antisera.

C. Lysogenic conversion

Lysogeny or lysogenic conversion involves the incorporation of genetic material of a bacteriophage into the DNA of a bacterium, with subsequent transmission of this viral genome to the bacterial progeny. The newly incorporated genetic material does not harm the bacterium but may be associated with a new capacity to produce a toxin, as has been described for scarlet fever–causing strains of *Streptococcus pyogenes,* for *Corynebacterium diphtheriae,* and for some alpha- and beta-hemolysin-producing strains of *S. aureus* (Kreiswirth *et al.*, 1982; Schutzer *et al.*, 1983). It has recently been demonstrated that 11 of 12 strains of TSS-associated *S. aureus* were lysogenized by one or a common bacteriophage compared to the presence of the same bacteriophage(s) in only one of 18 control *S. aureus* strains. A laboratory strain of *S. aureus* could be lysogenized by the bacteriophage from 2 of the TSS-associated strains (Schutzer *et al.*, 1983). It has not yet been determined whether this lysogenic conversion is associated with the production of PEC or SEF and how it is related to the chromosomal fragment that has been cloned in *E. coli* (Kreiswirth *et al.*, 1983).

D. Other animal models utilizing
TSS-associated *S. aureus* strains

Several additional animal models have been utilized to demonstrate the biologic effects of TSS-associated *S. aureus* strains. Beef heart infusion broth culture filtrates of TSS-associated strains were obtained from 16-hour-old cultures. These culture filtrates were found to be significantly less toxic than those from control strains for both chick embryos and rabbits observed for up to 12 hours after injection (Barbour, 1981). Most deaths occurred within 60 min and were strongly correlated with the presence of a protein resembling alpha toxin in both isoelectric point and molecular weight. In this model, the TSS-associated strains were not lethal up to 12 hours after injection and appeared not to produce a protein with the characteristics of alpha toxin.

In contrast, log-phase cultures of TSS-associated *S. aureus* strains grown in beef heart dialysate were lethal in 17 of 33 rabbits when injected into sub-cutaneous polyethylene infection chambers (Scott *et al.*, 1983); no deaths occurred in 10 rabbits injected with control strains. Fever, diarrhea and labored breathing occurred in most cases, and all deaths occurred within 48 hours. In this model, there was no evidence of a dose-response relationship when the initial inocula ranged from 1.5×10^7 to 4.8×10^9 CFU/animal. This finding suggests disease may result when a critical threshold of toxin is produced by relatively few organisms. In these same experiments, rabbit mortality occurred despite a normal leukocyte infiltrate into the chambers.

E. Other extracellular products of TSS-associated strains of *S. aureus*

Epidermal toxin is a heat-stable, acid-resistant, trypsin- and pronase-sensitive toxin of molecular weight 60,000, which is elaborated by 73% of TSS-associated *S. aureus* isolates compared to 18% of control strains (Kapral, 1982). In newborn mice, it causes a positive Nikolsky's sign and extensive cellular destruction beneath the germinal layer with an intact granular layer, a pattern distinctly different from the granular cell layer cleavage induced by exfoliatin toxin (Melish and Glasgow, 1970).

Almost all TSS-associated *S. aureus* strains show decreased hemolysis of sheep blood compared to control strains, particularly when hemolytic activity is measured in a liquid medium (Schlievert *et al.*, 1982). This difference in hemolysis is less striking when bovine, rabbit or human blood in agar is used (Barbour, 1981; Chow *et al.*, 1983). In addition, vaginal TSS *S. aureus* strains produce significantly less lipase and nuclease than control strains of *S. aureus* (Schlievert *et al.*, 1982). These findings may explain, in part, the relative noninvasive nature of these organisms in TSS (Lentino *et al.*, 1981).

TSS-associated *S. aureus* strains are not significantly different from non-TSS strains in their production of fibrinolysin and extracellular protein A, but do exhibit a marked increase in protease production, particularly when hemoglobin is used as a substrate (Barbour, 1981; Lawellin *et al.*, 1983). This finding suggests that TSS strains may produce a hemoglobin-specific protease.

Proteins 1 and 2 are additional extracellular products of TSS-associated *S. aureus* isolated from sonicated whole-cell suspensions and identified through the use of a binding assay to TSS patient convalescent antiserum. Proteins 1 and 2 were associated with 78% of TSS strains, as compared to 25% of control strains (Cohen and Falkow, 1981).

F. Bacteriophage lysis patterns

A majority of TSS-associated *S. aureus* strains are lysed by group I bacteriophage, particularly types 29 and 52, although some are lysed only by bacteriophages of other groups or are nontypable (Altemeier *et al.*, 1981; Davis *et al.*, 1980; Todd *et al.*, 1978). In one study, 145 of 248 TSS strains (58%) had the 29 or 29/52 phage type, compared to 10 of 86 control strains (Altemeier *et al.*, 1982). In a retrospective review of *S. aureus* obtained from patients with surgical wounds, strains lysed by phage 29, phage 52, or both increased in prevalence from 4.1% of 2593 strains in 1960 to a peak of 27.4% of 365 strains in 1970. Over this time the production of PEC by these strains (phage type 29/52) increased from 1 in 10 strains (10%) in 1971 to a peak of 22 in 26 strains (85%) in 1979 and then decreased to 6 in 21 strains (29%) in 1981 (Altemeier *et al.*, 1982).

V. PREVALENCE OF CERVICO–VAGINAL *S. AUREUS* COLONIZATION AND FACTORS AFFECTING COLONIZATION

The emergence of TSS has led to renewed interest in the cervico–vaginal flora, the normal prevalence of *S. aureus* in this flora and factors affecting changes in the flora.

A. Normal cervico–vaginal flow

The composition of the vaginal microbial flora changes with the stage of life (Larsen and Galask, 1982) and during the menstrual cycle (Bartlett *et al.*, 1977; Brown, 1982). Facultative lactobacillus species found in 17–96% of female patients dominate the facultative genital tract flora; anaerobic lactobacilli are most prevalent during the reproductive years and particularly during pregnancy (Larsen and Galask, 1982). Lactobacilli predominate in a low vaginal pH; whether the lactobacilli create the acidic environment or are selected for in this acidic environment is unclear. During the menstrual cycle the vaginal pH changes from an acidic pH of 4.2 midcycle to a pH of 6.6 with the onset of menses (Wagner and Ottesen, 1982; Noble *et al.*, 1982). This change correlates with a 100-fold decrease in the number of facultative genital tract bacteria present during the premenstrual week (Bartlett *et al.*, 1977) and a marked decrease in the number of anaerobic lactobacilli during menses (Brown, 1982). Although anaerobic organisms clearly dominate the vaginal flora by quantitative analysis, having a mean concentration 10-fold greater than the aerobes (Bartlett *et al.*, 1977), it is unclear as to which group causes the variation in the anaerobic:aerobic ratio seen with menses. Thus, during the week prior to the onset of menses, there is a significant 100-fold relative increase in anaerobic:facultative ratio, which changes abruptly with the onset of menses such that the facultative organisms then outnumber the anaerobes during menses and for the first postmenstrual week (Bartlett *et al.*, 1977; Brown, 1982).

Although estrogen has been shown to have a small suppressive effect on the anaerobic flora (Larsen and Galask, 1980), the overall influence of the hormonal changes of menses on the vaginal flora has not been well examined.

B. Prevalence of *S. aureus* and factors responsible for changes
of *S. aureus* in the cervico–vaginal flora

Early investigators have reported *S. aureus* to be isolated from cervical or vaginal cultures of fewer than 5% of women of reproductive age (Bartlett *et al.*, 1977; Corbishley, 1977; Sautter and Brown, 1980); more recent studies have noted a higher prevalence (Brown, 1982; Larsen and Galask, 1982; Martin *et al.*, 1982; Smith *et al.*, 1982).

The prevalence of *S. aureus* in genital cultures was evaluated prospectively in a group of 600 women being seen for routine pregnancy-related or problem-associated visits (Linnemann *et al.*, 1982). Of 175 individuals seen for a routine visit, 20 (7%) had a positive labial or vaginal culture for *S. aureus*, and 9 (3%) had a positive vaginal culture only. Three of the 20 isolates produced SEF. This represents approximately 1% of women seen for a routine exam. A significant trend was found between age and *S. aureus* colonization, with decreasing colonization occurring with increasing age. In addition, a significantly large number of black women were colonized compared to white women, and these differences were not explained by differences in age, socioeconomic status, or other medical problems. The highest colonization rates were found in postpartum women; 14 of 81 postpartum women (17%) had positive genital cultures, compared to 41 of 519 other women (8%). The association between colonization and postpartum women was significant after correction for confounding variables (Linneman *et al.*, 1982). The reasons for this increase in postpartum colonization are not clear.

Staphylococcus aureus may be isolated more frequently during menses than midcycle (Larsen and Galask, 1982; Sanders *et al.*, 1982; Smith *et al.*, 1982). In one study, *S. aureus* was isolated from the cervix of 9 of 52 women (17%) during menstruation and 3 of 52 women (5.8%) during the midcycle (Smith *et al.*, 1982). No subjects had negative menstrual cultures and positive midcycle cultures, and there was no significant difference in the rate of isolation of *S. aureus* between users of tampons and users of pads. In an associated study, 24% of the cultures taken from menstruating women using sea sponges were positive for *S. aureus*, compared to 5.2% of those taken from women using tampons. Women using sea sponges were also more likely to be colonized with *E. coli*, *Klebsiella* or other Enterobactteriaceae (Smith *et al.*, 1982).

Nasal carriage of *S. aureus* may be another factor that may predispose to genital carriage of *S. aureus*. Anterior nares cultures were positive in 15 (38%) of 29 women with positive genital cultures. When the isolates could be typed, they were always of the same phage type in both sites (Linneman *et al.*, 1982). Thus, in this study as in others (Guinan *et al.*, 1982), an association was found between *S. aureus* vaginal colonization and colonization of the labia minora and anterior nares.

Other factors felt to increase the likelihood of vaginal *S. aureus* colonization were described in a series of studies from the Centers for Disease Control

(Guinan *et al.*, 1982); those factors included a history of a genital herpes infection, insertion of tampons without using an applicator, and the use of a specific tampon brand. Systemic antibiotics used within 2 weeks prior to culture protected against *S. aureus* colonization. In addition, no single contraceptive method was signifiantly associated with *S. aureus* vaginal colonization in any one study, but colonization rates ranged from 3% in women with hysterectomies and tubal ligations to 18% in those who used diaphragms. Vaginal *S. aureus* colonization does not correlate with the use of oral contraceptives, use of tampons or napkins (Linneman *et al.*, 1982; Smith *et al.*, 1982), finger insertion of tampons, day of menstrual cycle culture, sexual activity or douching within 24 hours prior to the examination, diabetes, genital herpes simplex virus infection, or antibiotics received within 7 days of culture (Linneman *et al.*, 1982). The latter finding appears to conflict with the CDC data.

The explanation for the effect of age, race, postpartum status and presence of menses on *S. aureus* genital colonization is not clear.

C. Prevalence of SEF- and PEC-producing *S. aureus* in other populations

Up to 17–30% of non-TSS-associated strains of *S. aureus* produce PEC or SEF, suggesting that SEF-producing strains may be present in as many as 30% of individuals colonized with *S. aureus* (Bergdoll *et al.*, 1981; Schlievert *et al.*, 1982). Vergeront *et al.* (1983) have demonstrated that 60% of persons over the age of 10 and 90% of persons over the age of 25 have antibody to SEF. These data suggest that the prevalence of colonization with SEF-producing *S. aureus* strains in childhood may be high or that intermittent colonization with these strains may be frequent. It is of interest that the incidence of reported TSS in children is very low (Reingold *et al.*, 1982c). Apparently, most individuals acquire anti-SEF antibody at an early age, without developing TSS. Schlievert *et al.* (1982) found that 11 of 22 healthy children had anterior nares cultures positive for *S. aureus*, and 4 of these strains produced PEC. Linneman *et al.* (1982) found that in families of women with vaginal strains of SEF-producing *S. aureus*, 3 of 18 family members were colonized with SEF-producing *S. aureus*. Although TSS may have occurred within 24 hours in both a husband and wife (Fischer *et al.*, 1981), and nosocomial acquisition has been suggested (Reingold *et al.*, 1982b), the organisms associated with TSS appear not to be unusually transmissible. This may simply reflect the high degree of immunity to the toxin present in most individuals.

VI. PATHOLOGY

Substantial clinical evidence suggests that TSS is a toxin-mediated disease. This evidence includes negative bacterial cultures of blood, urine and CSF; systemic involvement with multisystem dysfunction; rapid onset and rapid recovery of many patients without antibiotics; subclinical inflammation in surgically infected wounds; and the absence of development of antiteichoic acid antibody during convalescence. The pathologic findings support this evidence of a toxin-mediated multisystem disease, as there is a total absence of tissue invasion by bacteria and minimal evidence of an acute inflammatory reaction in most organs. The most striking histopathologic findings felt to be unrelated to hypoperfusion, and therefore potentially due to the direct effects of toxin, have been found in the vagina, cervix, heart, muscle, liver, esophagus, lymph nodes, skin and kidney (Abdul-Karim *et al.*, 1981; Blair *et al.*, 1982; Larkin *et al.*, 1982; Paris *et al.*, 1982; Wick *et al.*, 1982).

A.   Genital tract

In fatal TSS, the mucosa of the cervix and vagina shows evidence of extensive inflammation, ulceration and desquamation. A characteristic vaginal lesion consisting of capillary vasodilatation and thrombosis with ulceration and inflammation of the mucosa but without deep-tissue bacterial invasion has been described (Larkin *et al.*, 1982). The vaginal ulcers are unusual and characteristic, as the layer of separation occurs beneath the basal layer in distinction to the separation within the granular cell layer that occurs in the staphylococcal scalded skin syndrome (Melish and Glasgow, 1970). In addition, this subbasal-layer vacuolization and separation is different from the previously described vaginal lesions found in association with tampon usage. In this latter instance, insertion of a superabsorbent tampon produced smaller ulcers characterized by epithelial layering, dessication and musocal detachment above the basal layer (Friedrich and Siegesmund, 1980). The presence of the characteristic subbasal ulcerations in one patient with menstrual TSS who had never used tampons and the identification of similar lesions on the bladder and esophagus have led to the suggestion that these ulcerations may be a direct result of the toxin (Larkin *et al.*, 1982).

In fatal cases, endometrial tissue was normal (Paris *et al.*, 1982) or showed hemorrhage and necrosis compatible with menstruation or prolonged shock (Larkin *et al.*, 1982); no organisms were identified in the endometrial tissue (Paris *et al.*, 1982). Severe congestion, hemorrhage and edema characterized the ovaries. The Fallopian tubes were congested with evidence of mild acute salpingitis, but there was no intraluminal blood or evidence of chronic pelvic inflammatory disease (Larkin *et al.*, 1982).

B.   Myocardium and muscle

The myocardium has been described as normal in the majority of fatal cases of TSS (Paris *et al.*, 1982). In one group of patients, heart valves were available from 4 of 12 patients, and all showed myxoid degeneration (Paris *et al.*, 1982). In another series of 8 autopsies, all patients had evidence of focal round-cell infiltration of the myocardium with variable degrees of edema, hemorrhage and congestion. Small foci of early myocardial fiber damage and myocardial capillary microthrombi were present in each of 3 patients. No heart valves were available for study (Larkin *et al.*, 1982).

Despite the impressive clinical findings of muscle tenderness and weakness, histopathologic examination of muscle sections have demonstrated normal findings or have shown only edema, focal hemorrhage, congestion, focal fiber necrosis or a mild acute inflammatory infiltrate (Larkin *et al.*, 1982; Paris *et al.*, 1982).

C. Liver

The overall liver size is normal. Varying degrees of triaditis or periportal lymphocytic inflammation have been the most consistent finding, although centrilobular congestion and necrosis and mild cellular degeneration have been described in most cases. Cytoplasmic vacuolization and fatty metamorphosis of hepatocytes is present in most patients (Ishak and Rogers, 1981). Acute cholangitis, bile stasis and intrasinusoidal acidophilic bodies were found in only a few cases (Larkin *et al.*, 1982).

D. Spleen and lymph nodes

In both the spleen and lymph nodes, the most characteristic findings have been lymphocyte depletion, inactive hypocellular hypoplastic lymphoid follicles, and edema and marked histocytosis in the interfollicular areas (Larkin *et al.*, 1982; Paris *et al.*, 1982). Considerable hemophagocytosis has been described in the spleen, lymph nodes, and bone marrow (Larkin *et al.*, 1982).

E. Skin

Sections of skin have been normal with a perivascular lymphocytic infiltrate and bullae that separate at the basement membrane (Abdul-Karim *et al.*, 1981; Paris *et al.*, 1982). There has been no evidence of vasculitis (Larkin *et al.*, 1982). In one patient, there were no immune globulin or complement deposits in the epidermis, basement membrane or dermovasculature (Larkin *et al.*, 1982).

F. Kidneys

Although acute tubular necrosis felt to be the result of hypoperfusion has been well described in fatal cases of TSS, earlier pathologic changes may be due to a direct effect of the toxin. A mononuclear interstitial nephritis appeared to be the result of progression of an initial perivasculitis of the adventitia of renal venules (Paris *et al.*, 1982).

G. Lungs

The well-described pathologic lung changes are most consistent with the diagnosis of shock lung or adult respiratory distress syndrome. These changes may be solely related to hypoperfusion and massive fluid replacement or they may, in part, be toxin mediated (Larkin *et al.*, 1982; Paris *et al.*, 1982).

H. Cause of death

The cause of death and factors predicting a fatal outcome in TSS have not always been clear. In one group of 9 patients, noncardiogenic pulmonary edema was the only clinical development that was predictive of a fatal outcome. In this group of patients, 7 died of a refractory cardiac ventricular arrhythmia, 1 of an acute respiratory arrest and 1 as a result of a coagulation defect (Larkin *et al.*, 1982).

VII.   PATHOGENESIS

Numerous theories have been advanced to explain the recent increase in incidence of TSS, its association with menses and tampons, and the sequence of events which promotes *S. aureus* toxin production and dissemination (Davis *et al.*, 1982b).

PEC- and SEF-producing strains of *S. aureus* are not new (Altemeier *et al.*, 1982), and antibody to SEF was prevalent in a general population as far back as 1960 (Vergeront *et al.*, 1983). Thus, the recent increase in incidence of TSS must be the result of other newly introduced co-factors.

Theories relating to the ability of the staphylococcus to proliferate and produce toxin under conditions associated with TSS have been advanced. One theory suggests that tampons induce or stimulate bacterial growth or toxin formation. In one study, tampons did not enhance the growth of PEC-producing *S. aureus* isolates in nutrient broth or human blood (Broome *et al.*, 1982). On the other hand, another study noted that tampon type may increase the amount of SEF produced *in vitro* by up to 300-fold (Lee and Crass, 1983).

Another proposed explanation for the role of tampons is that they may remove vaginal substrates that normally act to inhibit the growth of *S. aureus* (Davis *et al.*, 1982b). The anaerobic lactobacilli, present in high concentrations in the vagina in midcycle and in low numbers during menses, may inhibit the growth of *S. aureus* as they do the growth of *N. gonorrhea* (Sanders *et al.*, 1982). *In vitro*, the inhibitory effect of some lactobacilli is enhanced by the presence of other substrates. It has been suggested that tampons may remove these substrates, thus nullifying the inhibitory effect (Sanders *et al.*, 1982).

A third theory relates to a demonstrated transient decrease in the bactericidal activity of blood polymorphonuclear cells (PMN) during menses (Berger *et al.*, 1982). It has been suggested that this relative decrease may lead to decreased staphylococcal killing. In a separate study, no difference was noted in the bactericidal activity of PMNs against TSS and control strains of *S. aureus* grown in the presence of Rely® tampons (Bassaris *et al.*, 1981). In addition, there were no differences in the ability of TSS strains to adhere to vaginal epithelial cells obtained from 5 healthy women and 5 women who had recently recovered from TSS. These studies suggest that the pathogenesis of TSS may be unrelated to alterations in the adherence of *S. aureus* to vaginal epithelial cells or to the resistance of TSS *S. aureus* strains to killing by PMNs.

A fourth theory suggests that aerobic Gram-negative bacteria that may be part of the vaginal flora utilize cellulase to break down the carboxymethylcellulose present in some tampons into reducing sugars. These sugars might then enrich the vaginal microenvironmental encouraging growth of pathogenic organisms (Tierno *et al.*, 1983). However, it has been noted (Bonventre, 1983) that the minimal degradation of a relatively inert carboxymethylcellulose in menstrual fluid that is generally already rich in glucose and other potential nutrients could not explain the increased frequency of TSS among tampon users. Furthermore, high glucose concentrations have been found to inhibit PEC production (Schlievert and Blomster, 1983).

Endotoxin has been postulated to play a role in TSS pathogenesis (Fumarola, 1979; Schlievert, 1982). Many of the clinical findings in TSS are the same as those described for endotoxin or Gram-negative shock in both humans and animals. Perhaps SEF or PEC plus endotoxin in some way causes further impaired clearance of endotoxin by the reticuloendothelial system, thus allowing it to enter the circulation (Schlievert, 1983). The enhanced susceptibility to endotoxin in rabbits following the administration of PEC suggests that endotoxin may be an important mediator in TSS (Schlievert, 1982).

Additional theories regarding TSS pathogenesis relate to the direct role of tampons. It has been suggested that tampon-associated cervico–vaginal ulcerations may enhance toxin absorption. However, the chronic ulcers produced by long-term continuous use of tampons (Barrett *et al.*, 1977; Jimerson and Becker, 1980) and the superficial microulcerations described following the brief insertion of tampons in healthy women are very different histologically from the ulcerations found in TSS, as previously noted. In addition, the intact vaginal mucosa is a very absorptive surface, and there is no need to invoke a role of superficial mucosal ulceration to explain toxin absorption.

Finally, it has been suggested that reflux of infected menstrual blood into the peritoneal cavity may result in peritonitis and massive peritoneal absorption of toxin (Fuller *et al.*, 1980). The absence of clinical findings of peritonitis, the absence of blood in the peritoneum and Fallopian tubes, and the absence of *S. aureus* in the endometrium at autopsy have ruled out this proposed mechanism (Larkin *et al.*, 1982; Paris *et al.*, 1982).

VIII. CLINICAL FEATURES

A. Clinical presentation of severe confirmed disease

Toxic-shock syndrome comprises a spectrum of toxin-mediated multisystem organ damage with massive capillary vasodilatation and leakage. Prolonged hypotension following the loss of intravascular volume may result in ischemic organ damage, further enhancing the spectrum of multisystem involvement.

The incubation period of TSS is best defined in patients who develop the disease postoperatively (Bartlett *et al.*, 1982; Reingold *et al.*, 1982a). In 13 such patients, the median interval between the surgical procedure and the onset of TSS was 2 days. In menstrual TSS the peak days of onset are days 2 to 4 of active bleeding (Davis *et al.*, 1982a).

The onset of illness is usually abrupt, with symptoms and signs of fever, chills, malaise, headache, sore throat, myalgias, muscle tenderness, fatigue, vomiting, diarrhea, abdominal pain and orthostatic dizziness or syncope (P. J. Chesney *et al.*, 1981; Fisher *et al.*, 1981; McKenna *et al.*, 1980; Shands *et al.*, 1980; Todd *et al.*, 1978; Tofte and Williams, 1981a). During the next 24 to 48 hours, diffuse erythema, severe watery diarrhea often with incontinence, decreased urine output, edema of the face, hands and feet, and cyanotic extremities may be noted. The patient rapidly becomes somnolent, confused, irritable, and sometimes agitated, manifestations which may be the result of cerebral ischemia, edema or a direct effect of the toxin.

Fever, generalized erythroderma ("sunburned appearance"), muscle tenderness and abdominal tenderness are often noted on initial physical examination in conjunction with peripheral cyanosis, edema of the hands and feet, somnolence, confusion, disorientation, a low or unobtainable blood pressure, conjunctival injection and subconjunctival hemorrhages, and beefy-red, edematous pharynx and tongue. In menstrual TSS, cervico–vaginal erythema, edema and discharge and ulcerations may be noted along with a normal uterine and adnexal examination. Edema and erythema of the perineum and inner thighs may be noted. In cases not menstrually related, the focus of toxin-producing *S. aureus* may be a postoperative wound, a pustule, or a deep-tissue infection, or it may not be immediately obvious. Such sites frequently show no obvious evidence of inflammation (Bartlett *et al.*, 1982; Reingold *et al.*, 1982).

A multitude of abnormal laboratory data are found initially. The most impressive initial findings include a marked preponderance of immature and mature PMNs in the peripheral white blood cell count, thrombocytopenia, sterile pyuria increases in CPK, creatinine, blood urea nitrogen, prothrombin time, total bilirubin and other measures of liver function, and decreases in the total serum protein, albumin, calcium, and phosphorus (P. J. Chesney *et al.*, 1981). Many of these laboratory abnormalities are reflections of shock and organ failure (Davis *et al.*, 1982a), but some may be attributed to the direct action of the toxin. In menstrual TSS, cultures of the cervix or vagina will be positive for *S. aureus* more than 85% of the time (Davis *et al.*, 1982a; Shands *et al.*, 1980).

B. Hospital course

Hemodynamic monitoring of hypotensive patients with TSS has shown an initial increase in cardiac output, a subsequent fall with cardiac dysfunction, and a marked and often prolonged (up to 10 days) decrease in systemic vascular resistance (Bastian *et al.*, 1981; Fisher *et al.*, 1981). Thus, careful attention to monitoring of cardiovascular function, rapid administration of volume expanding fluids, and where necessary inotropic vasopressor agents may effectively restore circulating blood volume. Rapid volume expansion in these hypotensive patients frequently results in adult respiratory distress syndrome and pulmonary edema, serious complications that develop within 12–36 hours. Other serious complications frequently present in the first 24–48 hours include acidosis, hyponatremia and associated electrolyte disorders, acute renal failure, disseminated intravascular coagulation, myocardiopathy with arrhythmias, and hypocalcemia.

Once the hypovolemia has been corrected, and the life-threatening complications addressed, the subsequent hospital course is usually one of fairly rapid resolution. Characteristically, the fever abates within 48–72 hours. The erythroderma generally lasts only a few hours to days, and the muscle pain and weakness resolve over 7–10 days. Many patients experience painful oral ulcerations and glossitis within the first few days of hospitalization. Extensive edema and a brisk diuresis may be noted 48–72 hours after admission. Fine facial and truncal desquamation may begin after several days, whereas the characteristic peripheral (finger–toe–palm and sole) full thickness desquamation usually does not become apparent until 10–21 days after disease onset. Seven to 10 days after onset, more than 50% of patients have developed an extremely pruritic total-body maculopapular rash (P. J. Chesney *et al.*, 1981, 1982; Deetz *et al.*, 1981). This rash, which is usually warm to the touch and accompanied by extensive edema, may be associated with a low-grade fever. Although frequently attributed to a drug hypersensitivity reaction, patients who never received a penicillin type of antiobiotic have developed the rash and some patients have been continued on beta-lactamase-resistant penicillins or other antibiotic with resolution of the rash.

C. Outcome

Death associated with TSS may occur as late as 15 days after hospitalization and has been attributed most often to refractory cardiac arrhythmias, irreversible respiratory failure and bleeding due to coagulation defects (Larkin *et al.*, 1982). The only clinical development that could be used to predict a fatal outcome in one study was noncardiogenic pulmonary edema (Larkin *et al.*, 1982). An initial serum creatinine of ≥ 3 mg/dl was found to correlate with more severe disease and prolonged hospitalization in another study (Chesney *et al.*, 1982).

After discharge, prolonged fatigue, muscle weakness and pain are noted by most patients. In addition, other sequelae have been attributed to TSS (Chesney *et al.*, 1982; Rosene *et al.*, 1982). Although some of these such as chronic renal failure, gangrene and telogen effluvium appear to be clearly related to a prolonged period of hypotension, others—such as the neuropsychologic abnormalities, prolonged myalgias and weakness, and carpal tunnel syndrome—are less easily explained. Abnormalities such as impaired memory and poorly sustained concentration have been found in patients who did not require any therapy other than intravenous fluids to restore their blood pressure (Rosene *et al.*, 1982). Findings that relate primarily to the neuromuscular system result in speculation that the TSS-associated toxin has a direct effect on nerve or muscle tissue.

D. Diagnosis

In the absence of a specific diagnostic test, the diagnosis of TSS is considered to be confirmed when all the clinical criteria for the case definition are met. A probable case is one criterion short of being confirmed. In every instance, aggressive attempts should be made to find the focus of *S. aureus,* including cultures of mucous membranes, especially the cervix and vagina in menstrually associated cases, and other sites that may not appear to be obviously infected. Isolates of *S. aureus* should be saved and examined for their ability to produce either SEF or PEC. Acute and convalescent sera should also be examined for the presence of antibody to SEF or PEC. The presence of a high titer of antibody to SEF during the acute phase of illness would be highly unusual in TSS (Bergdoll *et al.*, 1981; Stolz *et al.*, 1982). Subsequent to the acute episode, the patient should be followed carefully for the detection of desquamation, which may occur even in mild cases.

E. Therapy

The most important aspect of the management of acutely ill patients with TSS is that of early aggressive supportive care (P. J. Chesney *et al.*, 1981; Fisher *et al.*, 1981; Todd *et al.*, 1978; Tofte and Williams, 1981a). The rapid restoration of intravascular volume and adequate tissue perfusion, using fluids and vasopressors if necessary, is the top priority. In order to achieve this goal, adequate monitoring of central venous pressure, cardiac output and pulmonary wedge pressure is mandatory in severe cases to monitor fluid balance and to detect early evidence of cardiac dysfunction. Pulmonary edema and acute respiratory disease syndrome (ARDS), which are almost inevitable following massive fluid replacement, should be managed early and aggressively with oxygen, artificial ventilation and positive end expiratory pressure.

Despite the presence of disseminated intravascular coagulation and marked thrombocytopenia, bleeding is usually not a problem and specific therapy is rarely necessary. Acute renal failure usually responds to rapid fluid administration, and in some cases hemodialysis may be necessary for a short period of time (R. W. Chesney *et al.*, 1981).

Hypocalcemia is thought to be related to both the low serum protein and the extraordinary high levels of serum calcitonin present (Chesney *et al.*, 1983). Very few patients have developed tetany; this suggests calcium may not need to be administered routinely. In one TSS case report, the administration of calcium resulted in the rapid resolution of prolonged hypotension, suggesting that low calcium concentrations may potentiate the activity of the toxin (Nusser *et al.*, 1981).

Although most critically ill TSS patients have received large doses of methylprednisolone or dexamethasone, the efficacy of these drugs for TSS has not been established. It has been suggested that steroids may be beneficial in reducing the length of fever and severity of fever if given early enough (Todd *et al.*, 1982).

Specific therapy for TSS involves the eradication of *S. aureus* and removal of TSS-associated toxin. With the exception of the rare patient who has a bacteremia or *S. aureus* bacteriuria, the use of antibiotics is not critical to recovery from the acute episode. Rather, specific antimicrobial therapy appears to be most crucial for eradication of the organism and prevention of recurrences. The importance of eradicating the focus of infection by removal of foreign bodies (tampons) and drainage and irrigation of abscesses, wounds and infected cavities has not been evaluated prospectively, but theoretically appears to be a very important aspect of management. Irrigation of such areas for removal of preformed toxin has also been suggested.

Systemic removal and inactivation of toxin may be best accomplished by rapidly restoring renal function. Staphylococcal enterotoxins, exoproteins comparable in size to PEC and SEF, have been shown to be broken down in the renal parenchyma of monkeys and rapidly excreted by the kidneys (Normann *et al.*, 1969; Normann, 1971). Impaired renal function may lead to decreased clearance or breakdown of toxin with continuing toxin recirculation. One report documented the rapid response of a patient with prolonged and refractory hypotension to acute hemodialysis (Fraley *et al.*, 1981).

Theoretically, administration of antitoxin may be useful for systemic inactivation of the toxin(s). Antibody to SEF has been found to be present in titers of 1:40,000 in an intravenous preparation of pooled human immune globulin (Chesney *et al.*, 1982). Using the analogies of other toxin-mediated diseases, such as tetanus and botulism, the early administration of immune globulin or a specific antitoxin might be an important aspect of therapy. Currently, such a recommendation cannot be made for TSS for several reasons: Koch's postulates have not yet been fulfilled for SEF or PEC, administration of immune globulin with specific antitoxin might result in the formation of harmful circulating immune complexes, and human studies documenting the efficacy and safety of this therapy have not yet been carried out.

F.   Recurrences

Recurrent TSS was first noted in Wisconsin in the Davis *et al.* (1980) study of 35 cases of menstrual TSS; 10 (28%) were noted to have recurrences. The incidence of recurrent TSS among nationally reported cases in 1980 also was approximately 30%. The majority of these recurrences occur during the first three menstrual periods following the acute illness, and all known recurrent episodes of TSS have been associated with menstrual TSS. Although the first episode is usually the most severe, mild episodes may precede a severe one (Davis *et al.*, 1980).

The rate of recurrence can be altered significantly through the use of antibiotics and discontinuing tampon use. The antibiotics are probably important for eradication of *S. aureus* colonization. Initially, Davis *et al.* (1980) found that patients who were treated with beta-lactamase-resistant antibiotics (BLRA) during their initial TSS episodes had a significantly lower rate of recurrence as compared to patients who did not receive BLRA during the initial episode. Data from the Tri-State TSS Study demonstrated that only 5 of 30 patients who received antistaphylococcal antibiotics during the initial episode and who discontinued tampon use after the initial episode (+AS/−tampon) had a recurrence by the fifth month after the initial episode, as compared to 12 of 18 patients who did not receive antistaphylococcal antibiotics during the initial episode and who continued to use tampons after the initial episode (Davis *et al.*, 1982a).

The rate of recurrences among Wisconsin patients with menstrual TSS has decreased from 65% (17/26) prior to 1980, to 20% (15/74) in 1980, and 0% (0/29) after 1980. Concomitantly, the percentage of patients in the +AS/−tampon category increased from 4% (1/26) prior to 1980, to 45% (27/60) in 1980, and 73% (19/26) after 1980 (J. P. Davis, personal observation; Stolz *et al.*, 1982). Thus, health education concerning the necessity for antistaphylococcal antibiotics and discontinuing tampon use have resulted in a dramatic decrease of the rate of recurrence of TSS.

Some patients do not develop antibody to the toxin following their illness and theoretically remain susceptible to TSS. This may account for the high rate of recurrences that have been noted with menstrual TSS. Serologic studies have demonstrated that fewer than 15% of patients with TSS have an acute anti-SEF titer of ≥1:5, determined by radioimmunoassay methods, in contrast to the general population where 90% of males and females more than 25 years of age have anti-SEF. In addition, only 45% of women with menstrual TSS develop an anti-SEF titer of ≥1:100 at 1 year after their initial illness (Stolz *et al.*, 1982; Vergeront *et al.*, 1983).

G. Recognition and management of mild cases of menstrual TSS

Recognition and careful management of patients with mild TSS is critical in order to prevent subsequent severe episodes (P. J. Chesney *et al.*, 1981; McKenna *et al.*, 1980; Tofte and Williams, 1981b). Recognition of such patients should start with a high index of suspicion for TSS in any woman experiencing an apparently infectious illness during menses. The presence of any combination of fever, headache, rash of any type, sore throat, diarrhea, vomiting, dizziness, syncope or myalgias should lead to examination of any vaginal discharge, cultures of the cervix and vagina for *S. aureus,* a urinalysis and urine culture, a complete blood count, and obtaining a serum to store for determination of the presence of antibody to SEF or PEC. If *S. aureus* is identified, the isolate should be saved for a determination of its ability to make SEF or PEC. If *S. aureus* is isolated from cervico–vaginal cultures of a menstruating patient, particularly from one using tampons who has a clinical picture compatible with some of the manifestations of TSS, discontinuation of tampon use should be recommended until it is certain that the patient is not susceptible to the TSS-associated toxin, and it may be appropriate to initiate therapy with a beta-lactamase-resistant antibiotic. Confirmation that the patient did have a mild case of TSS will depend on the subsequent development of desquamation and demonstration that the *S. aureus* isolate produced SEF or PEC and that there was no significant initial (acute phase) antibody titer to SEF or PEC.

Typically, patients with menstrual TSS do not develop anti-SEF antibody for up to several years after their initial episode and are thus presumably still at risk for recurrences (Stolz *et al.*, 1982). Thus, consideration should be given to repeating cultures and antibody determinations to determine whether a significant anti-SEF titer has been reached before tampon use is resumed.

Although the age, sex and race of patients with nonmenstrual TSS do differ from patients with menstrually associated TSS, the clinical manifestations do not differ (Reingold *et al.*, 1982b). TSS can clearly occur in any individual who has an infection due to a toxin-producing strain of *S. aureus* and who does not have antibody to SEF or PEC.

Table 2 Differential diagnosis of toxic-shock syndrome

Multi-system infections
    Septic shock with localized infection (meningococcus, gonococcus,
      pneumococcus, *H. influenzae* b)
    Leptospirosis
    Rubeola
    Rocky Mountain spotted fever
    Tick-borne typhus
    Viral syndrome (adeno- or enteroviruses)
    Legionnaires' disease
    Toxoplasmosis
Toxin-mediated infections
    Staphylococcal scalded skin syndrome
    Scarlet fever
    Gastroenteritis
Localized infections with abdominal pain and shock
    Urinary-tract infection
    Pelvic inflammatory disease
    Septic abortion
    Gastroenteritis
Noninfectious diseases
    Systemic lupus erythematosis
    Acute rheumatic fever
    Drug-related eruption (erythema multiforme, Stevens–Johnson
      syndrome)
    Juvenile rheumatoid arthritis
Multisystem illness, possibly infectious
    Kawasaki syndrome

H. Differential diagnosis

Although TSS has a relatively distinct constellation of clinical and laboratory findings, the differential diagnosis might include the entities listed in Table 2. The acute onset of disease with rapid progression to hypotension and multi-system involvement is most likely to be confused with sepsis and septic shock, meningococcemia, urinary-tract infection, leptospirosis, Rocky Mountain spotted fever, a fulminant viral syndrome, or a severe toxin-induced diarrhea.

Localized infections with septicemia and septic shock can usually be distinguished from TSS by the absence of erythroderma, conjunctivitis, subconjunctival hemorrhages and the generalized beefy-red erythema of all mucous membranes. In addition, few such patients have the profuse watery diarrhea present in moderate to severe TSS. Exclusion of this diagnosis is generally completed by the evaluation of the subsequent hospital course and absence of positive bacterial cultures of the blood and infected sites.

The rash, high fever and generalized toxicity may be seen in individuals with rubeola, viral syndromes due to the adenoviruses or enteroviruses, scarlet fever and the staphylococcal scalded skin syndrome. However, profuse diarrhea, evidence of multisystem involvement, generalized edema and rapid onset of hypotension would be unusual for all these entities. Other distinguishing clinical features of these diseases, such as cough with rubeola and purulent pharyngitis with scarlet fever, may be present. Finally, the results of bacterial and viral cultures should readily confirm the clinical impression.

Kawasaki syndrome is a multisystem disease that rarely occurs over the age of 7 years and is characterized by the onset of prolonged fever, lymphadenitis, conjunctivitis and rash with progression to erythema of mucous membranes, thrombocytosis, and characteristic peeling of the distal digits during the recovery phase. Prolongation of fever is an important distinguishing feature of Kawasaki syndrome, and patients with Kawasaki syndrome are rarely hypotensive. Myocardial or coronary artery injury may be present during the acute and convalescent stages. There is no known association of this disease with *S. aureus* or *Streptococcus pyogenes*. Although adult cases of Kawasaki syndrome have been reported recently (Everett, 1979; Milgrom *et al.,* 1980; Schlossberg *et al.,* 1979), most appear to have been cases of TSS.

Leptospirosis may present with fever, conjunctival injection, rash, headache and myalgias, but rarely does this disease progress to shock with evidence of severe multisystem involvement. Most cases of leptospirosis are diagnosed serologically.

Rocky Mountain spotted fever (RMSF) characteristically presents with the prodromal symptoms of frontal headache, fever, and myalgias (particularly of the gastrocnemius). About half the time a history of a tick bite during the preceding week can be elicited. After several days of the prodromal symptoms, a maculopapular rose-colored rash initially appears peripherally on the hands, feet, wrists and ankles. If treatment is delayed, the lesions may become petechial and then purpuric. Severe diarrhea, vomiting, and hypotension are not seen early in RMSF, although shock, disseminated intravascular coagulation and renal failure can occur later in the disease. The diagnosis may be difficult as 10% of patients with RMSF do not have an exanthem; RMSF is diagnosed serologically.

The arena viruses responsible for Lassa and dengue fever cause fulminant, potentially fatal viral infections associated with fever, rash, conjunctivitis and shock. Familiarity with the regions of endemic Lassa fever and dengue fever and careful travel histories should assist in the distinction of these illnesses from TSS.

Stevens–Johnson syndrome is usually due to an adverse drug reaction or infection and is associated with exfoliative dermatitis, mucous-membrane lesions, fever, and toxicity. Intestinal symptoms may be present due to an erosive enteritis. Corneal lesions are frequently present, and multisystem involvement with hypotension is uncommon.

IX. PREVENTION OF TSS

Theoretically, many TSS cases could be prevented by intermittent screening of individuals in "high-risk" groups for the absence of anti-SEF antibodies. Such individuals could then conceivably be intermittently screened for the presence of PEC- or SEF-producing *S. aureus*, and immunotherapy such as toxoid or passively administered antitoxin could be provided. However, the incidence of TSS does not warrant such an approach, nor are the reagents or techniques yet available to perform such tests. While discontinuing the use of tampons will clearly reduce the risk of menstrual TSS, other recommendations regarding tampon usage have not been well studied. Issues that merit further study include determination of what is a "safe tampon," and determination of the optimal pattern of tampon use, which considers the optimal frequency of change, optimal time of wearing, and optimal use of additional catamenial products.

Once an individual has had menstrual TSS, the recurrence risk is high enough that attempts to eradicate the organism with antibiotics should be made. Tampon use should be discontinued until a significant anti-SEF titer can be demonstrated.

Widespread health education efforts and media publicity pertaining to TSS have been beneficial. The case fatality rate among all cases of TSS reported to the CDC has decreased from 14.8% in patients with onsets prior to 1979, to 4.9% in patients with onsets in 1980, to 3.1% in patients with onsets in 1981 (Institute of Medicine, 1982; Reingold *et al.*, 1982c). In addition, the decreasing number of reported confirmed cases of TSS might reflect the actual prevention of cases or amelioration of signs and symptoms to such a degree that cases are not severe enough to meet the confirmed or probable case definition.

After media publicity on TSS in 1980, the pattern of catamenial product usage in the United States changed dramatically. During July to August 1980, prior to widespread publicity on Rely® tampons, 47.1% of catamenial units sold in the United States were tampons; during the next four months, tampon unit sales declined 25% and represented only 35.7% of all catamenial unit sales (Osterholm *et al.*, 1982b). In Minnesota, between October 1980 and June 1981, the percentage of market share of tampon units in the highest absorbency category dropped from 31.4% to 24.5% (Osterholm *et al.*, 1982b).

In California, a survey of adolescent women representing a diverse cultural/ethnic distribution demonstrated that roughly 34% changed their tampon usage habits and 28% stopped using tampons after publicity on TSS. Adolescent tampon users that shifted toward napkin use were more likely to have been Rely® brand tampon users or those individuals who for some reason felt more susceptible to TSS (Irwin and Millstein, 1982).

However, among controls in the Tri-State TSS Study, 70–75% of women in the 15-to-24-year age group, the group that had highest risk of developing TSS, continued to use tampons in the highest absorbency group 1 year after widespread publicity on menstrual TSS. This rate of use was higher than that found for the general public based on market research data. Generally, increases in tampon sales have been noted since January 1981 (Osterholm *et al.*, 1982b).

Health education efforts must continue to enhance the decision-making efforts of those at greatest risk of TSS. With this in mind, the Institute of Medicine Committee on TSS (Institute of Medicine, 1982) has recommended that:

1. Women who have already had TSS should be advised not to use tampons. Postpartum women should be informed that the use of tampons may increase TSS risk.
2. Women, especially adolescents, should be advised to minimize their use of high-absorbency tampons.
3. Physicians and other health professionals should be informed about the variations in presentation of non-tampon-associated cases that have occurred, should be alerted to the symptoms of TSS, and should be encouraged to report all definite and probable cases, as well as suspected cases. Physicians also should be advised that treatment of TSS patients with beta-lactamase-resistant antibiotics apparently decreases the chance of recurrence.

The United States Food and Drug Administration has mandated that warning labels discussing the risks and association of TSS with the use of tampons be included on the tampon packages (Food and Drug Administration, 1982). Tampon manufacturers in conjunction with consumers through the American Society for Testing and Materials (Philadelphia, PA) are currently involved in establishing standards for tampon labeling, absorbency assessment, and other factors concerning product safety.

X. UNRESOLVED PROBLEMS AND MAJOR RESEARCH NEEDS

Continued active surveillance of TSS is critical to determine long-term trends, evaluate the effectiveness of health education and control measures on the incidence of disease, and to clarify geographic and racial differences in incidence. Retrospective hospital chart reviews would also be important to determine some of these differences.

Development of an appropriate animal model is critical to define mechanisms of pathogenesis and determinants of host resistance and susceptibility in TSS. Human studies will be necessary to further clarify human susceptibility, the immune response, and further determine the efficacy of antibiotic therapy in TSS. Further animal and human work is necessary to determine how the specific organism associated with TSS accesses humans and becomes colonized. The mechanism by which tampons enhance the risk of TSS is not precisely known, nor is it clear what the effect of tampons are on the organism, toxin production, and on the bacterial flora of the vagina.

Finally, the development of a good useful clinical diagnostic test will ease the ability to screen for this disease, will obviate the need for a strict clinical case definition in some situations, and will enhance early diagnosis.

ACKNOWLEDGMENTS

From the Bureau of Community Health and Prevention, the Wisconsin Division of Health; and the Departments of Pediatrics and Preventive Medicine, the University of Wisconsin Center for Health Sciences, Madison, Wisconsin.

REFERENCES

Abdul-Karim, F. W., Lederman, M. D., Carter, J. R., Hewlett, E. L., Newman, A. J., and Greene, B. M. (1981). *Hum. Path.* **12,** 16.

Alcid, D. V., Kothari, N., Quinn, E. P., Geismar, L., and Glowinsky, L. Z. (1982). *Lancet* **1,** 1363–1364.

Altemeier, W. A., Lewis, S. A., Schlievert, P. M., and Bjornson, H. S. (1981). *Surg. Gynecol. Obstet.* **153,** 481–485.

Altemeier, W. A., Lewis, S. A., Schlievert, P. M., Bergdoll, M. S., Bjornson, H. S., Staneck, J. L., and Crass, B. A. (1982). *Ann. Intern. Med.* **96**(Part 2), 978–982.

Aranow, H. Jr., and Wood, W. B., Jr. (1942). *JAMA, J. Am. Med. Assoc.* **119,** 1491–1495.

Baehler, E. A., Dillon, W. P., Cumbo, T. J., and Lee, R. V. (1982). *Fertil. Steril.* **38,** 248–250.

Barbour, A. G. (1981). *Infect. Immun.* **33,** 442–449.

Barrett, K. F., Bledsoe, S., Greer, B. E., and Droegemueller, W. (1977). *Am. J. Obstet. Gynecol.* **144,** 386–388.

Bartlett, J. G., Onderdonk, A. B., Drude, E., Goldstein, C., Anderka, M., Alpert, S., and McCormack, W. M. (1977). *J. Infect. Dis.* **136,** 271–277.

Bartlett, P., Reingold, A. L., Graham, D. R., Dan, B. B., Selinger, D. S., Tank, G. W., and Wichterman, K. A. (1982). *JAMA, J. Am. Med. Assoc.* **247,** 1448–1450.

Bassaris, H. P., Venezio, F. R., Morlock, B. A., and Phair, J. P. (1981). *J. Infect. Dis.* **144,** 386–388.

Bastian, J., Carson, S., Conners, J., and Griswold, W. (1981). *Clin. Res.* **29**(2), 125A.

Bergdoll, M. S., Crass, B. A., Reiser, R. F., Robbins, R. N., and Davis, J. P. (1981). *Lancet* **1,** 1017–1021.

Berger, E. M., Bowman, C. M., Harada, R. N., and Repine, J. E. (1982). *Clin. Res.* **30**(1), 57A.

Blair, J. D., Livingston, D. G., and Vongsnichakul, R. (1982). *Am. J. Clin. Pathol.* **78,** 372–376.

Bonventre, P. F. (1983). *Lancet* **1,** 873–874.

Broome, C. V., Hayes, P. S., Ajello, G. W., Feeley, J. C., Gibson, R. J., Graves, L.

M., Hancock, G. A., Anderson, R. L., Highsmith, A. K., Mackel, D. C., Hargrett, N. T., and Reingold, A. L. (1982). *Ann. Intern. Med.* **96**(Part 2), 959–962.

Brown, W. J. (1982). *Ann. Intern. Med.* **96**, 931–934.

Centers for Disease Control (1980a). *Morbid. Mortal. Week. Rep.* **29**, 229–230.

Centers for Disease Control (1980b). *Morbid. Mortal. Week. Rep.,* **29**, 441–445.

Centers for Disease Control (1981). *Morbid. Mortal. Week. Rep.* **30**, 25–33.

Centers for Disease Control (1982a). *Morbid. Mortal. Week. Rep.* **31**, 201–204.

Centers for Disease Control (1982b). *Morbid. Mortal. Week. Rep.* **32**, 18.

Chesney, P. J., Davis, J. P., Purdy, W. K., Wand, P. J., and Chesney, R. W. (1981). *JAMA, J. Am. Med. Assoc.* **246**, 741–748.

Chesney, P. J., Crass, B. A., Polyak, M. B., Wand, P. J., Warner, T. F., Vergeront, J. M., Davis, J. P., Tofte, R. W., Chesney, R. W., and Bergdoll, M. S. (1982). *Ann. Intern. Med.* **96**(Part 2), 847–851.

Chesney, R. W., Chesney, P. J., Davis, J. P., and Segar, W. E. (1981). *Am. J. Med.* **71**, 583–588.

Chesney, R. W., McCarron, D. M., Haddad, J. G., Hawker, C. D., DiBella, F. P., Chesney, P. J., and Davis, J. P. (1983). *J. Lab. Clin. Med.* **101**, 576–585.

Chow, A. W., Gribble, M. J., and Bartlett, K. H. (1983). *J. Clin. Microbiol.* **17**, 524–528.

Cobb, W. B., Helms, W. B., and Hoseley, P. L. (1982). *N. Engl. J. Med.* **306**, 1422–1423.

Cohen, M. L. and Falkow, S. (1981). *Science* **211**, 842–844.

Corbishley, C. M. (1977). *J. Clin. Pathol.* **30**, 745–748.

Davis, J. P., and Vergeront, J. M. (1982). *J. Infect. Dis.* **145**, 449–457.

Davis, J. P., Chesney, P. J., Wand, P. J., LaVenture, M., and the Investigative and Laboratory Team (1980). *N. Engl. J. Med.* **303**, 1429–1435.

Davis, J. P., Osterholm, M. T., Helms, C. M., Vergeront, J. M., Wintermeyer, L. A., Forfang, J. C., Judy, L. A., Rondeau, J., Schell, W. L., and the Investigative Team (1982a). *J. Infect. Dis.* **145**, 441–448.

Davis, J. P., Vergeront, J. M., and Chesney, P. J. (1982b). *Ann. Intern. Med.* **96**(Part 2), 986–991.

Deetz, T. R., Reves, R., and Septimus, B. (1981). *N. Engl. J. Med.* **304**, 174.

De Nooij, M. P., Van Leeuwan, W. J., and Notermans, S. (1982). *J. Hyg.* **89**, 499–505.

de Saxe, M., Wieneke, A. A., De Azevedo, J., and Arbuthnott, J. P. (1982). *Ann. Intern. Med.* **96**(Part 2), 991–996.

DeYoung, P., Martyn, J., Wass, H., Harth, L., Crichton, E., and Reynolds, C. (1982). *Can. Med. Assoc. J.* **127**, 611–612.

Dunnet, W. B., and Schallibaum, E. M. (1960). *Lancet* **2**, 1227–1229.

Everett, E. D. (1979). *J. Am. Med. Assoc.* **242**, 542–543.

Fischer, C. J., Horowitz, B. Z., and Nolan, S. M. (1981). *West. J. Med.* **135**, 175–182.

Fisher, R. F., Goodpasture, H. C., Peterie, J. D., and Voth, D. W. (1981). *Ann. Intern. Med.* **94**, 156–163.

Food and Drug Administration. (1982). *FDA Drug Bull.* **3**, 19–20.

Fraley, D. S., Bruns, F. J., Segel, D. P., and Adler, S. (1981). *Ann. Intern. Med.* **95**, 124.

Friedrich, E. G., and Siegesmund, K. A. (1980). *Obstet. Gynecol.* **55**, 149–156.

Fuller, A. F., Jr., Swartz, M. N., Wolfson, J. S., and Salzman, R. (1980). *N. Engl. J. Med.* **303**, 881.

Fumarola, D. (1979). *Lancet* **1**, 221.

Guinan, M. E., Dan, B. B., Guidotti, R. J., Reingold, A. L., Schmid, G. P., Bettoli, E. J., Lossick, J. G., Shands, K. N., Kramer, M. A., Hargrett, N. T., Anderson, R. L., and Broome, C. V. (1982). *Ann. Intern. Med.* **96**(Part 2), 944–947.

Helgerson, S. D., and Foster, L. R. (1982). *Ann. Intern. Med.* **96**(Part 2), 909–911.
Helms, C. M., Lengeling, R. W., Pinsky, R. L., Myers, M. G., Koontz, F. P., Klassen, L. W., and Wintermeyer, L. A. (1981). *Am. J. Med. Sci.* **282**, 50–60.
Ikejima, T., Dinarello, C. A., Gill, M. D., and Wolff, S. M. (1983). *Clin. Res.* **31**, 496A.
Institute of Medicine (1982). "Toxic Shock Syndrome: Assessment of Current Information and Future Research Needs." Nat. Acad. Sci., Washington, D.C.
Irwin, C. E., Jr., and Millstein, S. G. (1982). *Am. J. Public Health* **72**, 464–467.
Ishak, K. G., and Rogers, W. A. (1981). *Am. J. Clin. Pathol.* **76**, 629–626.
Jimerson, S. D., and Becker, J. D. (1980). *Obstet. Gynecol.* **56**, 97–99.
Kapral, F. A. (1982). *Ann. Intern. Med.* **96**(Part 2), 972–974.
Kehrberg, M. W., Latham, R. H., Haslam, B. T., Hightower, A., Tanner, M., Jacobson, J. A., Barbour, A. G., Nobel, V., and Smith, C. B. (1981). *Am. J. Epidemiol.* **114**, 873–879.
Kreiswirth, B. N., Novick, R. P., Schlievert, P. M., and Bergdoll, M. (1982). *Ann. Intern. Med.* **96**(Part 2), 974–977.
Kreiswirth, B. N., Lofdahl, S., Betley, M. J., O'Reilly, M., Schlievert, P. M., Bergdoll, M. S., and Novick, R. P. (1983). *Nature* **305**, 709–712.
Larkin, S. M., Williams, D. N., Osterholm, M. T., Tofte, R. W., and Posalaky, Z. (1982). *Ann. Intern. Med.* **96**(Part 2), 858–864.
Larsen, B., and Galask, R. P. (1980). *Obstet. Gynecol.* **55**, 1005–1135.
Larsen, B., and Galask, R. P. (1982). *Ann. Intern. Med.* **96**(Part 2), 926–930.
Lawellin, D. W., Frano-Bulf, A., Vasil, M. L. and Todd, J. K. (1983). *Abstr. Annu. Meet. Am. Soc. Microbiol.* Abst. B194, p. 156.
Lee, A. C., and Crass, B. A. (1983). *Abstr. Annu. Meet. Am. Soc. Microbiol.* Abst. B27, p. 59.
Lentino, J. R., Rytel, M. W. and Davis, J. P. (1981). *N. Engl. J. Med.* **305**, 641–642.
Linneman, C. C., Staneck, J. L., and Hornstein, S. (1982). *Ann. Intern. Med.* **96**(Part 2), 940–944.
McKenna, U. G., Meadows, J. A., III, Brewer, N. S., Wilson, W. R., and Perrault, J. (1980). *Mayo Clin. Proc.* **55**, 663–672.
Martin, R. R., Buttram, V., Besch, P., Kirkland, J. J., and Petty, G. P. (1982). *Ann. Intern. Med.* **96**(Part 2), 951–953.
Melish, M. E., and Glasgow, L. A. (1970). *N. Engl. J. Med.* **282**, 1114–1119.
Melish, M. E., Chen, F. S., and Murata, S. M. (1982). *Clin. Res.* **31**(1), 122A.
Milgrom, H., Palmer, E. L., Slovin, S. F., Morens, D. M., Freeman, S. D., and Vaughan, J. H. (1980). *Ann. Intern. Med.* **92**, 467–470.
Minnesota Department of Health. (1980). *Dis. Control Newsl.* **7**(8).
Murphy, P. A., Simon, P. L., and Willoughby, W. F. (1980). *J. Immunol.* **124**, 2498–2503.
Noble, V. S., Jacobson, J. A. and Smith, C. B. (1982). *Am. J. Obstet. Gynecol.* **144**, 186–189.
Normann, S. J. (1971). *Lab. Invest.* **25**, 126–132.
Normann, S. J., Jaeger, R. F. and Johnsey, R. T. (1969). *Lab. Invest.* **20**, 17–25.
Notermans, S., and Dufrenne, J. B. (1982). *Antonie van Leeuwenhoek* **48**, 447–455.
Nusser, R., Rowe, P., Frierson, J. G., and Murphy, C. (1981). *Ann. Intern. Med.* **95**, 124–125.
Osterholm, M. T., and Forfang, J. R. (1982). *J. Infect. Dis.* **145**, 458–464.
Osterholm, M. T., Davis, J. P., Gibson, R. W., Mandel, J. S., Wintermeyer, L. A.,

Helms, C. M., Forfang, J. C., Rondeau, J., Vergeront, J. M., and The Investigative Team (1982a). *J. Infect. Dis.* **145**, 431–440.

Osterholm, M. T., Davis, J. P., Gibson, R. W., Forfang, J. C., Stolz, S. J., Vergeront, J. M., and the Investigative Team (1982b). *Ann. Intern. Med.* **96**(Part 2), 954–958.

Paris, A. L., Herwaldt, L. A., Blum, D., Schmid, G. P., Shands, K. N., and Broome, C. V. (1982). *Ann. Intern. Med.* **96**(Part 2), 852–857.

Peterson, P. K., Schlievert, P. M., Conroy, W., Kelly, J. A., Spika, J., and Quie, P. G. (1983). *J. Infect. Dis.* **147**(2), 358.

Quimby, F. W., Olstad, M., and Weiner, E. (1984). *Fed. Proc.* **43**, 378.

Reingold, A. L., Dan, B. B., Shands, K. N., and Broome, C. V. (1982a). *Lancet* **1**, 1–4.

Reingold, A. L., Hargrett, N. T., Dan, B. B., Shands, K. N., Strickland, B. Y., and Broome, C. V. (1982b). *Ann. Intern. Med.* **96**(Part 2), 871–874.

Reingold, A. L., Hargrett, N. T., Shands, K. N., Dan, B. B., Schmid, G. P., Strickland, B. Y., and Broome, C. V. (1982c). *Ann. Intern. Med.* **96**(Part 2), 875–880.

Rosene, K. A., Copass, M. K., Kastner, L. S., Nolan, C. M., and Eschenbach, D. A. (1982). *Ann. Intern. Med.* **96**(Part 2), 865–870.

Sanders, C. C., Sanders, W. E., Jr., and Fagnant, J. E. (1982). *Am. J. Obstet. Gynecol.* **142**, 977–982.

Sautter, R. L., and Brown, W. J. (1980). *J. Clin. Microbiol.* **11**, 479–484.

Schlech, W. F., Shands, K. N., Reingold, A. L., Dan, B. B., Schmid, G. P., Hargrett, N. T., Hightower, A., Herwaldt, L. A., Neill, M. A., Band, J. D., and Bennett, J. V. (1982). *JAMA J. Am. Med. Assoc.* **248**, 835–839.

Schlievert, P. M. (1982). *Infect. Immun.* **36**, 123–128.

Schlievert, P. M. (1983). *J. Infect. Dis.* **147**, 391–398.

Schlievert, P. M., and Blomster, D. A. (1983). *J. Infect. Dis.* **147**, 236–342.

Schlievert, P. M., Shands, K. N., Dan, B. B., Schmid, G. P., and Nishimura, R. D. (1981). *J. Infect. Dis.* **143**, 509–516.

Schlievert, P. M., Osterholm, M. T. and Kelly, J. A. (1982). *Ann. Intern. Med.* **96**(Part 2), 937–940.

Schlossberg, D., Kandra, J., and Kreiser, J. (1979). *Arch. Dermatol.* **115**, 1435–1436.

Schrock, C. G. (1980). *JAMA, J. Am. Med. Assoc.* **243**, 1231.

Schutzer, S. E., Fischetti, V. A., and Fabsiskie, J. B. (1983). *Science* **220**, 316–318.

Scott, D. F., Kling, J. M., Kirkland, J. J., and Best, G. K. (1983). *Infect. Immun.* **39**, 383–387.

Shands, K. N., Schmid, G. P., Dan, B. B., Blum, D., Guidotti, R. J., Hargrett, N. T., Anderson, R. L., Hill, D. L., Broome, C. V., Band, J. D., and Fraser, D. W. (1980). *N. Engl. J. Med.* **303**, 1436–1442.

Smith, C. B., Noble, V., Bensch, R., Ahlin, P. A., Jacobson, J. A., and Latham, R. H. (1982). *Ann. Intern. Med.* **96**(Part 2), 948–951.

Stallones, R. A. (1982). *Ann. Intern. Med.* **96**(Part 2), 917–920.

Stevens, F. A. (1927). *JAMA, J. Am. Med. Assoc.* **88**, 1957–1958.

Stolz, S. J., Davis, J. P., Vergeront, J. M., Crass, B. A., Bergdoll, M. S., Chesney, P. J., and Wand, P. J. (1982). *Intersci. Conf. Antimicrob. Agents Chemother., 22nd* Abst. 371.

Tierno, P. M., Hana, B. A., and Davies, M. B. (1983). *Lancet* **1**, 615–618.

Todd, J., Fishaut, M., Kapral, F., and Welch, T. (1978). *Lancet* **2**, 1116–1118.

Todd, J. K., Ressman, M., Caston, S. A., and Wiesenthal, A. M. (1982). *Intersci. Conf. Antimicrob. Agents Chemother., 22nd* Abst. 368.

Tofte, R. W., and Williams, D. N. (1981a). *Ann. Intern. Med.* **94**, 149–156.

Tofte, R. W., and Williams, D. N. (1981b). *JAMA, J. Am. Med. Assoc.* **246,** 2163–2167.

Vergeront, J. M., Evenson, M. L., Crass, B. A., Davis, J. P., Bergdoll, M. S., Wand, P. J., Noble, J. H., and Petersen, G. K. (1982). *J. Infect. Dis.* **145,** 456–459.

Vergeront, J. M., Stolz, S. J., Crass, B. A., Davis, J. P., Bergdoll, M. S., Wand, P. J., Noble, J. H., and Petersen, G. K. (1983). *J. Infect. Dis.* **148,** 692–698.

Wagner, G., and Ottesen, B. (1982). *Ann. Intern. Med.* **96**(Part 2), 921–923.

Wick, M. R., Bahn, R. C., and McKenna, U. G. (1982). *Mayo Clin. Proc.* **57,** 583–589.

Wiesenthal, A. M., Ressman, M., Caston, S. A., and Todd, J. K. (1982). *Intersci. Conf. Antimicrob. Agents Chemother., 22nd* Abst. 537.

2 The acquired immune deficiency syndrome

DONALD ARMSTRONG

The acquired immune deficiency syndrome (AIDS) is an appalling disease seen regularly in certain large cities in the United States and Canada, but also now recognized in Europe.

The immune deficiency, which is acquired by certain individuals at risk (Table 1), results in the development of opportunistic infections and neoplasia. The opportunistic infections (OI) are due to organisms which take advantage of a defect in the thymus-derived lymphocyte, mononuclear phagocyte arm of the immune defense, and they are listed in Tables 2–5. The neoplasms that have occurred have usually been Kaposi's sarcoma (KS), but others that appear in some of the high-risk groups are B cell lymphomas, including Burkitt's and squamous-cell carcinomas of the anus and mouth. These are mainly seen in homosexual men, and the lymphomas have been unusually aggressive, including involvement of the brain.

I. EPIDEMIOLOGY

AIDS was first recognized in New York City, Los Angeles and San Francisco in 1981, when homosexual men were noted to develop KS and OI, and intravenous drug addicts were also developing OI. Reports first appeared in the Centers for Disease Control (CDC), U.S. Public Health Service publication, *Weekly Morbidity and Mortality Reports* (1981) and subsequently in journals (Gottlieb *et al.*, 1981; Masur *et al.*, 1981; Siegal *et al.*, 1981). The CDC established a task force to work with city and state health departments and with physicians seeing the patients. In New York City a working group of such physicians was established by the Commissioner of Health and has been meeting on a monthly basis since. These meetings include reports by representatives from CDC on the international and national epidemiology, reports from the N.Y.C. Department of Health members on cases in the Greater New York City Area, including New Jersey, and reports from members of various groups in the area studying the disease. The meetings are large (50 or more people) and the discussions are lively. Because we believed the CDC definition (Centers for Disease Control, 1982) to be imprecise, we attempted to establish our own definition of AIDS. A committee was appointed. Disagreement abounded. The committee was disbanded. A working definition will appear in another publication (Armstrong, 1983), but it has become apparent that hairsplitting is unnecessary. The immune deficiency is unique in that it is clearly progressive. Thus the Kaposi's sarcoma is progressive, and the opportunistic infections are not only difficult to treat, but occur one after the other and tend to recur. The CDC definition will suffice until the agent or a specific immune defect is found. It is important that we do not label as AIDS the symptoms and signs we do not understand occurring in high-risk groups. An example is lymphadenopathy. Of more than 100 people in high-risk groups with lymphadenopathy that we have followed, 90% have not developed AIDS. It *is* imprecise to label as AIDS lymphadenopathy or any other set of signs or symptoms that are nonspecific. Table 1 lists those groups of people who have or may have developed AIDS. The types of people at risk plus clusters of cases among homosexual men suggest an infectious agent which is passed by sexual contact between men, by inoculated blood products, and by intimate contact of children with infected parents. This epidemiological pattern suggests an agent such as hepatitis B, hepatitis non-A or non-B or cytomegalovirus (CMV). It is not entirely clear that AIDS is spread by blood transfusions, but evidence appears to be mounting that it is. It does not appear as prevalent as hepatitis B. Against the suggestion of a highly cell-associated virus such as cytomegalovirus is the fact that the agent survives the preparation of factor VIII concentrate for hemophiliacs. Cytomegalovirus has survived storage in blood for weeks (Armstrong *et al.,* 1971), however, and remains among the leading candidates for an etiological or contributing agent. Other candidates include retroviruses, delta virus, para-

Table 1   Risk groups for AIDS

People at risk for AIDS
   Homosexual men
   Intravenous drug abusers
   Hemophiliacs receiving factor VIII concentrate
Apparently at risk for AIDS
   Spouses of above
   Children of above
   Haitians other than above?
   Central African residents?
   Blood-product recipients

---

voviruses, adenoviruses, papovaviruses and unknown or previously undescribed agents. Retroviruses such as the human T cell leukemia virus (HTLV) have received considerable attention recently as candidate causes of AIDS. A number of patients with AIDS have antibody, some have infection of the T cells, and a retrovirus of cats can cause an immune deficiency syndrome as well as feline leukemia (Essex *et al.*, 1983; Gallo *et al.*, 1983; Barre-Sinoussi *et al.*, 1983; Francis, 1983). These facts plus the mysterious presence of the HTLV in southern Japan, the United States and the Caribbean has attracted considerable attention to the retroviruses. Some strongly object to claiming retroviruses as leading potential causal agents (Black and Levy, 1983).

An explanation of the appearance of this disease in 1981 on the basis of known viruses requires a change in the action of a virus or the introduction of a previously unrecognized agent. One hypothesis is that CMV was rapidly passed in the bath houses and gay bars of these cities so that a particularly virulent strain was selected that exaggerates the immunosuppression previously noted during self-limited CMV infections. Another hypothesis is that an unusual strain of a known virus or of an unknown agent has been introduced from a society where it occurred rarely and went unnoticed by the medical profession until it was passed among promiscuous homosexual men and i.v. drug abusers in areas where it was recognized.

The epidemic rages rather than wanes. In New York City during the summer of 1982, one new case was seen every other day. During the autumn this increased until by January 1983 a new case was seen every day, and this was reflected in reports of increased numbers nationwide. If subclinical infection occurs leaving individuals immune, it has not been noted yet by a decrease in the epidemic curve.

II.   OPPORTUNISTIC INFECTIONS

The organisms causing the opportunistic infections that have been reported and those we anticipate will be seen are listed with comments in Tables 2–5. The organisms are facultative or obligate, intracellular parasites that tend to cause latent infections, which then recrudesce and disseminate in people who are immunosuppressed. We expect to see these organisms infecting patients with leukemias and lymphomas, which alter T cell function, or in organ and bone-marrow transplant recipients, whose T cell function we deliberately suppress. The patterns of infectious diseases that develop in the AIDS patients most resemble those seen in bone-marrow transplant recipients when their neutrophile counts are normal.

The immune defects that are most regularly documented in the AIDS patients are listed in Table 6. Not one of them is specific, and all are seen in other conditions. Whether a constellation of immune defects or certain levels of immune deficiency will eventually be found specific remains to be proven, but is doubtful. A specific test such as low NK activity or low levels of IF production by NK cells may be predictive, but it is most likely that the agent must be found and a diagnostic test developed on that basis before we will have a marker for AIDS.

We have seen 166 patients with AIDS at Memorial Sloan–Kettering Cancer Center. Of these, 127 had Kaposi's sarcoma and 39 had opportunistic infections. Some data are presented below concerning these patients. Most have been cared for primarily by J. W. M. Gold, B. Safai, P. Myskowski and S. Krown. A number of other members of our staff, however, have contributed measurably to their care.

III. VIRAL INFECTIONS

The viruses most commonly infecting patients with AIDS are listed in Table 2. It is most likely that the agent responsible for AIDS is a virus. Other types of agents such as spirochetes or difficult-to-grow intracellular parasites of various types could be responsible and should be investigated. The agent causes a decrease in

Table 2 Viruses

Organisms	Syndromes	Comment
Cytomegalovirus	Encephalitis Pneumonia Hepatitis Colitis Adrenalitis Disseminated	Found in almost all patients; liver, lungs and colon frequent sites of severe disease, and biopsy usually needed to document

Herpes simplex virus	Skin ulcers:
	  Persistent
	  Recurrent
	  Disseminated
		HSV-2 perineal lesion frequently an early occurrence; respond to antiviral therapy, but recur

Varicella–zoster virus	Local, severe Disseminated	Occasionally appear especially severe
Papovavirus	Central nervous system	Progressive multifocal leucoencephalopathy, one of major CNS diseases
Adenoviruses	Colonization Disseminated	Regularly isolated, rarely cause symptomatic disease; high serotypes similar to bone-marrow transplant patients

helper T cells and perhaps in an earlier stem-cell lymphocyte, so that natural killer cells are also affected. This results in the profound, persistent and progressive immune defect, and the neoplasms or opportunistic infections occur.

Cytomegalovirus is found most often among the viruses that infect AIDS patients and is the virus most often causing disseminated disease (Gold and Armstrong, 1983; Armstrong, 1983). It has been present in the disseminated form in 27 of our 35 autopsied patients, and antibody is present in all patients we have tested for it, with no exception. The syndromes most often seen are listed in Table 2. These must be reactivation infections in every case in most of the high-risk groups. Sexually active homosexuals are regularly exposed to CMV, as are i.v. drug abusers. In the other groups at risk, the degree of exposure is less certain but is probably high. With the techniques presently available it is not known how many different strains of CMV there are and whether reinfection occurs, so that differentiating new from recrudescent infection is not possible unless the patient is antibody-negative when first seen. We have not seen this in any of the AIDS patients.

Encephalitis is clinically not specific for CMV, but virus has been found in the brain at postmortem associated with a subacute encephalitis. Typical intranuclear inclusions should be seen, or staining of multiple cells with specific anti-CMV antigen reagents can detect infection. Some patients with the subacute encephalitis show neither (Snider *et al.*, 1983). CMV has not been isolated from CSF.

Pneumonia is one of the most common manifestations of severe CMV infection. In the AIDS patients it has frequently been accompanied by *Pneumocystis carinii* pneumonia, and together they can progress rapidly and result in fulminant respiratory insufficiency and death. The diagnosis of CMV pneumonia is best made by lung biopsy with histopathology, immunoperoxidase staining and culture. Typical cells with intranuclear inclusions on bronchial washings suggest the diagnosis, but the absence of such cells does not rule it out. Culture of bronchial washings or lavage fluid may yield the virus, but it could be due to contamination of the bronchoscope by saliva containing CMV. Unfortunately, when the diagnosis is established, there is no treatment.

Hepatitis is common in CMV infections and is usually mild. Modest elevations in SGOT and alkaline phosphatase levels occur. It can progress in a subacute fashion and may be responsible for persistent fever and weight loss. Diagnosis is by liver biopsy.

Colitis due to CMV has been subacute and persistent, and in addition acute cases have occurred. The diagnosis must be made by biopsies of the colonic lesions, which are otherwise not specific clinically. Just as with pneumonia and hepatitis, there is no treatment.

Disseminated CMV infections are frequently found at autopsy in AIDS patients. It is also frequently found along with other disseminated infections such as mycobacteriosis. Pneumonias are a common part of the dissemination and, in combination with other infections, are often the cause of death. Adrenal involvement, with necrosis, is also common.

Cytomegalovirus appears to be one of the common denominators of AIDS. Terminal dissemination is common and not treatable.

Herpes simplex infections that are clinically significant occur almost as often as CMV. The HSV-2 infections are more likely to be localized to the perineal area, persistent and severe (Siegal *et al.,* 1981; Gold and Armstrong, 1984). The diagnosis is easy to establish, for the virus is readily isolated and produces typical cytopathic effect in cell cultures in 24–48 hours. If the lesions are persistent and painful or progressive, acyclovir has produced responses. We have seen CMV retinitis progress rapidly while the patient was receiving acyclovir for a herpes simplex ulcer and would proceed with more caution in such a setting in the future.

Herpes zoster appears to occur more frequently in AIDS patients than in the general population, with dissemination in some cases, but rarely life threatening.

Epstein–Barr virus (EBV) has infected all our patients with AIDS, as determined by antibody studies. There is no evidence that EBV produces severe infections in these patients, but indirect implication accrues through the aggressive Burkitt cell lymphomas recently observed.

Adenoviruses have been repeatedly isolated from stool and urine of AIDS patients. The latter is an unusual site for adenovirus to be found, and the adenoviruses are unusual in that they are of high serotypes—31 through 34—which are quite rare but have been described in bone-marrow transplant recipients, and indeed in the urine and even disseminated as well as in the stool. The adenovirus isolates and infections appear, then, to be similar to those found in our bone-marrow transplant recipients.

Progressive multifocal leukoencephalopathy has been documented in a number of cases. The symptoms are typical of this disease with multifocal signs, waxing and waning, but ultimate progression to death. Diagnosis is suggested by computerized axial tomography (CAT) scan showing loss of white matter, but should be documented by brain biopsy. Improvement during Ara-C administration has been reported, but controlled studies are lacking (Bauer *et al.,* 1973).

IV. BACTERIAL AND MYCOBACTERIAL INFECTIONS

These infectious agents are listed in Table 3.

Mycobacterium tuberculosis causes what has been described as unusually severe disease in Haitian patients. This has appeared as a miliary, disseminated tuberculosis or tuberculous meningitis responding poorly to therapy. It is recommended that at least three drugs such as isoniazid, rifampin and ethambutol be used, because of the severity of the disease and potential resistance among organisms from Haiti (Roberts, 1984).

Table 3 Bacteria and mycobacteria

Organism	Comments
Mycobacterium tuberculosis	Unusual resistance may be seen in isolates from Haitians
Mycobacterium avium-intracellulare	Serotypes similar; some may grow slowly (8 weeks)
Mycobacterium fortuitum	
Nocardia asteroides	Found in brain abscess, mixed with *Salmonella*
Salmonella species	Non-*typhi* species likely to produce typhoidal syndrome. Recurs
Listeria monocytogenes	Bacteremias reported
Brucella species	Not yet reported

Mycobacterium avium-intracellulare (MAI) is one of the most common disseminated infections in AIDS (Zakowski *et al.*, 1982). Of our first 35 patients who came to autopsy, 17 have had it. An antemortem diagnosis was not often made, but in almost every instance where an isolate was identified—whether from sputum, urine or stool—the patient had disseminated disease. Acid-fast bacilli can frequently be seen on smear as well as isolated from stools, and they may also be seen and isolated from tissue such as bone marrow, liver biopsy or lymph-node biopsy where there is no evidence of granuloma formation and even little evidence of any inflammatory reaction. When the gastrointestinal tract is involved it may cause a syndrome resembling Whipples' disease with malabsorption and weight loss, and on biopsy of the bowel large, foamy PAS-positive macrophages are seen that are packed with MAI (Gold *et al.*, 1983). Quantitative blood cultures in some cases have revealed counts as high as 28,000 or 1800 CFU/ml blood. Decreases to the 100 range have been recorded on therapy, but when the patients died they still had disseminated MAI at postmortem (Wong *et al.*, 1983). The epidemiology of this disease in AIDS patients is unknown. The source—whether water or particulate environmental matter such as dirt or dust—is uncertain, and the portal of entry, whether respiratory or gastrointestinal, is equally uncertain. In a number of cases the gastrointestinal tract is the most heavily involved and appears to be the portal of entry. Prevention is therefore difficult. Whether early treatment would give better results is unknown, and which drugs to use is uncertain. The most effective drugs *in vitro* are ansamycin and clofazamine. Others that have been used are ethambutol, ethionamide, cycloserine and pyrazamide. The isolates are less often sensitive *in vitro* to these. Isonazide is usually used in addition, despite uniform *in vitro* resistance. Most isolates have been serotype 4, while in the general population in the past we have seen more serotypes 1 or untypable isolates, in addition to type 4.

An optimal treatment regimen has not been developed. There is a real question whether any of the AIDS patients have shown more than a minimal response.

Mycobacterium fortuitum has been found in 1 of our 35 patients at autopsy, along with MAI, both disseminated.

Nocardia asteroides has been observed (Louria, 1983) in 1 patient with AIDS who had a mixed *N. asteroides* and *Salmonella* species brain abscess.

Salmonella species which are non-*typhi* have caused bacteremic syndromes in 3 of our patients. All responded to appropriate therapy, but tended to relapse.

Legionella species infections that were especially severe have been observed and should be anticipated.

Listeria monocytogenes has occurred as a bacteremic illness in two of our AIDS patients and in another observed in New York City (J. Kislak and A. Loquerquist, personal communication). Whether the attack rate is higher than in the general population remains to be seen.

Brucella species have not been reported complicating AIDS, but they, just as *Listeria* and the rest of the organisms mentioned, should. They all take advantage of defects in T lymphocyte function.

V. FUNGAL INFECTIONS

The fungal infections are listed in Table 4. *Candida* species, mostly *C. albicans,* but a few isolates of *C. tropicalis,* have been the cause of one of the most frequent infections seen in AIDS patients. These have been oral and pharyngeal candidiasis or thrush. This type of infection rarely if ever disseminates, but it can cause the patient considerable discomfort and trouble in eating.

Candida esophagitis is also exceedingly common, but exact figures are not available. This illness creates even greater difficulty in eating and swallowing. There have been no convincing reports of dissemination of the *Candida* infection

Table 4 Fungi

Organisms	Comment
Candida species	Most disease is of the mucous membranes and esophagus; most isolates are *C. albicans,* but *C. tropicalis* has been identified
Cryptococcus neoformans	Pneumonias as well as meningitis seen; should look for antigen in serum as well as cerebrospinal fluid
Histoplasma capsulatum	Seen in nonendemic areas in those with travel in endemic areas in the past; disseminated, so should stain and culture marrow for diagnosis
Aspergillus species	Reported, but apparently very uncommon
Coccidioides immitis	Not yet reported
Blastomyces dermatitidis	Not yet reported

from these sites. The 3 cases of disseminated candidiasis we have seen were in hospitalized patients and were probably intravenous catheter associated. It appears then that *Candida* infections are primarily local but very persistent. They may respond to local treatment with agents such as nystatin liquid "swish and swallow" or clotrimazole troches, but some patients have required systemic therapy, and oral ketoconazole has been effective in some.

Cryptococcus neoformans has been seen regularly in most series. We have seen 1 case. The diagnosis should not be difficult, because antigen as well as organisms appear plentiful in serum or urine as well as cerebrospinal fluid. Patients have responded well to the combination of amphotericin B and 5-fluorocytosine.

Histoplasma capsulatum in disseminated form has been reported in New York City in patients not in the endemic area at the time they developed the illness.

It is likely we will see such recrudescent, disseminated disease with *C. immitis* and *Blastomyces dermatitidis* in addition to *H. capsulatum*.

Aspergillus species have been reported in a patient or two with AIDS in lists from the CDC. If it occurs as a true opportunistic infection, it is rare.

VI. PARASITIC INFECTION

Table 5 lists common parasitic infections.

Pneumocystis carinii pneumonia is probably the single most common infection bringing the patients to the physicians (*Candida* oral or esophageal infection seems almost as frequent). The disease may present as bothersome dry cough or

Table 5 Parasites

Organism	Comments
Pneumocystis carinii	Unusually large numbers of organisms seen, regardless of stain; toluidine blue on bronchoalveolar lavage effective in our experience; prolonged therapy necessary (≥ 4 weeks)
Toxoplasma gondii	Brain abscess and encephalitis common; antibody response may be poor, especially IgM; rising titers in cerebrospinal fluid suggests diagnosis; prolonged therapy necessary (≥ 4 months)
Cryptosporidia sp.	Illness varies from mild, self-limited diarrhea to cholera-like syndrome, unresponsive to any therapy; organisms seen by sugar floatation or Zeihl–Neelsen stain
Strongyloides stercoralis	Not yet reported

just dyspnea on exertion, or a fulminant pneumonia may occur. Since its occurrence has become well known in high-risk groups, the diagnosis is usually made early by bronchoscopy with washings, lavage or biopsy. Open-lung biopsies are seldom necessary, since the organisms are so abundant that less invasive procedures readily yield what is needed for diagnosis. The methenamine silver stain remains the definitive one; however, more rapid stains with excellent yields include the Gram–Weigart and toluidine blue. The more fulminant cases have been in mixed pneumonias with CMV. Treatment with sulfamethoxazole–trimethoprim (co-trimoxazole) has resulted in good responses in our experience (close to 70%), but recurrence has been more frequent than we are used to seeing in other immunocompromised hosts. We have seen 51 episodes in 43 patients. When recurrences were treated, only 1 patient responded. Because of the recurrences and sometimes slow responses, we have treated our patients for a minimum of 3 weeks. We would like to administer subsequent prophylactic therapy with co-trimoxazole, but so many patients have developed adverse reactions, manifest usually by rash, that we are loath to continue even low-dose co-trimoxazole. Prophylaxis with pentamidine has not been tried, and results of treatment have varied. Usually pentamidine is given after co-trimoxazole has failed, or after a reaction, so that it is not fair to compare the efficacy of the two drugs. We have given them together in some cases with a good response.

Toxoplasma gondii is a frequent cause of central nervous system (CNS) disease in AIDS patients (6 cases among 166 at risk in our series), usually presenting as a brain abscess or encephalitis. Lesions are usually evident on CT scan with ring enhancement on contrast, but this is not invariable. Patients may or may not develop an IgG antibody response, and in one case the rise appeared only in the cerebrospinal fluid (CSF) (Wong *et al.*, 1984). No IgM response is the rule, and this is in sharp contrast to other immunocompromised hosts with CNS toxoplasmosis. Diagnosis thus depends on the clinical picture alone or this plus a brain biopsy. A therapeutic trial in the former situation where a brain biopsy must be avoided seems reasonable. Recurrences are the rule after the usual recommended 6-week course of therapy. We have seen this twice, while 2 other patients have responded to long-term therapy of 4 months or longer. Sulfadiazine at 2–4 g/day plus pyrimethamine at a loading dose of 75 mg followed by 25 mg/day along with folinic acid (10 mg/day) has resulted in gratifying responses.

Cryptosporidia species have caused remarkably severe diarrhea in AIDS patients. In contrast, we have seen 2 patients with *Cryptosporidia* in the stool and only mild, intermittent diarrhea. One patient had a cholera-like syndrome, producing up to 15 liters/day of liquid stool. The diagnosis can be made on finding oocysts by using a sugar flotation method on ordinary preparations of stools for ova and parasites and by ordinary Ziehl Neelsen stains. A bowel biopsy should be done if stools are negative and the parasite is suspected. Protozoa, 2–3 μm in size, can be seen lining the brush border on hematoxylin and eosin and Giemsa stain. Both trophozoites and schizoites are apparent. Oral furazolidone, 150 mg 4 times daily, has been reported as efficacious. We have seen one notable failure, and bovine transfer factor also failed in this case. Spiramycin has not been successful in our experience. There is a veterinary coccidiostat called amprollium that has been effective in veterinary practice, but has not to my knowledge been effective in humans.

The hyperinfection syndrome due to *Strongyloides stercoralis,* which usually occurs in patients on high doses of corticosteroids, has not yet been recorded in AIDS patients. It should be anticipated.

VII. OTHER INFECTIONS

Severe infections with agents such as chlamydiae or mycoplasmas have not yet been reported. We might suspect severe chlamydial infection in the face of the T cell defect of AIDS, but they have not been reported.

VIII. IMMUNOLOGICAL ALTERATIONS IN AIDS

The immune alterations most often reported in AIDS patients are listed in Table 6. There is no consistent immune alteration that is specific for AIDS. The reversed T cell helper/suppressor ratio is seen in other diseases such as hepatitis B or cytomegalovirus infection and does not indicate AIDS. The defect in AIDS is a low helper T cell ratio. The suppressor cells may even be elevated. Until we have a more specific immunological marker or a specific agent for AIDS, the diagnosis must remain a clinical one based on the types of infections or neo-

Table 6　Immunological alterations in AIDS[a]

1. Lymphopenia
2. Anergy to skin-test antigens
3. Decreased total T cells
4. Decreased helper/inducer T cells
5. Normal to only slightly decreased suppressor T cells
6. Decreased natural killer-cell activity
7. Decreased interferon production by lymphocytes
8. Increased circulating alpha interferon (acid labile)
9. Decreased selected antibody response
10. Increased gamma globulin levels
11. Circulating immune complexes

[a] None is consistent or specific.

plasms the patients develop. Immunological data should continue to be collected, and patients should be studied for other more specific markers, but we must for the time being rest on a clinical diagnosis of AIDS. This should not include lymphadenopathy in high-risk individuals such as homosexual men or intravenous drug abusers. We have followed more than 100 high-risk individuals with lymphadenopathy, and only 10% have developed AIDS. The other 90% are doing well and are without evidence of AIDS. It is clear then that they should not be termed as having AIDS, pre-AIDS, AIDS-associated complex or anything else other than lymphadenopathy of unknown etiology.

IX. ETIOLOGY OF AIDS AND CONCLUSIONS

The epidemiology of AIDS from early in the epidemic suggested the presence of an infectious agent (Table 7)—one that was passed by sexual contact (in homosexual men) and by sharing intravenous needles. This closely approximated the epidemiology of hepatitis B and cytomegalovirus and therefore suggested delta virus and non-A, non-B hepatitis. As it became apparent that hemophiliacs, and probably spouses and children, were infected, this reinforced the first observations and called to mind other agents such as Epstein–Barr virus.

The frequent isolation of adenoviruses, especially of high serotypes, brings this agent along with parvoviruses to the front. It is interesting that canine parvovirus disease appeared in the 1970s, appearing to be a new viral disease among dogs, just as AIDS has among humans. Finally, retroviruses such as the human T cell leukemia virus have become prime candidates because they do infect T lymphocytes and cause neoplasia in human as well as apparent asymptomatic infection. In addition a retrovirus (feline leukemia virus) also causes a disease in cats that causes both immunosuppression, resulting in opportunistic infections, and neoplasia, manifest as a lymphoma or leukemia.

Table 7 Etiology of AIDS

An infectious agent
Multiple infectious agents
One or more infectious agents plus antigenic overload
A virus
Cytomegalovirus
Epstein–Barr virus
Retrovirus
Hepatitis B virus
Hepatitis non-A, non-B virus
Delta virus
Adenovirus
Parvovirus

The etiologic agent in AIDS remains to be identified. Not only must the agent be identified so that the epidemiology can be carefully delineated and a vaccine prepared, but the immunologic deficit must be pinpointed so that it can be reversed. If we isolated the agent today, it would still be years before a vaccine could be developed, safety tested, and inoculated into high-risk individuals. At the same time, the incubation period of up to 2 years or more will supply more years of cases, even after vaccination is accomplished. To stop the epidemic we must isolate the agent and the immune defect, so that we can protect against the former and develop means of correcting the latter.

REFERENCES

Armstrong, D. (1983). *In* "The AIDS Epidemic" (K. M. Cahill, ed.), pp. 63–71. St. Martin's Press, New York.

Armstrong, D. (1984). *In* "The Acquired Immune Deficiency Syndrome and Infections of Homosexual Men" (P. Ma and D. Armstrong, eds.), pp. 197–203. Yorke Medical Books.

Armstrong, D., Ely, M., and Steger, L. (1971). *Infect. Immun.* **3,** 159–163.

Barre-Sinoussi, F., Chermann, J. C., Rey, F., Nugeyre, M. T., Chamaret, S., Gruest, J., Dauguet, C., Axler-Blin, C., Vezinet-Brun, F., Rouzioux, C., Rozenbaum, W. and Montagnier, L. (1983). *Science* **220,** 868–871.

Bauer, W. R., Turel, J. R. and Johnson, K. P. (1973). *JAMA, J. Am. Med. Assoc.* **226,** 174–176.

Black, P. H., and Levy, E. M. (1983). *N. Engl. J. Med.* **309,** 856.

Centers for Disease Control (1981). *Morbid. Mortal. Week. Rep.* **30,** 305–308.

Centers for Disease Control (1982). *Morbid. Mortal. Week. Rep.* **31,** 508–513.

Essex, M., McLane, M. F., Lee, T. H., Falk, L., Howe, C. W. S., Mullins, J. I., Cabradilla, C. and Francis, D. P. (1983). *Science* **220,** 859–862.

Francis, D. P. (1983). *In* "The AIDS Epidemic" (K. M. Cahill, ed.), pp. 137–148. St. Martin's Press, New York.

Gallo, R. C., Sarin, P. S., Gelmann, E. P., Robert-Guroff, M., Richardson, E., Kalyanaraman, V. S., Mann, D., Sidhu, G. D., Stahl, R. E., Zolla-Pazner, S., Leibowitch, J. and Popovic, M. (1983). *Science* **220,** 865–867.

Gold, J. W. M. and Armstrong, D. (1984). *In* "The Acquired Immune Deficiency Syndrome and Infections of Homosexual Men" (P. Ma and D. Armstrong, eds.), pp. 294–301. Yorke Medical Books.

Gold, J. W. M., Weikel, C. L., Tapper, M. L., Kiehn, T. E., Lerner, C. W., Urmacher, C., Rotterdam, H. Z. and Armstrong, D. (1983). *Abstr., ICAAC, 1983.*

Gottlieb, M. S., Schroff, R., Schanker, H. M., Weisman, J. D., Fan, P. T., Wolf, R. A. and Saxon, A. (1981). *N. Engl. J. Med.* **305,** 1425–1431.

Louria, D. B. (1983). *In* "The AIDS Epidemic" (K. M. Cahill, ed.), pp. 72–85. St. Martin's Press, New York.

Masur, H., Michelis, M. A., Greene, J. B., Onorato, I., Vande Stouwe, R. A., Holzman, R. S., Wormser, G., Brettman, L., Lange, M., Murray, H. W. and Cunningham-Rundles, S. (1981). *N. Engl. J. Med.* **305,** 1431–1438.

Roberts, R. B. (1984). *In* "The Acquired Immune Deficiency Syndrome and Infections of Homosexual Men" (P. Ma and D. Armstrong, eds.), pp. 302–316. Yorke Medical Books.

Siegal, F. P., Lopez, C., Hammer, G. S., Brown, A. E., Kornfeld, S. J., Gold, J. W. M., Hassett, J., Hirschman, S. Z., Cunningham-Rundles, C., Adelsberg, B. R., Parham, D. M., Siegal, M., Cunningham-Rundles, S. and Armstrong, D. (1981). *N. Engl. J. Med.* **305,** 1439–1444.

Snider, W. D., Simpson, D. M., Nielsen, S., Gold, J. W. M., Metroka, C. E. and Posner, J. B. (1983). Ann. Neurol. **14,** 403–418.

Wong, B., Kiehn, T. E., Edwards, F. F., Whimbey, E., Donnelly, H., Gold, J. W. M. and Armstrong, D. (1983). *Clin. Res.* **31,** 692A.

Wong, B., Gold, J. W. M., Brown, A. E., Lange, M., Fried, R., Grieco, M., Mildvan, D., Giron, J., Tapper, M. L., Lerner, C. W. and Armstrong, D. (1984). *Ann. Intern. Med.* **100,** 36–42.

Zakowski, P., Fligiel, S., Berlin, G. W. and Johnson, L. (1982). *JAMA, J. Am. Med. Assoc.* **248,** 2980–2982.

3 *Gardnerella vaginalis* and bacterial vaginosis

C. S. F. EASMON and C. A. ISON

I. INTRODUCTION

Genital infection caused by *Trichomonas vaginalis, Candida* spp. and *Neisseria gonorrhoeae* is readily diagnosed and treated. However, controversy still surrounds vaginal infection where none of these pathogens is isolated, so-called "nonspecific vaginitis." Gardner and Dukes (1954) reported the isolation of a small Gram-negative bacillus from 81 of 91 cases of nonspecific vaginitis. The following year they published a more extensive study, which confirmed the initial observation and examined the syndrome in more detail. Gardner and Dukes named the bacillus *Haemophilus vaginalis* because of its morphology, Gram reaction and apparent need for blood-containing media. They showed that male partners of infected women had a high rate of carriage and that the vaginitis could be initiated in normal volunteers with vaginal material taken from women with documented infection. They were, however, less successful with pure cultures of *H. vaginalis*.

Coincidentally, Leopold in 1953 had described a Gram-negative coccobacillus isolated from urine samples and cervical cultures. He did not associate the bacillus with vaginitis or any other pathology but suggested inclusion in the genus *Haemophilus*.

While these studies clearly established an association between *H. vaginalis*, vaginitis and possibly other infections, they proved to be the start of 25 years of controversy, both microbiological and clinical. The classification of the bacillus has been a major problem, being named successively *Haemophilus vaginalis, Corynebacterium vaginale* and *Gardnerella vaginalis*. The causative role of *G. vaginalis* in vaginitis claimed by Gardner and Dukes has been challenged by a number of workers on the basis that the organism is part of the normal vaginal flora that is not associated with nonspecific vaginitis (McCormack *et al.*, 1977) or more recently that obligate anaerobes may also be involved (Chen *et al.*, 1979; Spiegel *et al.*, 1980; Taylor *et al.*, 1982). Undoubtedly much of this confusion stems from a failure to standardise the clinical definition of the syndrome and laboratory methods (Taylor *et al.*, 1982; Amsel *et al.*, 1983).

The following questions remain unresolved.

1. Is the term vaginitis appropriate, given the absence of inflammatory cells?
2. Is nonspecific vaginitis a truly mixed infection with *G. vaginalis* and anaerobes working together?
3. Is neither the cause of the condition, both groups of organisms being present as markers?
4. Is *G. vaginalis* the sole cause of nonspecific vaginitis, with anaerobes merely being associated with the condition or is the converse true?
5. Is the condition sexually transmitted or merely associated with sexual activity?

In this chapter we shall review the microbiology and taxonomy of *Gardnerella vaginalis*, clinical syndromes with which it is associated, and their laboratory diagnosis and management, and attempt to answer some of these points.

II. BACTERIOLOGY OF *GARDNERELLA VAGINALIS*

A. Taxonomy

We start with taxonomy because the use of three names for a single organism over a 30-year period has led to considerable confusion. The Gram reaction of *G. vaginalis* varies depending on the strain used and the age of the culture. We have found that stock laboratory strains tend to be Gram-negative while many fresh clinical isolates are more Gram-positive.

Both Leopold (1953) and Gardner and Dukes (1955) considered *G. vaginalis* to be a small, predominantly Gram-negative bacillus. Its morphology and isolation on blood-containing medium suggested a member of the genus *Haemophilus*, and the term *Haemophilus vaginalis* was proposed and widely used. At the same time in France the term *Hermophilus haemolyticus vaginalis* was used by Wurch and Lutz (1955) and Lutz *et al.* (1956) for organisms associated with leukorrhoea. A member of the genus *Haemophilus* should require either haemin (X) or nicotinamide-adenine dinucleotide (V) or both as growth factors, and Dukes (1956) was unable to demonstrate this in *H. vaginalis*.

Lapage (1961) confirmed that the organism required neither X nor V factors and suggested that it might be a *Corynebacterium*. Dunkleberg and McVeigh (1969) were able to define the growth requirements more precisely and to show that neither X, V, blood, or serum was necessary for culture. With this pattern it clearly could not be a *Haemophilus,* but nevertheless the term *H. vaginalis* continued to be used.

Zinneman and Turner (1963) found a number of strains, including the type strain deposited by Gardner and Dukes, to be Gram-positive and suggested that the bacillus should be named *Corynebacterium vaginale.* This proposal was supported by the work of Dunkleberg and his colleagues, mentioned above. By the early 1970s both names were being widely used, adding to the confusion.

In fact, the name *Corynebacterium vaginale* was never accepted by a number of bacteriologists. Most *Corynebacteria* are catalase-positive, whereas *C. vaginale* is not. *Corynebacterium vaginale* does not contain arabinose in its cell wall and has no wall teichoic acid as do other *Corynebacteria.* DNA homology studies show *C. vaginale* does not have a G:C content similar to other *Corynebacteria.* As with members of the genus *Haemophilus,* there is little cross reactivity between *C. vaginale/H. vaginalis* and other corynebacteria (Redmond and Kotcher, 1963; Vice and Smaron, 1963).

Park and his colleagues (1968) suggested that a new genus was required for the organism. Greenwood and Pickett (1979) proposed a new genus *Gardnerella* (in honour of Gardner's pioneering work), based on analysis of cell-wall chemistry, electron microscopy and DNA hybridisation, and this was supported by an extensive taxonomic study by Piot *et al.* (1980). The term *Gardnerella vaginalis* has been widely accepted and is used henceforth in this chapter.

Gardnerella vaginalis (Greenwood and Pickett, 1980)

Gram-variable to Gram-negative bacilli with laminated cell walls
Acetic acid major end product of fermentation
Acid from dextrin, fructose, galactose, glucose, maltose, mannose, ribose, starch
Variable results from lactose, sucrose, xylose
Catalase, oxidase, indole, and urease negative
Noncapsulated, nonmotile
Facultatively anaerobic
DNA base composition 43 ± 1 mol% GC
Temperature: Optimum, 35–37°C
               Grows at 25 and 40°C
Haemolysis: Beta-haemolytic on human and rabbit blood
               Nonhaemolytic on sheep blood
pH: Grows best between 6 and 6.5
               Poor growth at 4.5
               No growth at 4.0
Type strain: 594 of Gardner and Dukes
               ATCC 14018 NCTC 10287

B. Isolation and identification

Gardnerella vaginalis is a facultative anaerove that will grow on most blood or chocolate agars at a temperature of 35–37°C to produce nondescript colonies in 48–72 hours. Although it will grow in air, growth is enhanced when in the presence of increased carbon dioxide or when anaerobic. Because of the close association between *G. vaginalis* and obligate anaerobes, particularly of the *Bacteroides oralis/melaninogenicus* group, we prefer to use a carbon dioxide atmosphere for primary isolation from vaginal samples.

Gardnerella vaginalis produces a diffuse beta-haemolysis on human and rabbit blood agar, but not on sheep or horse blood. This is a useful aid to identification. We have found growth to be better on human than on horse blood agar.

Early studies used blood or heated blood most often with Casman's agar or broth. However, Dunkleberg and McVeigh (1969) and Park *et al.* (1968) showed that *G. vaginalis* would grow on dextrose-starch agar without blood. From this was developed peptone starch dextrose (PSD) medium. In this medium the choice of peptone is critical, as not all contain the necessary purines, pyrimidines and B vitamins (Dunkleberg and McVeigh, 1969). Proteose peptone number 3 (Difco) and Myosate (BBL) have been recommended. On PSD agar, growth develops in 48 hours and the colonies are white. Dunkleberg *et al.* (1970) developed an identification system based on colonial morphology on PSD agar assessed with a dissecting microscope. This technique has been used successfully by others, but it is time consuming and requires considerable operator skill. We have found that growth on PSD agar is variable, some clinical isolates growing very much more slowly than others. Our experience of the medium has, however, been limited to work with pure cultures and not with primary isolates.

There have been a number of variations on the PSD theme. Smith (1975) omitted dextrose, used corn starch and added bromcresol purple as an indicator. Mickelsen *et al.* (1977) used a selective medium with 1% corn starch GC base, colistin and nalidixic acid. Starch-utilising colonies could be identified by the formation of a surrounding halo. Goldberg and Washington (1976) used a Columbia nalidixic acid colistin agar with corn starch reduced to only 0.1%. These latter media are the direct forerunners of the human blood agar media that are now being used and that are discussed below.

Gardnerella vaginalis grows well in liquid or semisolid media. Thioglycollate medium was used by both Leopold (1953) and Dukes and Gardner (1961). We have encountered the "puff-ball" appearance that they noticed. A large amount of extracellular material seems to be produced in thioglycollate, as we have found the optical density to be far greater than the bacterial count would suggest. Growth is enhanced by the addition of serum or cysteine hydrochloride. *Gardnerella vaginalis* grows well in PSD broth. With the addition of 5% serum, most broth media will support its growth. Liquid media have little role in routine diagnostic work, apart from their use in antibiotic sensitivity testing.

The real problems with *G. vaginalis* have been, first, to grow it rapidly in primary culture with a medium that is selective (to suppress other vaginal bacteria) and on which it can be readily distinguished and, second, to identify it simply and rapidly.

Although other workers had noted the diffuse beta-haemolysis produced by *G. vaginalis* on human or rabbit blood agar, Greenwood *et al.* (1977) were the first to exploit this characteristic as an aid to identification. Their vaginalis or V agar was composed of Columbia agar base (BBL), 1% proteose peptone number 3 (Difco), and 5% human blood. Smith (1979) found V agar to be comparable with his own starch/bromcresol agar. Shaw *et al.* (1981) found both V agar and a variant omitting the proteose peptone to be a very accurate means of identifying *G. vaginalis* when combined with Gram stain and morphology.

Spiegel *et al.* (1980), Totten *et al.* (1982), and Ison *et al.* (1983) used bilayer human blood agar plates with an antibiotic supplement of colistin or gentamicin, nalidixic acid and amphotericin b. Although colistin has been more widely used, we have found that gentamicin at a concentration of 4 mg/litre gives a more selective medium. The bilayer plate makes the diffuse beta-haemolysis more pronounced, as does the addition of Tween 80 (Totten *et al.*, 1982). Using single-layer plates, some strains of *G. vaginalis* produce alpha- rather than beta-haemolysis. One disadvantage of Tween 80 is that the blood in stored plates tends to lyse more rapidly.

While human blood agar plates are probably no better at growing *G. vaginalis* than other media, the beta-haemolysis produced by the organism does make them more convenient to use for primary isolation. Against this must be set the inconvenience of pouring bilayer plates and the problem of obtaining a steady supply of time-expired human blood.

1. Identification

Gardnerella vaginalis appears on Gram staining as a variable bacillus or coccobacillus. It is still not certain whether *G. vaginalis* is Gram-positive or negative. Harper and Davis (1982) found that it had a cell-wall amino acid composition of a Gram-positive bacterium. Greenwood and Pickett (1980), however, in their proposal for the creation of a new genus, defined it as Gram-negative to Gram-variable. Criswell *et al.* (1971) also claimed that *G. vaginalis* was Gram-negative on the basis of the wide range of amino acids found in the cell wall. Their work has been criticised because of their failure to detect diaminopimelic acid not only in the cell wall of *G. vaginalis* but also in *Escherichia coli* and *Bacillus megaterium,* species in which this key wall amino acid is known to exist.

Much has been made of carbohydrate fermentation reactions with starch, maltose and dextrose being those quoted normally. Although perhaps necessary for a reference laboratory, standard carbohydrate fermentation tests are difficult to carry out with absolute reliability. We agree with Taylor and Phillips (1983) that they are not suitable for the diagnostic laboratory. Yong and Thompson (1982) suggested the use of a rapid (4-hour) micro method for starch and raffinose fermentation and hippurate hydrolysis, based on the same principle as their tests for *Neisseria gonorrhoeae* (Yong and Prytula, 1978). We have no direct experience of this technique as opposed to more conventional tests, but if it proves to be more reproducible, it could be useful for the diagnostic laboratory and warrants further evaluation.

Hippurate hydrolysis is among the characteristics that Greenwood and Pickett (1979) and Jolly (1983) suggested for the differentiation of *G. vaginalis* from other oxidase/catalase-negative Gram-negative bacteria. In contrast, Taylor and Phillips (1983) did not find hippurate hydrolysis to be useful as a means of differentiating *G. vaginalis* from catalase-negative coryneforms. They suggested the use of growth in 2% (wt/vol) sodium chloride and on nutrient agar. *Gardnerella vaginalis* is oxidase- and catalase-negative and sensitive to hydrogen peroxide, but while these reactions may be useful, they are not specific.

The other group of tests that may be of value in the identification of *G. vaginalis* are antibiotic sensitivity patterns. Sensitivity to metronidazole and trimethoprim and resistance to sulphonamides appear to be most useful (Bailey *et al.*, 1979; Piot *et al.*, 1980; Taylor and Phillips, 1983).

In summary, diffuse beta-haemolysis on human blood but not sheep or horse blood agar, combined with Gram reaction and morphology, hippurate hydrolysis, and sensitivity to metronidazole and trimethoprim, will give a satisfactory identification of *G. vaginalis*. As growth of *G. vaginalis* from cases of nonspecific vaginitis is usually heavy on primary culture, it may be possible to use antibiotic discs on the primary plate. In practice, differential beta-haemolysis with Gram stain and morphology will be sufficient more than 85% of the time.

In none of this have we mentioned the use of serology. Several groups have raised antisera to *G. vaginalis* and have found them to provide a simple, highly specific means of identification by immunofluorescence (Redmond and Kotcher, 1963; Vice and Smaron, 1973; Svarva and Moeland, 1982). We too have done this, and the antisera raised can be used in ELISA and immunofluorescence tests. We are currently evaluating them as coagglutination reagents. The immunological approach may also give an effective, direct diagnosis of nonspecific vaginitis by detecting gardnerella antigen in vaginal samples. This will depend on *G. vaginalis* colonisation, the levels of *G. vaginalis* antigen in normal women and on the sensitivity of antigen detection, as well as the specificity of the antisera used. It is, however, an approach that needs investigation, as it combines speed with specificity. Unfortunately no antisera are currently commercially available for either the detection or identification of *G. vaginalis.* Only those groups with the interest in and facilities for antibody production have been able to use serology.

C. Antimicrobial susceptibility

McCarthy *et al.* (1979) determined the minimum inhibitory concentrations of 19 antimicrobial agents against 56 strains of *G. vaginalis.* All strains were very sensitive to penicillin, ampicillin, carbenicillin, and vancomycin, erythromycin and clindamycin (minimum inhibitory concentration, MIC < 1 mg/litre). Cephalosporins were less active than the penicillins. Of the aminoglycosides, streptomycin and gentamicin were the most active, tobramycin and particularly kanamycin less so. The MIC of chloramphenicol ranged from 0.25 to 2.0 mg/litre, while tetracycline showed a bimodal distribution, just over half the strains being inhibited by ≤ mg/litre while 43% had MICs between 16 and 64 mg/litre. All strains of *G. vaginalis* were highly resistant to nalidixic acid, colistin and sulphadiazine.

Ralph and Amatnieks (1980) examined the sensitivity of ten gardnerella strains to the nitroimidazole metronidazole and its two principal metabolites. Using a broth dilution technique, unlike most other facultative species they found metronidazole to have significant activity against *G. vaginalis,* the media MIC being 8 mg/litre. The hydroxy metabolite was more active, with a median MIC of only 2 mg/litre. Phiefer *et al.* (1978) found a similar range of MICs for metronidazole but did not investigate the activity of the hydroxy metabolite. Tinidazole and its hydroxy metabolite appear to be even more active (Shanker and Munro, 1982; Shanker *et al.,* 1982).

The observations on *G. vaginalis* and metronidazole were also noticed by Balsdon and Jackson (1981) and Easmon *et al.* (1982). The latter looked at the levels of metronidazole and its metabolites in the serum and urine of volunteers given either 400 mg or 2 g metronidazole orally (Flagyl) and compared these with the MIC of metronidazole and metabolites for a range of *G. vaginalis* isolates. MICs were done by agar dilution method both anaerobically and aerobically. As well as confirming the greater activity of the hydroxy metabolite against *G. vaginalis,* Easmon *et al.* (1982) found that this activity was less affected by incubation aerobically than was that of the parent compound. With the 400-mg dose of metronidazole, urine levels of both active agents exceeded the MIC of *G. vaginalis,* while plasma levels did not reach MIC for even the most sensitive gardnerella isolate. With the 2-g dose, plasma concentrations did exceed the MIC of the more sensitive strains.

The treatment of nonspecific vaginitis will be covered in another section. It is, however, worth noting here the correlation between *in vitro* activity and clinical efficacy. Metronidazole and ampicillin, the most widely used agents, are clearly active *in vitro* against *G. vaginalis.* Erythromycin, one of the most active agents *in vitro,* is however of little use clinically, this being ascribed to the relatively low pH of the vagina (Durfee *et al.,* 1979). The other agents used have been tetracycline and local sulphonamides. A number of strains of *G. vaginalis* are sensitive to the former, but all are highly resistant to the latter. Dunkleberg (1977) suggested that the efficacy of sulphonamides might be due to the acidic nature of the local preparation rather than to the direct antimicrobial activity of the drug.

III. CLINICAL SYNDROME

Although the term nonspecific vaginitis is widely used, this is more because of uncertainty about its aetiology and pathogenesis than because it is an appropriate name. In fact, it is a poor name for a disease that is a well-defined clinical entity associated with particular groups of bacteria and that is not characterised by vaginal inflammation. Its similarity to nonspecific genital infection, which has a quite different aetiology, is confusing. Vaginosis is now preferred to vaginitis by many workers. Blackwell and Barlow (1982) have used anaerobic vaginosis, while Mårdh (1982) has suggested that it is really an amidosis. Balsdon (1982) was more specific with *Gardnerella vaginalis* syndrome. Bacterial vaginosis is perhaps the most appropriate term, and at this time it is used synonymously with nonspecific vaginitis.

The clinical features of the syndrome are as follows. There is a thin homogeneous vaginal discharge, which is often grey or grey-green in colour and may be frothy. There is a genital "fishy" malodour, which may not always be apparent to the woman, but may be more so to her sexual partner. Many women complain of increased malodour after menstruation or sexual intercourse. There is a vaginal pH of 5 or higher. There is a positive amine test on the addition of 10% potassium hydroxide to the vaginal discharge. Vaginal or vulval irritation are uncommon, and there is little or no vaginal inflammation. Clue cells (epithelial cells covered with small bacilli) are seen on microscopic examination of a wet preparation of the discharge. On Gram staining both clue cells and large numbers of Gram-variable bacilli are seen and lactobacilli are usually absent. Table 1 gives a comparison of the types of discharge found in the common vaginitides.

Bacterial vaginosis is the mildest and probably the most common of the three common vaginitides. Candidal, trichomonal and gonococcal infection must be excluded, as should intrauterine infection. Because of its mild course and the surrounding bacteriological confusion, bacterial vaginosis is still overlooked and underreported.

Since the thorough description by Gardner and Dukes (1955) of the syndrome

Table 1 Characteristics of vaginal discharges

Characteristic	Normal	Trichomoniasis	G. vaginalis vaginosis	Candidiasis
Volume	0 to +	+ to +++	0 to +++	0 to ++
Consistency	Curdy	Homogeneous	Homogeneous	Curdy or thrush patches
Colour	White or slate	Grey or green-ish	Grey	White or slate
Odour	0	+ to +++	+ to ++	0
Frothiness	0	+ (10%)	+ (7%)	0
pH	3.8–4.2	5.5–5.8	5.0–5.5	4.0–5.0

nearly 30 years ago, there has been some heated debate over its prevalence and aetiology, but much of this has arisen from a failure to standardise clinical and laboratory diagnostic criteria. The main clinical debate has been whether to use symptoms or more objective criteria for diagnosis. Many women who fulfil the latter do not initially complain of symptoms. Often, however, after successful treatment they realise that what they considered ''normal'' was in fact far from being so. Holmes' group in Seattle have been strong advocates of the use of criteria other than symptoms. They recently reviewed the use of sets of criteria for the diagnosis of nonspecific vaginitis (Amsel *et al.*, 1983). These were:

1. A thin homogeneous discharge with a milk-like consistency.
2. A vaginal pH higher than 5.
3. Release of a fishy amine odour on addition of 10% potassium hydroxide to discharge.
4. Abnormal amines detected by chromatography.
5. Clue cells.

They proposed the use of numbers 1, 2, 3 and 5 and that a diagnosis of bacterial vaginosis should be made on the finding of three of the four. Symptoms should not be considered. Blackwell and Barlow (1982) came to similar conclusions.

We analysed a group of 100 women and 29 controls selected on the basis of symptoms, using the criteria already mentioned, with bacteriology for *G. vaginalis* and anaerobes and analysis of nonvolatile fatty acids. We found that the use of the four criteria gave a much closer correlation with bacteriological and chromatographic findings than did the use of symptoms (Ison *et al.*, 1983) and would support the general adoption of the criteria proposed by Amsel and his colleagues.

IV. LABORATORY DIAGNOSIS

The diagnostic criteria discussed in the previous section can be carried out easily in a sexually transmitted disease clinic where there are experienced medical, technical and nursing staff. In other situations—e.g., in busy antenatal or gynaecology clinics—lack of experience may be a problem, particularly when looking for clue cells. Here the diagnostic bacteriology laboratory may be of use, the only problem being how far it is reasonable to go.

A Gram stain of the vaginal discharge for Gram-variable bacilli and clue cells is essential. Culture for *G. vaginalis* is debatable. Modern selective bilayer human blood agars (Spiegel *et al.*, 1980; Totten *et al.*, 1982; Ison *et al.*, 1982) will detect small numbers of *G. vaginalis* in 36–48 hours. A simple identification based on differential haemolysis, hippurate hydrolysis and possibly sensitivity to metronidazole, trimethoprim and sulphonamides should be sufficient to differentiate *G. vaginalis* from coryneforms and other similar bacteria. Carbohydrate tests are difficult to perform reliably and are not suitable for routine laboratory use.

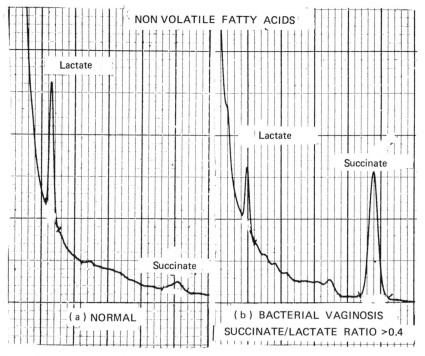

Fig. 1 Gas-liquid chromatography of vaginal washings from (a) normal woman showing high lactate and low succinate peaks, and (b) woman with bacterial vaginosis showing reversal of succinate/lactate ratio.

Against the use of culture must be weighed the availability of human blood and the inconvenience of preparing bilayer plates. The isolation of *G. vaginalis* on this medium, particularly a scanty growth, may be of little significance, as women without bacterial vaginosis carry *G. vaginalis* (Amsel *et al.*, 1983; Ison *et al.*, 1983).

Biochemical techniques have been tried in an attempt to give a rapid definitive diagnosis. Spiegel *et al.* (1980) analysed the pattern of nonvolatile fatty acids (NVFA) in vaginal washings. Whereas in normal samples lactate was the main NVFA present with only low levels of succinate, in women with bacterial vaginosis the succinate was increased (Fig. 1). A succinate/lactate ratio of 0.4 or greater was diagnostic of bacterial vaginosis. This was confirmed by Piot *et al.* (1982) (using a ratio of 0.3 rather than 0.4) and by ourselves (Ison *et al.*, 1983), although we found that the predictive value of a negative test was low at 58%. Chen *et al.* (1979, 1982) detected the diamines putrescine and cadaverine in vaginal washings by thin-layer chromatography.

While these two techniques are useful research tools and may be valuable in monitoring the success of antimicrobial therapy, they do not replace the simple clinical/laboratory criteria that we believe should remain the basis for diagnosing bacterial vaginosis. Any new technique specific for *G. vaginalis* must now take account of its undoubted position as part of the normal vaginal flora in some women.

V. AETIOLOGY AND PATHOGENESIS

Despite the original work of Gardner and Dukes in 1954 and 1955 and their subsequent reports, the aetiology of gardnerella-associated vaginosis has remained controversial. Gardner (1980), in a review of vaginitis, reaffirmed his belief that *G. vaginalis* was the sole aetiological agent. The opposite extreme is represented by the work of McCormack *et al.* (1977), who not only found *G. vaginalis* in women without vaginitis but also claimed that there was no evidence of close association between organism and infection. The persistent use of the term nonspecific vaginitis, or more recently bacterial vaginosis, even in papers that accept an aetiological role for *G. vaginalis*, is perhaps the clearest indication of continuing uncertainty.

An important factor in this confusion has been the lack of standardisation of clinical definition and laboratory techniques (Gardner, 1980; Taylor *et al.*, 1982; Amsel *et al.*, 1983). Should vaginitis be defined in terms of symptoms, or should the more objective criteria advocated by Spiegel *et al.* (1980) and Amsel *et al.* (1983) be used? Recent reports using selective human blood media have in general shown far higher levels of *G. vaginalis* colonisation in "normal" women than earlier work.

Proof of pathogenicity using Koch's postulates requires the regular isolation of the organism from the site of infection, its passage in pure culture for several generations to remove any host material, reproduction of the disease by re-inoculation into the host (or a suitable model), and isolation of the organism from the infected site. There are, of course, limits to this approach, which was really aimed at single pathogens of well-defined virulence. The concepts of a mixed infection and of a pathogen that may at the same time be part of the normal flora of the site involved make its application more difficult.

Perhaps the first point to consider is the evidence of true infection. *Gardnerella*-associated "vaginitis" is marked by an absence of inflammatory cells in the discharge and minimal signs of vaginal or vulval inflammation. For this reason the term vaginosis has been suggested as being more appropriate. The clue cell suggests that *G. vaginalis* can adhere readily to epithelial cells, but no one knows whether adherence plays any part in the disease process or indeed whether *G. vaginalis* adheres to intact vaginal epithelium *in vivo*. The main symptoms relate to the smelly discharge, rather than to tissue damage.

Clay (1982) has reviewed the odour of gardnerella-associated vaginosis. A major part is due to the presence of certain diamines, notably putrescine and cadaverine (Chen *et al.*, 1979, 1982). These diamines are produced by the decarboxylation of amino acids; this is not done by *G. vaginalis* (Chen *et al.*, 1979). Thus, one of the principal symptoms and signs of bacterial vaginosis is not attributable to *G. vaginalis*.

With the exception of McCormack *et al.* (1977), it is generally agreed that there is a close association between bacterial vaginosis and the isolation of *G. vaginalis*. However, recent studies where human blood agar has been used have shown that *G. vaginalis* is found in 25–40% of women with no signs of vaginitis (Table 2). The differences in the results of the same group (Pheifer *et al.*, 1978; Spiegel *et al.*, 1980; Amsel *et al.*, 1982) with changes in media are striking. This certainly supports McCormack's view that *G. vaginalis* is part of the normal vaginal flora. The key factor may be the numbers of organisms present. Spiegel *et al.* (1980) found differences in the total count of *G. vaginalis* in controls and women with vaginosis.

Table 2 *Gardnerella vaginalis* association with bacterial vaginosis

Reference	Bacterial vaginosis (%)	Controls (%)
Gardner and Dukes (1955)	129/138 (93)	0/78 (0)
Pheifer *et al.* (1978)	17/18 (94)	1/18 (6)
Taylor *et al.* (1982)	23/35 (66)	3/23 (13)
Amsel *et al.* (1983)	41/44 (93)	64/160 (40)
Ison *et al.* (1983)	90/100 (90)	10/29 (35)

Although there is a close association between *G. vaginalis* and bacterial vaginosis, this is equally true of another group of organisms, the obligate anaerobes. Of these, bacteroides of the *Melaninogenicus oralis* group, particularly *B. bivius,* together with peptostreptococci, are most prominent (Pheifer *et al.,* 1978; Spiegel *et al.,* 1980; Taylor *et al.,* 1982). Unlike *G. vaginalis,* these anaerobes will produce putrescine and cadaverine (Chen *et al.,* 1979). *In vitro,* a nutritional and environmental balance is achieved between *G. vaginalis* and anaerobes, resulting in a higher final pH and survival of both bacterial groups. This has been proposed as the basis of a mixed infection where the two groups of organisms work together to produce the signs (and symptoms) of vaginosis (Chen *et al.,* 1979). It is an attractive hypothesis. Gardner (1980) has criticised it on the grounds that no single anaerobic species has the high rate of association of *G. vaginalis,* but this is perhaps to take a rather naive view of the way anaerobic populations work together.

Seventy years ago, Curtis (1913) isolated motile Gram-negative curved bacilli from the vagina in women with abnormal discharges. They were strict anaerobes with up to six flagella. Moore (1954) studied two types of curved anaerobic rods from the vagina. One type had a single flagellum, the other up to six flagella. In late 1981 and early 1982, several groups reported the isolation of curved motile Gram-negative anaerobes from the vaginal secretions of patients with bacterial vaginosis (Hjelm *et al.,* 1981; Skarin *et al.,* 1981; Spiegel *et al.,* 1981; Phillips and Taylor, 1982; Holst *et al.,* 1982; Sprott *et al.,* 1982). Those described by Skarin and by Spiegel have many of the characteristics of *Wolinella succinogenes.* Sprott *et al.* (1983) recently characterised two types of curved rod, one short, one long, which are distinct from each other and from *Wolinella* spp. Both types of bacilli were isolated from 18 of 86 patients with a vaginal discharge but only from 2 of 33 patients without a discharge. While the discovery or rediscovery of these curved rods has been of considerable microbiological interest, their link to the causation of vaginosis is unknown. A variety of anaerobic bacteria coexist with *G. vaginalis,* but no one species is particularly associated with vaginosis.

Gardner and Dukes (1955) attempted to fulfil Koch's postulates by inoculating volunteers either with the vaginal contents of women with proven gardnerella-associated vaginosis or with pure cultures of *G. vaginalis.* Eleven of 15 women given the former developed vaginosis from which *G. vaginalis* could be isolated. However, only 1 of 13 women given a large inoculum of pure *G. vaginalis* developed the disease. Later work from the same group suggested that the age of the culture might be important. Twelve-hour cultures of *G. vaginalis* were more effective at producing vaginosis in volunteers than were 24-hour cultures of the same strain (Criswell *et al.,* 1969). This work provides the best evidence for the pathogenicity of *G. vaginalis* in vaginosis. The numbers are, however, small, and the inocula used were very high (10^{10} CFU).

A good animal model for bacterial vaginosis is needed, but there is no report in the literature of any attempt to develop such a model. In collaboration with colleagues at the Clinical Research Centre and the National Institute for Medical Research, we attempted to induce vaginosis with *G. vaginalis* in three primate species (chimpanzee, pigtail macacque and tamarin). With chimpanzees we were unsuccessful, although we did use stock laboratory strains rather than fresh clinical isolates. We also failed to infect 4 tamarins with 24-hour broth cultures of fresh clinical isolates of *G. vaginalis* (inoculum 3×10^6 CFU). We were, however, successful in colonising pigtail macaques with a similar inoculum of the same organism. This success was repeated with a second strain of *G. vaginalis*, and the bacteria persisted in the vagina for several weeks. However, none of the monkeys developed an abnormal discharge and we saw no clue cells in the vaginal samples. The physiology and microbiology of the vagina in the pigtail macacque differs from the human state. It has an oestrus cycle and has a vaginal pH of about 7. A wide variety of obligate anaerobes were present, among which *Bacteroides fragilis* was prominent. Analysis of nonvolatile fatty acids of vaginal washings was of little value because of the presence of large amounts of succinate even before inoculation with *G. vaginalis*. The raised pH and anaerobic flora may account for the ease with which we established colonisation with *G. vaginalis* using an inoculum some 4 logs less than that of Criswell *et al.* (1969). The pigtail macacque is not a good model for the study of vaginitis in humans, but it may be worth looking at other easily kept small primates such as marmosets.

Another way of evaluating the relative contributions of *G. vaginalis* and anaerobes would be to use differential antimicrobial therapy. With most facultative bacteria, metronidazole would help to distinguish their role from that of the anaerobes, but *G. vaginalis* is moderately sensitive to metronidazole and even more so to one of its major breakdown products, the hydroxy metabolite (Ralph and Amatnieks, 1980). It is also very sensitive to clindamycin, another useful antibiotic with considerable activity against anaerobes.

There is, of course, the possibility that neither *G. vaginalis* nor anaerobes cause bacterial vaginosis and that they are both merely useful markers.

Gardnerella vaginalis and anaerobes are present in most cases of bacterial vaginosis. They are also present in trichomonal vaginitis and in cases of gonorrhoea, and the vaginal pH is raised in both conditions (Table 3) (Taylor *et al.*, 1982; Ison *et al.*, 1983). There is a clinical association between *G. vaginalis* and gonorrhoea and in female contacts of men with nonspecific urethritis (Balsdon, 1982). A suitable stimulus (possibly nonmicrobiological) could change the conditions in the vagina so as to allow the overgrowth of anaerobes and *G. vaginalis* commonly present as part of the normal flora, albeit sometimes in small numbers.

This still leaves the mechanism of pathogenicity. If *G. vaginalis* is the primary pathogen in bacterial vaginosis, adherence must play a key role in the causation

Table 3 Microbiological and biochemical findings in different types of female genital tract infection

Cause of vaginitis	Total tested	% Positive				
		$S/L > 0.4^a$	G. vaginalis	Anaerobes	Amines	pH > 4.5
Nonspecific	100	78	90	92	85	68
Trichomonas vaginalis	54	69	93	83	80	63
Gonorrhoea	17	82	88	88	83	59
Candida	51	14	55	47	31	12
Controls	29	14	35	61	31	6

[a] Succinate/lactate ratio.

of disease, as it is a superficial infection. The presence of clue cells reinforces this. However, it is not known whether G. vaginalis adheres to intact vaginal epithelium in vivo, whether this adherence causes exfoliation or whether the organism merely adheres to exfoliated cells.

Several groups have looked at the adherence of G. vaginalis to exfoliated vaginal epithelial cells. Mårdh and Weström (1976) found the adherence of G. vaginalis, Neisseria gonorrhoeae and group B streptococci to these cells to be far higher than that of Lactobacillus acidophilus and other aerobic and anaerobic commensals. Unlike Candida (Mead, 1974) and N. gonorrhoeae (Braude et al., 1978), Sobel et al. (1981) found no link between adherence of Gardnerella and particular times in the menstrual cycle. Tompkins et al. (1982), however, did show a lesser adherence of G. vaginalis before and a greater adherence during menstruation.

The adherence of G. vaginalis has been assessed using microscopy to count adherent bacteria. Little analysis of the phenomenon has yet been carried out.

Adherence is mannose resistant (Sobel et al., 1982), but there are conflicting reports as to the effect of pH (Sobel et al., 1981; Tompkins et al., 1982). In an attempt to reproduce conditions in vivo, particularly to take account of possible variations in the surface of epithelial cells, Sobel et al. (1982) used a noncontinuous multilayer culture system grown from vaginal explants. Electron microscopy showed considerable variation in the adherence of G. vaginalis to different cells, with increased adherence to mature cells and decreased adherence in areas of active mitosis. Cell variability, surface receptors and the effect of hormones all need to be analysed more fully with respect to the adherence of G. vaginalis to vaginal epithelium.

We have started to analyse the adherence of G. vaginalis to both human red blood cells and vaginal epithelial cells using radiolabelled G. vaginalis by the methods of Lambden et al. (1979). Adherence to red blood cells has proved useful in the study of the mechanisms of adherence of a number of microbial pathogens (Evans et al., 1977). Our studies are at a very early stage, but with this technique the adherence of G. vaginalis to human red cells is mannose resistant and inhibited by galactose and galactosamine. There is considerable strain variability, an observation which is reproducible. Adherence to epithelial cells is also mannose resistant and partially inhibited by galactose.

VI. EPIDEMIOLOGY

Whilst there seems little doubt that gardnerella-associated vaginosis is linked to sexual activity, it is still unclear whether or not it is a sexually transmitted disease. If we assume that G. vaginalis plays an active role in the disease, there are two points that have to be considered. First, is G. vaginalis part of the normal vaginal flora? Second, what is the precise role of the male partner in the epidemiology of the disease?

Table 2 compares isolation rates of *G. vaginalis* from "normal" women and those with vaginosis. Whereas in earlier studies *G. vaginalis* was rarely isolated, our own results tally with those of Amsel *et al.* (1983), Spiegel *et al.* (1980) and McCormack *et al.* (1977) in finding *G. vaginalis* in over one-third of normal women. Three of these studies used highly selective bilayer human blood agar medium. Amsel *et al.* (1983) found this to be more sensitive than chocolate in detecting low numbers of *G. vaginalis.* There is, of course, a limit to the sensitivity of any cultural technique, and the percentage of women without vaginosis who carry *G. vaginalis* may be even greater than so far described.

Much has been made of the failure to isolate *G. vaginalis* from sexually inexperienced women (Kummel, 1963; Karpovskaya, 1970, 1971), but as these studies did not use the sensitive cultural techniques now available, they are difficult to evaluate. The differences in isolation rates of *G. vaginalis* in studies carried out by Holmes' group in Seattle using different media are, however, telling (Pheifer *et al.*, 1978; Spiegel *et al.*, 1980; Amsel *et al.*, 1983).

Of male consorts of women with gardnerella-associated vaginitis, 80–90% show asymptomatic urethral colonisation with *G. vaginalis* (Gardner and Dukes, 1955, Pheifer *et al.*, 1978). Leopold (1953) isolated *G. vaginalis* from the urines of men whose sexual partners were infected with the same organism. In contrast, Dawson *et al.* (1982) and Kinghorn *et al.* (1982) only found colonisation rates of 7–11% among unselected men. Urethral carriage of *G. vaginalis* can persist for at least 6 months (Gardner and Dukes, 1955). Both Gardner and Dukes and Pheifer *et al.* (1978) found that reinfection rates in women after successful treatment were lower among those women whose sexual partners used barrier contraceptives or who refrained from sexual intercourse. The use of the contraceptive sheath was associated with a lower incidence of *G. vaginalis* among women than the use of "nonbarrier methods" (Bramley *et al.*, 1981).

While this provides strong evidence of sexual transmission of *G. vaginalis,* it is not conclusive. The little evidence we have of vaginal installation of *G. vaginalis* showed that even an inoculum of 10^{10} CFU of a young culture did not invariably produce infection (Criswell *et al.*, 1969). No quantitative work has been done on male carriage, but it is likely that any sexually transmitted inoculum would be many orders of magnitude lower than 10^{10} CFU. If *G. vaginalis* is a vaginal commensal that multiplies to cause vaginosis given the correct conditions, the presence of semen in the vagina after sexual intercourse could provide such a stimulus. This would account for the observations on contraceptive sheaths and vaginosis. The association between male carriage and gardnerella-associated vaginosis could be viewed as continual reinoculation of the male urethra. Male carriage of *G. vaginalis* is not on its own proof of sexual transmission from male to female.

Conclusive proof of sexual transmission requires the following: proof that *G. vaginalis* is wholly or partly responsible for this type of vaginitis; a clear demonstration that it can induce infection at those levels of inoculum that would be transmitted during intercourse; an effective typing system, which would show that strains of *G. vaginalis* in sexual partners were probably identical; well-controlled studies showing the eradication of male carriage by antibiotic and the superiority of treating male partners, as well as their consorts, in terms of preventing infection.

VII. MANAGEMENT

Although it has been claimed that *Gardnerella*-associated bacterial vaginosis is a self-limiting condition (Dattani *et al.*, 1982), most workers would agree with Gardner and Dukes that when diagnosed it requires specific antimicrobial therapy (Balsdon *et al.*, 1980).

Gardner and Dukes originally recommended local sulphonamide creams. Heltai and Taleghany (1959) were able to cure vaginosis but not to eradicate *G. vaginalis*. *G. vaginalis* is, as mentioned earlier in this chapter, highly resistant to sulphonamides, and the success of these preparations may relate to the acidic base of the cream. Other agents used locally include hexetidine gel (Gardner and Dukes, 1957), neomycin (Spitzbart, 1967) and povidone iodine (Dattani *et al.*, 1982).

Topical therapy has increasingly been replaced by systemic antimicrobial therapy. Seven-day courses of tetracycline (500 mg q.d.s.), ampicillin (500 mg q.d.s.), cephalosporins [cephradine (250 mg q.d.s.) and cephalexin (500 mg q.d.s.)], and metronidazole (500 mg b.d.) have all been used with varying degrees of success (Gardner, 1980). Erythromycin, despite its marked *in vitro* activity against *G. vaginalis,* is ineffective *in vivo*.

Two published trials have established the efficacy of metronidazole for *Gardnerella*-associated vaginosis. Pheifer *et al.* (1978) reported that a regimen of metronidazole (500 mg b.d.) for 7 days eradicated *G. vaginalis* from all 81 women treated by the end of the course. Eighty of 81 showed clinical improvement. At 2–5 weeks later, *G. vaginalis* could be cultured from 8 of 57, and 9 had a recurrence of signs and/or symptoms. In contrast, sulphonamide cream failed to eradicate the organism, while doxycycline (100 mg b.d.) and ampicillin (500 mg q.d.s.) for 7 days were far less effective in achieving microbiological or clinical cure. Balsdon *et al.* (1980) found a 7-day course of metronidazole (Flagyl) (400 mg b.d.) superior to oxytetracycline (500 mg b.d.). Spiegel *et al.* (1980) also found oral metronidazole to be very effective. It is not clear whether the efficacy of metronidazole in this condition is due to its effect on the obligate anaerobes usually found with *G. vaginalis* (Spiegel *et al.*, 1980) or to the combined effect of the parent compound and its hydroxy metabolite on *G. vaginalis* (Ralph and Amatnieks, 1980; Easmon *et al.,* 1982).

Apart from initial cure, the other problems are recurrence and treatment of male contacts. With metronidazole, Pheifer *et al.* (1978) found relapse rates of over 50% in those women who had sexual intercourse with a new or untreated partner and only 4% in those without such exposure.

Gardner (1980) recommended treatment of male contacts with the same systemic agent, as is done for trichomoniasis. The excretion of metronidazole and its hydroxy metabolite (and for that matter ampicillin) in the urine suggests that this would be effective in dealing with urethral carriage in the male. Although studies are in progress, there are no properly controlled reports published showing the effect of treatment of male partners on recurrence rates. This information is badly needed, not only for clinical purposes, but also for the light it may shed on the role of the male carrier and the importance of sexual transmission.

If metronidazole and related agents are taken as the current treatment of choice for this type of vaginosis, the question of dose regimen must be considered. Most studies have used 400 or 500 mg b.d. for 5 to 7 days. There may be advantages to a single 2-g dose if this can be shown to be effective. This may be particularly useful for treatment of asymptomatic male carriers if this is shown to be necessary.

VIII. *G. VAGINALIS* IN EXTRAVAGINAL SITES

A. Urinary tract

Leopold (1953) isolated *G. vaginalis* from the urine of a number of men. McFadyen and Eykyn (1968) isolated *G. vaginalis* from 159 of 1000 urine samples taken from women by suprapubic aspiration. McDowall *et al.* (1981) found *G. vaginalis* to be the organism most commonly isolated from the urine of pregnant women in whom routine culture was negative. *Gardnerella vaginalis* has also been found in urine from renal transplant patients (Birch *et al.,* 1981) and has been incriminated as one cause of the urethral syndrome (Maskell *et al.,* 1979), and there is one report of *G. vaginalis* urinary tract infection in a man (Abercrombie *et al.,* 1978). We have recently been looking at midstream urines with a raised cell count taken from pregnant women in which no bacteria were isolated on routine culture. When those patients on antimicrobial therapy were excluded, 40% of the urines were found to contain $\geq 10^5$ colony forming units of *G. vaginalis*. This is only a preliminary study. We did not use suprapubic aspiration, neither did we look for other fastidious urinary pathogens, nor take parallel vaginal samples, but the results, taken with other published work, do suggest that the role of *G. vaginalis* in lower urinary-tract infections should be examined more closely.

B. Urethritis and balanoposthitis

Urethral carriage of *G. vaginalis* is usually asymptomatic, gardnerella-associated urethritis in one group with "clue cells" has been reported, but since other causes of nonspecific urethritis such as *Chlamydia trachomatis* and *Ureaplasma urealyticum* were not excluded, the pathogenic role of *G. vaginalis* in these cases must remain doubtful (Dunkleberg and Woolvin, 1963; Sylvestre and Ethier, 1963). Kinghorn *et al.* (1982) have reported several cases of noncandidal balanoposthitis in which *G. vaginalis* was isolated in combination with obligate anaerobes, mirroring the situation found in bacterial vaginosis.

C. Perinatal infections

Gardnerella vaginalis has been occasionally isolated from blood and other samples associated with intra- and postpartum pyrexia and postabortal sepsis (Edmunds, 1959; Rotheram and Schick, 1969; Regamey and Schoenknecht, 1973; Monif and Baer, 1974). It has also been reported in cases of neonatal infection (Platt, 1971).

D. Other sites

Gardnerella vaginalis has been isolated from abdominal wounds and fluid Bartholin's cysts and even from pharyngeal culture (Malone *et al.*, 1975; Gardner, 1980).

IX. CONCLUSIONS

Recent work has confirmed the original observations of Gardner and Dukes (1955) that bacterial vaginosis is a distinct clinical entity. Although a mild condition, it is probably the commonest form of vaginal infection. As many women do not complain of symptoms, both diagnosis and cure should be based on signs such as the nature of the discharge, the presence of clue cells, a raised vaginal pH and a positive amine test. Metronidazole and related nitroimidazoles appear to be the most effective antibiotics for this condition. Although treatment of the male partner is advocated by many, conclusive proof of its efficacy is awaited.

The placing of *G. vaginalis* in a new genus has resolved much of the bacteriological confusion. Some problems, however, still remain. Is *G. vaginalis* Gram-positive or Gram-negative? Why is it so much more sensitive to nitroimidazoles and their metabolites than most other facultative organisms? Can the organism be biotyped or serotyped?

There are even more unresolved questions concerning the aetiology, pathogenesis and epidemiology of bacterial vaginosis. Both *G. vaginalis* and anaerobes are closely associated with this type of vaginosis, but a similar association exists between these organisms in trichomonal vaginitis, in gonorrhoea and possibly in chlamydial and mycoplasma infections too. Are *G. vaginalis* and anaerobes producing a mixed infection, or are they merely markers of some other change in vaginal ecology? Whatever its pathogenic potential, *G. vaginalis* must now be regarded as a part of the normal vaginal flora. It would be interesting to know if some cases of postgonococcal genital infection in women were associated with *G. vaginalis* and anaerobes.

This is a sexually associated disease certainly, a sexually transmitted disease possibly. Male partners of women with gardnerella-associated vaginosis certainly have a high rate of urethral carriage, but this alone is not proof of sexual transmission. This is especially so if *G. vaginalis* in small numbers is part of the normal flora of the vagina, for then it is no longer necessary to ascribe reinfection to sexual transmission from male to female. Vaginosis has been induced in volunteers with *G. vaginalis* but not with complete success, even at very high inocula.

Clinically it is to be hoped that the recent interest in bacterial vaginosis will benefit the women who suffer from this common condition. It is a distinct clinical entity, and the use of a more suitable name such as bacterial vaginosis might improve its status and encourage a more aggressive approach to treatment. Scientifically there are enough questions left unanswered about both *G. vaginalis* and vaginosis to keep those who are interested in either busy for many years.

ACKNOWLEDGMENT

Our own work on *G. vaginalis* is supported by a grant from the Medical Research Council.

REFERENCES

Abercrombie, G. F., Allen, J., and Maskell, R. (1978). *Lancet* **1,** 766.
Amsel, R., Totten, P. A., Spiegel, C. A., Chen, K. C. S., Eschenbach, D., and Holmes, K. K. (1983). *Am. J. Med.* **74,** 14–22.
Bailey, R. K., Voss, J. L., and Smith, R. F. (1979). *J. Clin. Microbiol.* **9,** 65–71.
Balsdon, M. J. (1982). *Eur. J. Clin. Microbiol.* **1,** 288–293.
Balsdon, M. J., and Jackson, D. (1981). *Lancet* **1,** 1112.
Balsdon, M. J., Pead, L., Taylor, G. E., and Maskell, R. (1980). *Lancet* **1,** 501–504.
Birch, D. F., D'Apice, A. J. F., and Fairley, K. F. (1981). *J. Infect. Dis.* **144,** 123–127.
Blackwell, A., and Barlow, D. (1982). *Br. J. Vener. Dis.* **58,** 387–393.
Blackwell, A., Fox, A. R., Phillips, I., and Barlow, D. (1984). *Lancet* **1,** 1379–1382.
Bramley, H. M., Dixon, R. A., and Jones, B. M. (1981). *Br. J. Vener. Dis.* **57,** 62–66.
Braude, A. I., Corbeil, L. B., Levine, S., Ho, J., and McCutchan, J. A. (1978). *In*

"Immunobiology of *Neisseria gonorrhoeae*" (G. F. Brooks, E. C. Gotschlich, K. K. Holmes, W. D. Sawyer, and F. E. Young, eds.), pp. 328–337. Am. Soc. Microbiol., Washington, D.C.

Chen, K. C. S., Forsyth, P. S., Buchanan, T. M., and Holmes, K. K. (1979). *J. Clin. Invest.* **63**, 828–835.

Chen, K. C. S., Amsel, R., Eschenbach, D. A., and Holmes, K. K. (1982). *J. Infect. Dis.* **145**, 337–345.

Clay, J. C. (1982). *Eur. J. Clin. Microbiol.* **1**, 317–319.

Criswell, B. S., Ladwig, C. L., Gardner, H. L., and Dukes, C. D. (1969). *Obstet. Gynecol.* **33**, 195–199.

Criswell, B. S., Marston, J. H., Stenback, W. A., Black, S. H., and Gardner, H. L. (1971). *Can. J. Microbiol.* **17**, 865–869.

Curtis, A. H. (1913). *J. Infect. Dis.* **12**, 165–169.

Dattani, I. M., Gerken, A., and Evans, B. A. (1982). *Br. J. Vener. Dis.* **58**, 32.

Dawson, S. G., Ison, C. A., Csonka, G., and Easmon, C. S. F. (1982). *Br. J. Vener. Dis.* **58**, 243–245.

Dukes, C. D. (1956). *Bacteriol. Rev.* **20**, 275.

Dukes, C. D., and Gardner, H. L. (1961). *J. Bacteriol.* **81**, 277–283.

Dunkleberg, W. E. (1977). *Sex. Transm. Dis.* **2**, 69–75.

Dunkleberg, W. E., and McVeigh, I. (1969). *Antonie Van Leeuwenhock* **35**, 129–145.

Dunkleberg, W. E., and Woolvin, S. C. (1963). *Mil. Med.* **128**, 1098–1101.

Dunkleberg, W. E., Skaggs, R., and Kellogg, D. S. (1970). *Appl. Microbiol.* **19**, 47–52.

Durfee, M. A., Forsyth, P. S., Hale, J. A., and Holmes, K. K. (1979). *Antimicrob. Agents Chemother.* **19**, 47–52.

Easmon, C. S. F., Ison, C. A., Kaye, C. M., Timewell, R. M., and Dawson, S. G. (1982). *Br. J. Vener. Dis.* **58**, 246–249.

Edmunds, P. N. (1959). *J. Obstet. Gynaecol. Br. Emp.* **66**, 917–926.

Evans, D. G., Evans, D. J., and Tjoa, W. (1977). *Infect. Immun.* **18**, 330–337.

Gardner, H. L. (1980). *Am. J. Obstet. Gynecol.* **137**, 385–390.

Gardner, H. L., and Dukes, C. D. (1954). *Science* **120**, 853.

Gardner, H. L., and Dukes, C. D. (1955). *Am. J. Obstet. Gynecol.* **69**, 962–976.

Gardner, H. L., and Dukes, C. D. (1957). *Obstet. Gynecol.* **9**, 610–612.

Gibbons, R. J., Spirell, D. M., and Skobe, Z. (1976). *Infect. Immun.* **13**, 238–246.

Goldberg, R. I., and Washington, J. A. (1976). *J. Clin. Microbiol.* **4**, 245–247.

Greenwood, J. R., and Pickett, M. J. (1979). *J. Clin. Microbiol.* **9**, 200–204.

Greenwood, J. R., and Pickett, M. J. (1980). *Int. J. Syst. Bacteriol.* **30**, 170–178.

Greenwood, J. R., Pickett, M. J., Martin, W. J., and Mack, E. G. (1977). *Health Lab. Sci.* **14**, 102–106.

Harper, J. J., and Davis, G. H. G. (1982). *Int. J. Syst. Bacteriol.* **32**, 48–50.

Heltai, A., and Taleghany, P. (1959). *Am. J. Obstet. Gynecol.* **77**, 144–148.

Hjelm, E., Hallén, A., Forsum, U., and Wallin, J. (1981). *Lancet* **2**, 1353–1354.

Holst, E., Skarin, A., and Mårdh, P. A. (1982). *Eur. J. Clin. Microbiol.* **1**, 310–316.

Ison, C. A., Dawson, S. G., Hilton, J., Csonka, G. W., and Easmon, C. S. F. (1982). *J. Clin. Pathol.* **35**, 550–554.

Ison, C. A., Easmon, C. S. F., Dawson, S. G., Southerton, G., and Harris, J. R. W. (1983). *J. Clin. Pathol.* **36**, 1367–1370.

Johnson, A. P., Ison, C. A., Hetherington, C. M., Osborn, M. F., Southerton, G., London, W. T., Easmon, C. S. F., and Taylor-Robinson, D. (1984). *Br. J. Exp. Pathol* (in press).

Jolly, J. L. S. (1983). *J. Clin. Pathol.* **36**, 476–478.

Karpovskaya, O. G. (1970). *Vestnik Dermatol. I. Venerol.* **44**, 51–54.

Karpovskaya, O. G. (1971). *Akush. Ginekol.* **47**, 33–35.

Kinghorn, G. R., Jones, B. M., Chowdhury, F. H., and Geary, I. (1982). *Br. J. Vener. Dis.* **58**, 127–129.

Kummel, J. (1963). *Arch. Gynekol.* **199**, 5.

Lambden, P. R., Heckels, J. E., James, L. T., and Watt, P. J. (1979). *J. Gen. Microbiol.* **114**, 305–312.

Lapage, S. P. (1961). *Acta Pathol. Microbiol. Scand.* **52**, 34–54.

Leopold, S. (1953). *U.S. Armed Forces Med. J.* **4**, 263–266.

Lutz, A., Grootten, O., and Wurch, T. (1956). *Rev. Immunol.* **20**, 132–138.

McCarthy, L. R., Mickelsen, P. A., and Grover-Smith, E. (1979). *Antimicrob. Agents Chemother.* **16**, 186–189.

McCormack, W. M., Hayes, C. H., Rosner, B., Evrard, J. R., Crockett, V. A., Alpert, S., and Zinner, S. H. (1977). *J. Infect. Dis.* **136**, 740–745.

McDowall, D. R. M., Buchanan, J. D., Fairley, K. F., and Gilbert, G. L. (1981). *J. Infect. Dis.* **144**, 114–122.

McFadyen, I. R., and Eykyn, S. J. (1968). *Lancet* **1**, 1112–1114.

Malone, B. H., Schreiber, M., Schneider, N. J., and Holdeman, L. V. (1975). *J. Clin. Microbiol.* **2**, 272–275.

Mårdh, P. A. (1982). *Eur. J. Clin. Microbiol.* **1**, 285–287.

Mårdh, P. A., and Weström, L. (1976). *Infect. Immun.* **13**, 661–666.

Maskell, R., Pead, L., and Allen, J. (1979). *Lancet* **1**, 1058–1059.

Mead, P. B. (1974). *In* "Infectious Diseases in Obstetrics and Gynaecology" (G. R. G. Monif, ed.), pp. 242–267. Harper & Row, New York.

Mickelsen, P. A., McCarthy, L. R., and Magnum, M. E. (1977). *J. Clin. Microbiol.* **5**, 488–489.

Monif, G. R. G., and Baer, H. (1974). *Am. J. Obstet. Gynecol.* **121**, 1041–1045.

Moore, B. (1954). *J. Pathol. Bacteriol.* **67**, 461–473.

Park, C. H., Fauber, M., and Cook, C. B. (1968). *Am. J. Clin. Pathol.* **49**, 590.

Pheifer, T. A., Forsyth, P. S., Durfee, M. A., Pollock, H. M., and Holmes, K. K. (1978). *N. Engl. J. Med.* **298**, 1429–1434.

Phillips, I., and Taylor, E. (1982). *Lancet* **1**, 221.

Piot, P., Van Dyck, E., Goodfellow, M., and Falkow, S. (1980). *J. Gen. Microbiol.* **119**, 373–396.

Piot, P., Van Dyck, E., Godts, P., and Vanderheyden, J. (1982). *Eur. J. Clin. Microbiol.* **1**, 301–306.

Platt, M. S. (1971). *Clin. Pediatr. (Philadelphia)* **10**, 513–516.

Ralph, E. D., and Amatnieks, Y. E. (1980). *Sex. Transm. Dis.* **7**, 157–160.

Redmond, D. L., and Kotcher, E. (1963). *J. Gen. Microbiol.* **33**, 89–94.

Regamey, C., and Schoenknecht, F. D. (1973). *JAMA, J. Am. Med. Assoc.* **225**, 1621–1623.

Rotheram, E. B., and Schick, S. F. (1969). *Am. J. Med.* **46**, 80–89.

Shanker, S., and Munro, R. (1982). *Lancet* **1**, 167.

Shanker, S., Toohey, M., and Munro, R. (1982). *Eur. J. Clin. Microbiol.* **1**, 298–300.

Shaw, C. E., Forsyth, M. E., Bowie, W. R., and Black, W. A. (1981). *J. Clin. Microbiol.* **14**, 108–110.

Skarin, A., Spiegel, C. A., Westrom, L., Holmes, K. K., and Mårdh, P. A. (1981). *Abstr. Int. Meet. Sex. Transm. Dis., 4th, 1981*, p. 8.

Smith, R. F. (1975). *Health Lab. Sci.* **12**, 219–224.

Smith, R. F. (1979). *J. Clin. Microbiol.* **9**, 729–730.

Sobel, J. D., Schneider, J., Kaye, D., and Levison, M. E. (1981). *Infect. Immun.* **32**, 194–197.

Sobel, J. D., Myers, P., Levison, M. E., and Kaye, D. (1982). *Infect. Immun.* **35**, 697–701.

Spiegel, C. A., Amsel, R., Eschenbach, D., Schoenknecht, F., and Holmes, K. K. (1980). *N. Engl. J. Med.* **303**, 601–607.

Spiegel, C. A., Skarin, A., Mårdh, P. A., and Holmes, K. K. (1981). *Abstr. Int. Meet. Sexually Transmitted Dis., 4th, 1981,* p. 8.

Spitzbart, H. (1967). *Dtsch. Gesundheitswes.* **22,** 1225–1227.

Sprott, M. S., Pattman, R. S., Ingham, H. R., Short, G. R., Narang, H. K., and Selkon, J. B. (1982). *Lancet* **1,** 54.

Sprott, M. S., Ingham, H. R., Pattman, R. S., Eisenstadt, R. L., Short, G. R., Narang, H. K., Sisson, P. K., and Selkon, J. B. (1983). *J. Med. Microbiol.* **16,** 175–182.

Svarva, P. L., and Moeland, J. A. (1982). *Acta Pathol. Microbiol. Scand., Sect. Microbiol. B:* **90B,** 453–455.

Sylvestre, L., and Ethier, J. (1963). *Can. Med. Assoc. J.* **89,** 1218–1220.

Taylor, E., and Phillips, I. (1983). *J. Med. Microbiol.* **16,** 83–92.

Taylor, E., Barlow, D., Blackwell, A. L., and Phillips, I. (1982). *Lancet* **1,** 1376–1379.

Tompkins, L. S., Oberg, J., and Holmes, K. K. (1982). *Abstr. ICAAC, 1982* No. 462, p. 148.

Totten, P. A., Amsel, R., Hale, J., Piot, P., and Holmes, K. K. (1982). *J. Clin. Microbiol.* **15,** 141–147.

Vice, J. L., and Smaron, M. F. (1973). *Appl. Microbiol.* **25,** 908–916.

Wurch, T., and Lutz, A. (1955). *Rev. Fr. Gynecol. Obstet.* **50,** 289–294.

Yong, D. C. T., and Prytula, A. (1978). *J. Clin. Microbiol.* **8,** 643–647.

Yong, D. C. T., and Thompson, J. S. (1982). *J. Clin. Microbiol.* **16,** 30–33.

Zinnemann, K., and Turner, G. C. (1963). *J. Pathol. Bacteriol.* **85,** 213–219.

4 Trichomoniasis

GEORGE W. CSONKA and S. L. SQUIRES

I. INTRODUCTION

A. Definition

Trichomoniasis is a common condition with more than 19,000 new patients reported annually from the venereal disease clinics in the United Kingdom. It is caused by the protozoon *Trichomonas vaginalis*. The infection is localised in the genital tract and considered to be sexually transmitted, causing a persistent vaginitis in the female and more rarely urethritis in the male. It can be asymptomatic in the male and less commonly also in the female. The parasite is cosmopolitan in its distribution, and it has been estimated that 10% or more of the sexually active population may be infected.

B. History

Trichomonas vaginalis was first described in 1836 by Donné, who isolated it from a patient with vaginitis. He believed at first that the organism was also responsible for syphilis and gonorrhoea but changed his mind when he found the protozoon also in healthy women. In 1894, Marchand and independently Miura (1894) and Dock (1896) observed trichomonads in male urethritis. Treatment of the condition was unsatisfactory due to the absence of a specific therapy until 1959, when oral metronidazole was first used by Durel *et al.* in the treatment of human trichomoniasis.

II. THE TRICHOMONADS

A. In man

These organisms are found in man, where they may be one of three species (Table 1):

Medical Microbiology, 4
ISBN 0-12-228004-0

1. *Trichomonas vaginalis Donné* (the only species inhabiting the genitourinary tract)
2. *Trichomonas hominis* (in the intestinal tract)
3. *Trichomonas tenax* (in the mouth)

Of these three, *T. vaginalis* is the only one considered to be pathogenic. However, *T. hominis* is often present in diarrhoeal conditions, and may be associated with *Entamoeba histolytica* or *Giardia lamblia*. All three exist only in the trophozoite stage and resemble one another morphologically, but *T. vaginalis* is larger.

B. In animals

Other strains of trichomonads infect a variety of animals where they can be of significant economic importance, e.g., causing abortion in cattle (*T. foetus*), infection of pigeons by *T. columbiae,* and blackhead in turkeys by *Histomonas meleagridis*, previously described as a trichomonad, which caused serious losses in turkey breeding until the introduction of dimetridazole. A number of strains of trichomonads are known to infect reptiles, fish and amphibians.

C. Morphology

The shape of the organism is commonly oval, round or pyriform (Fig. 1) but may vary depending on the environment. On average it is 10–13 μm in length and 7–10 μm in width. Variations in size have been frequently reported, ranging from giant forms of up to 100 μm (Whittington, 1957) to less than 9 μm (Mekki and Ivic, 1979). Winston (1974) has suggested that the size of the parasite is reflected in the clinical condition. In his studies, three-quarters of the patients had small trichomonads with an average diameter of less than 16 μm. Half of these complained of acute vaginal discharge and irritation; most also had marked inflammatory changes in the desquamated vaginal squamous cells. Patients carrying large parasites of 16 μm or greater were usually asymptomatic. The organism seen in culture is also large.

Table 1 Species of *Trichomonas*

Man	Animals	Birds
T. vaginalis	T. foetus	T. columbiae
T. hominis	T. suis	T. gallinarum
T. tenax	T. muris	H. meleagridis
(T. elongata,		
T. flageata)		

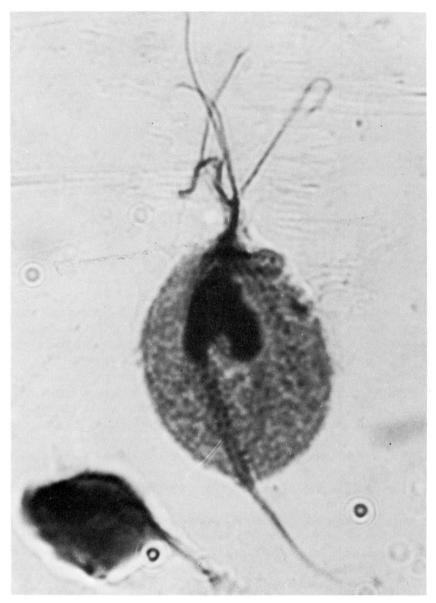

Fig. 1   Trichomonas vaginalis.

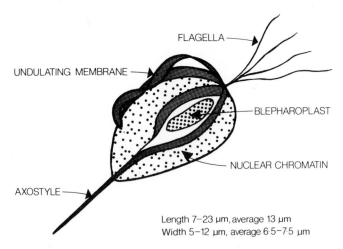

Fig. 2   The morphology of *Trichomonas vaginalis*.

Trichomonads divide by binary fission, and are motile, propelled by four rapidly thrashing anterior flagella that impart a characteristic jerky and twisting movement; the smaller organisms are more actively motile than the large ones. The protozoon has a large nucleus, vacuoles and a rigid axostyle, which passes through the entire cytoplasm and protrudes as a spine posteriorly. It originates from the blepharoplast, from which arises also an undulating membrane (Fig. 2).

Recognition of the parasite can on occasion be difficult, either due to its tendency to cling to cellular material [Figs. 3(a) and 3(b)], or when there are morphological abnormalities of shape and flagella such as the multiflagellated "amoeboid" forms and absence of flagella or numerous flagella arising around the circumference of the body (Fig. 4). By general consent, the use of wet-mounted unstained preparations is considered preferable to fixed preparations stained with Romanowski stain, acridine orange, neutral red, etc., as fixing and staining causes distortion and loss of fine detail, making recognition difficult. In cervical smears stained by the Papanicolaou method, trichomonads appear green, and positive results may sometimes be obtained when wet-mounted films fail. Most success is claimed for cultures using modern media when heavy growth becomes visible after overnight incubation.

Trevoux *et al.* (1976) described "round" forms, which he named "pseudo-cysts." Verges (1979) found that 22% of his patients carried such round forms. John and Squires (1978), using scanning electron microscopy, found that among trichomonads isolated from women who had previously been infected a number of times, there were large forms with abnormal morphology (Figs. 5–7). These may have been organisms that had failed to divide by binary fission.

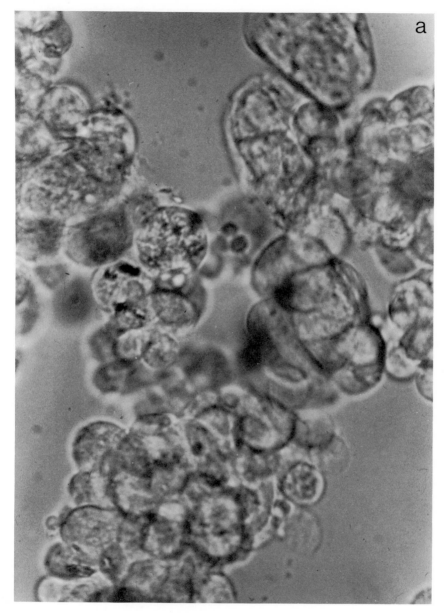

Fig. 3 (a) The growth of *Trichomonas vaginalis* organisms. (b) Clinging to cellular material and to each other (continued).

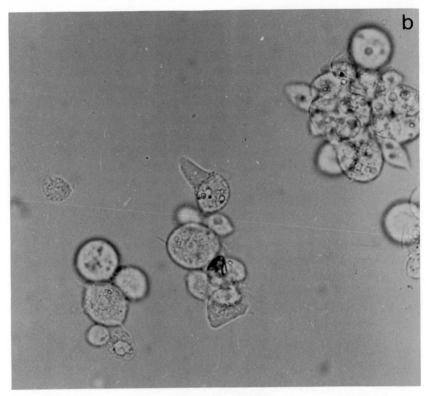

Fig. 3   (Continued.)

D.   Cultivation

The first recorded growth of the parasite was in 1915, when Lynch had some success using broth which had been acidified. Following this, many attempts were made to get axenic cultures. The next advance was made by Adler and Pulvertaft (1944), who added a crude penicillin filtrate to the medium and thus eliminated contaminating bacteria. This work had not been published earlier due to wartime censorship. In 1945, a similar method was published by Johnson, Trussell, and Jahn, who also used penicillin to suppress bacterial overgrowth. More recent culture media contain meat extract with liver solubles, buffered saline to maintain the osmotic pressure, and reducing agents such as ascorbic acid.

In 1957, at a symposium held in Reims, a number of media were described. Several were based on the medium first reported by Bushby and Copp (1955), which consisted of a watery extract of liver with the addition of meat broth. This medium had certain disadvantages in its preparation that led Squires and McFad-

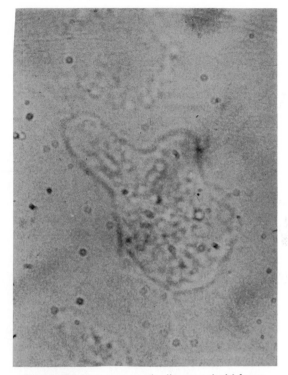

Fig. 4 Trichomonas vaginalis, amoeboid form.

zean (1962) to prepare a modification using commercially available freeze-dried aqueous liver and meat extracts. In this medium, heavy growth could be obtained in 24 hours even from a minimal inoculum (Fig. 8).

More recently, Linstead (1981) has described a semidefined medium based on the CMRL 1066 tissue culture medium, which was modified by lowering the redox potential by the addition of high concentrations of ascorbate and replacing serum by bovine albumin and cholesterol. These modern culture methods give very reliable results. Using them, Fouts and Kraus (1980) identified *T. vaginalis* by culture in 131 women, while the wet mount was positive in only 66. It is generally found that wet mounts are about 80% as sensitive as cultures in acute cases, but far less sensitive in asymptomatic vaginal infections. Thus, culture is the most sensitive and specific method, followed by wet mounts, with fixed stained specimens being a poor third.

For routine use we suggest that a fresh vaginal swab preparation be made with saline and examined microscopically without delay, preferably by the dark-field method when numerous motile trichomonads are usually seen. If a culture service is available and the wet mounted preparation is negative, a swab should be

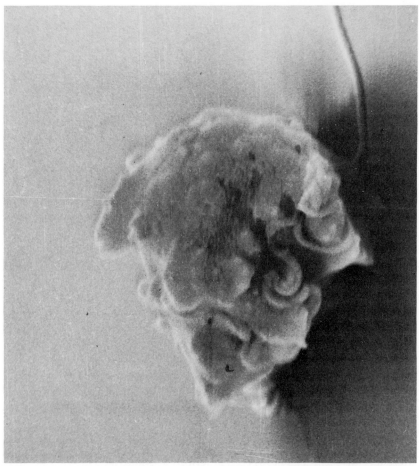

Fig. 5 Trichomonas vaginalis by scanning electron microscopy, abnormal form, ×1200.

Culture medium for *T. vaginalis*[a]

Dehydrated liver infusion	18 g
Dextrose	20 g
Calcium pantothenate (0.5% solution)	1 ml
Trypsin digest broth	to 1000 ml
Adjust medium to pH 6.5, sterilise at 5 psi	for 15 min
Before use, add 10% horse serum.	

[a] From Squires and McFadzean (1962).

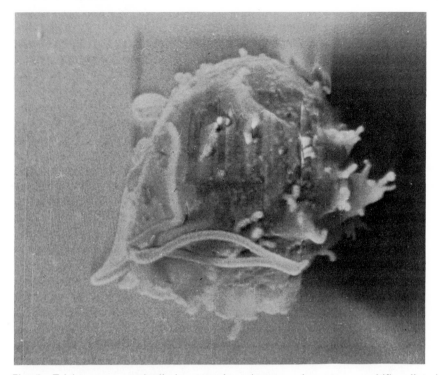

Fig. 6 *Trichomonas vaginalis* by scanning electron microscopy, multiflagellated, ×1200.

placed in a tube of suitable medium and incubated at 36.5°C for 24 hours. Growth occurs at the bottom of the tube and is then examined microscopically. The combination of direct microscopy and culture can be expected to give optimal results. Culture is of special importance when there is apparent treatment failure that needs further investigation.

Trichomonas vaginalis may remain viable in culture diluted with physiological saline or in undiluted discharge for many hours at room temperature. Tap water kills the organism in minutes, since it does not tolerate hypotonicity. Dessication and temperature over 45°C are instantly lethal (World Health Organization, 1981).

1. Transport medium

For specimens that must be transported from the clinic to the laboratory, the use of a nonnutritional semisolid medium such as described by Stuart (1946) is useful. Fastidious organisms, including *T. vaginalis,* will survive up to 24 hours in such media at room temperature.

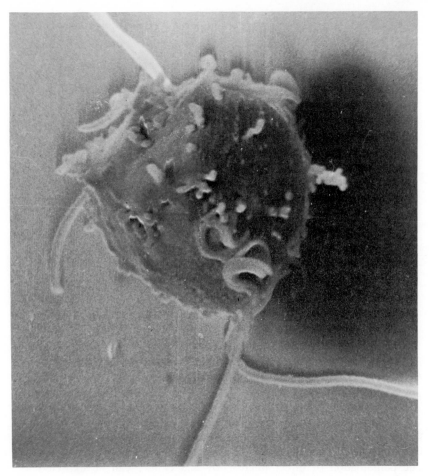

Fig. 7 Trichomonas vaginalis by scanning electron microscopy, multiflagellated,
×1200.

Stuart medium (pH 7.4)

Component	g/litre
Sodium glycerophosphate	10.0
Sodium thioglycollate	1.0
Calcium chloride	0.1
Methylene blue	0.002
Agar	2.0

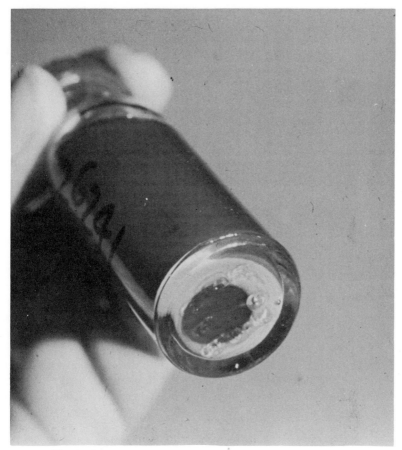

Fig. 8 Growth of *Trichomonas vaginalis* in liquid medium.

2. Tissue culture

Heath (1981), using conventional light microscopy along with the scanning electron microscope, examined the effect of growth of *T. vaginalis* on mammalian cell cultures using RK13, rabbit kidney cells. Within 6 hours of inoculation, some 10% of the cells were destroyed. The parasites adhered to the cells, developed an amoeboid appearance, and moved over the cell culture.

Other workers have used a variety of cell lines, HeLa cells, chick fibroblasts, human synovial cells and chick embryo explants. The cytotoxicity observed is thought by some to be a direct result of contact by the parasite, whilst others believe the effect to be due to a toxic substance produced by the trichomonad.

E. Antigenic properties

Protozoa are usually weak antigens, and it is obvious from the reinfection rate that any immunity arising from infection is not sufficiently effective to destroy the parasite. However, both common and specific antibodies of *T. vaginalis* and *T. foetus* were shown by McDonald and Tatum (1948) by agglutination and cross-absorption tests. Schoenherr (1959) used complement fixation and precipitin reactions. McEntegart *et al.* (1958) applied the fluorescent antibody technique to differentiate microscopically between human and bovine genital trichomonads. A number of serotypes were demonstrated by various authors (Hoffman and Gorczynski, 1964; Teras, 1966; Rõigas, 1975). Local antibodies were shown to be present in vaginal secretions by Pierce (1946) and more recently by John (1980). Systemic antibodies were first reported by Riedmüller (1932) and confirmed by John (1980).

F. Immunoprotection

Three-quarters of mice immunised with killed *T. vaginalis* were protected against challenge inoculation (Nakabayashi, 1952; Baba, 1958). Jaakmees *et al.* (1966) noted that mice were protected by the intraperitoneal administration of human sera from infected patients, but that this protection tended to disappear with time and was completely absent after 6 months. Mason (1979) found antitrichomonal immunoglobulins of the IgG class in the sera of 90% of women with proven *Trichomonas* vaginitis, versus 17% in controls, and considered that the combined effect of local and systemic antibodies may have a moderating influence on the infection. Gillin and Sher (1981) reported that lysis of the protozoa by serum is caused by activation of the alternative complement pathway. Serum deficient in C3 or C8 did not cause lysis of the parasite, nor did serum heated to 56°C.

Rein *et al.* (1980) and Mantovani *et al.* (1981) demonstrated by *in vitro* studies that human polymorphonuclear neutrophils and monocytes are cytotoxic to *T. vaginalis* under aerobic conditions. This is not easy to correlate with clinical experience, as in trichomonas vaginitis there are abundant polymorphs present in the vagina without demonstrable effect; one explanation might be that the comparatively anaerobic milieu of the vagina does not provide a suitable environment for cytotoxic activation.

III. EPIDEMIOLOGY

A. Prevalence

Trichomonas vaginalis is one of the commonest causes of specific vaginitis. Its distribution is worldwide. The figure of about 19,000 new cases reported yearly occurring in women attending the clinics for sexually transmitted diseases (STD) in the United Kingdom is similar to that for gonorrhoea. In the United States, incidences of up to 10% have been found in healthy women (Naguib *et al.*, 1966) and over 30% in women attending STD clinics (Fouts and Kraus, 1980). In an unpublished series of 350 women from factories in North London attending a well-women clinic that included screening for STD in its programme, the incidence for *Trichomonas* vaginitis was 3.4% and it was the commonest genital infection. Keighley (1971) studied the incidence in prostitutes in an English prison and found that of 476 prostitutes examined for evidence of a venereal disease, 51% carried *T. vaginalis*. The figures are generally higher in the lower socioeconomic groups, in gynaecological and antenatal patients, and in those seeking advice in STD clinics.

B. Age

Infection has rarely been reported in female neonates who have been exposed to infected mothers during birth and in prepubertal girls following close contact with their mothers. The incidence rises to its maximum during the second and third decade, and declines in older women. In males the infection is also most common in the second and third decade but extends to older patients more readily than in women.

C. Sex

From the available data it appears that trichomoniasis is about 10 times more common in women than men. However, as the majority of men who are sexual contacts of women with trichomoniasis are asymptomatic and have no cause to seek medical advice, the true incidence of men with infestation is not known. Explanation for the apparent difference between the sexes must take into account anatomical differences, the less congenial environment of the male urethra compared with the vagina for the parasite, the frequent disturbance due to the urethral urinary stream, and the reputed antitrichomonal action of prostatic secretions. The reported incidence of trichomoniasis in men varies significantly between observers, which may be a reflection of the time allowed to examine the specimen and also the time relationship to sexual contact with trichomoniasis. Thus Whittington (1957) found it present in 19%, versus 70% reported by Block *et al.* (1959). These figures may be misleading, as none of the authors repeated these tests over a period of time to see whether the presence of the parasite was transient or persistent. John (1980) found *T. vaginalis* in the urethra of 38% of male sexual contacts of vaginal trichomoniasis *provided the tests were performed within 4 days of sexual contact*. With prolonged interval, the proportion of negative tests rose. This indicates that in a number of men the infection was self-limited. In a small study of our own, 4 men who were contacts of *Trichomonas* vaginitis developed urethritis with trichomonads in the secretions. The parasite disappeared spontaneously in 3 men within 2 weeks, but the urethritis persisted and responded to tetracycline; in the fourth man, trichomonads were still present after 2 weeks and could be cleared together with the urethritis following treatment with metronidazole.

A further problem in assessing the involvement of men with trichomoniasis is the fact that *T. vaginalis* is notoriously difficult to culture from the male urethra. There is also some evidence that the trichomonads may be present in a stage of their development when they are atypical and more difficult to recognise in the usual wet-mounted preparation. The inhibiting effect of the prostatic fluid on *T. vaginalis,* possibly related to its zinc content, may be a further factor (Krieger and Rein, 1982).

D. Race

In several reports from the United States there was a significantly higher prevalence of *Trichomonas* vaginitis in nonwhite women compared with white women. Trussell (1946) reported a 45.2% incidence in his series of nonwhite women versus 23.5% in white women, and Burch *et al.* (1959) recorded 60.9% and 8.1% respectively, a difference that was also noted in this country by John (1980).

E. Transmission

It is generally assumed that in the majority of women and in all the men the infection is sexually transmitted by an infected partner. There are problems in accepting sexual transmission on direct evidence as so often the male sexual partner is apparently uninfected, and some of the difficulties surrounding the diagnosis of trichomoniasis in the male have been outlined. Sexual transmission is supported by circumstantial evidence such as:

1. Simultaneous treatment of symptomatic women and their asymptomatic male contacts has been shown by many observers to reduce the incidence of further attacks in the women.
2. The optimal age of trichomoniasis in both sexes is in the second and third decade as is usually characteristic of other sexually transmitted disease (STD).
3. Contact tracing has established extensive chains of infection (Anonymous, 1977).
4. Other STDs, especially gonorrhoea, are not infrequently present with trichomonal vaginitis.
5. Trichomonal vaginitis in married women sometimes closely follows extramarital intercourse.

6. The incidence of trichomoniasis is higher in promiscuous women.
7. *Trichomonas vaginalis* has been isolated in homosexual consorts.
8. Experimental infection by inoculation of *T. vaginalis* cultures into the vagina of human volunteers resulted in clinical trichomoniasis (Asami and Nakamura, 1955).

It is feasible that occasional nonsexual transmission of trichomoniasis occurs in females, as the organism remains viable outside the body for hours, possibly even a day, provided it is in a moist environment such as moist flannels, towels and perhaps toilet seats. Infection of infants during birth and of very young girls by close contact with their infected mothers is another possible asexual route of transmission.

IV. PATHOLOGY

A. Pathogenicity

Although the parasite is firmly established as being the cause of symptomatic vaginitis, the organism can exist in the vagina without producing any symptoms or signs, especially in older women. It has been proposed that in such cases *T. vaginalis* is a saprophyte and becomes pathogenic only when the vaginal epithelium becomes inflamed for any reason. There is rather better evidence that *T. vaginalis* strains differ in pathogenicity (Kulda *et al.*, 1970). Other factors suggested from animal experiments include host immunity, endocrine status, and local genital abnormalities. Host factors play a role in man in determining the severity of an attack, since menstruation and pregnancy are associated with acute episodes. The most compelling evidence for assuming primary pathogenicity of *T. vaginalis* is the prompt clinical and microbiological response to specific trichomonicidal therapy.

B. Histology

Trichomonas vaginalis can cause some of the most marked inflammatory reactions of the vaginal and cervical lining, and as these changes include temporary cervical epithelial hyperplasia and metaplasia with polymorphonuclear infiltration and increased vascularity with local extravasation of blood, assessment of the cervical smear by Papanicolaou stain must be postponed for 3 months after successful treatment, when these changes will be reversed. In the vagina, trichomonads can be found in clusters around degenerating epithelial cells, which are followed by polymorphonuclear neutrophils. The colour of the discharge is due to myeloperoxidase pigment of the polymorphonuclear leucocytes. Up to 700,000 polymorphs/mm^3 may be present in the discharge. Phagocytosis and pinocytosis (i.e., ingestion of small particles and large molecules) is an essential characteristic of trichomonads. The parasite is in turn phagocytosed by macrophages and polymorphs. In asymptomatic patients these changes may be minimal or absent.

V. CLINICAL PICTURE

The incubation period is difficult to establish, as the chain of infection is often obscure. The generally accepted range is wide and lies between 3 and 21 days. In our experience it is commonly 7 days or less.

A. Women

The clinical spectrum ranges from the acute severe attack to the asymptomatic carrier state. In the severe case, the onset is acute and frequently follows sexual intercourse. There is a florid vaginitis and vulvitis with purulent, frothy, offensive yellow-green discharge and the patient complains of soreness and irritation. In the most severe cases the vaginal wall and vulva are oedematous with excoriation and intertrigo of the adjacent skin with extreme discomfort. Such patients will also complain of dyspareunia, frequency and dysuria. On examination there is copious discharge and the vagina and cervix may show punctate haemorrhagic spots ("strawberry" appearance). Even gentle examination may be too painful. In the less severe attack, the onset may be insidious with slight to moderate mucopurulent vaginal discharge, which, however, contains trichomonads and numerous polymorphs. The vaginal pH tends to become alkaline (pH above 4.5). Colposcopy shows abnormally dilated vessels, as well as an increased density of vessels on the cervical and vaginal wall. These changes are less marked in candidiasis and absent in nonspecific vaginitis (Pheifer *et al.,* 1978).

Complications reported include involvement of Skene's glands, Bartholin's ducts, urethritis and cystitis. Several authors, impressed by the endocervical hyperplasia, suggested that a later sequel might be an increased incidence of cervical carcinoma. However, the experience of many observers, including our own, shows that there is prompt reversal of these changes after successful treatment, and there is as yet no compelling evidence that trichomoniasis leads to cervical malignancy. The possibility that trichomonads carry herpes virus that may lead to an oncogenic process later on has not been excluded. Our own experiments have demonstrated mycoplasmas within *T. vaginalis.*

From the continent of Europe, a number of reports claim that *T. vaginalis* may cause a variety of systemic lesions affecting the skin, mouth, joints, liver, kidneys and intestinal tract. The majority affected were women, and although trichomonads were not found in the extragenital sites, metronidazole was said to be effective in clearing all lesions. Kolman (1973) reported many such cases in a monograph. Our own impression is that there is insufficient scientific ground for assuming the existence of trichomonal extragenital lesions, and the case reports are uncritical and often sketchy. However, one should not ignore this possibility out of hand, and one should investigate any case in which this appears to be even remotely likely (Csonka, 1974).

B. Men

Trichomoniasis in men, unlike the disease in women, is commonly asymptomatic, although the exact ratio of symptomatic to asymptomatic cases is unknown. It is probable that even asymptomatic men are infectious. The clinical spectrum includes:

1. Asymptomatic carriers with the parasite persisting in the urethra and, some believe, also in the prostate.
2. True *Trichomonas* urethritis, with mucopurulent secretion that is commonly minimal and confined to scanty early-morning discharge. This conditions responds rapidly to the nitroimidazoles.
3. Nongonococcal urethritis (NGU) with the transient presence of *T. vaginalis* in the discharge. It appears that here *T. vaginalis* is not pathogenic, and disappearance of the parasite after metronidazole does not clear the urethritis.

In practice, therefore, the parasite will disappear together with urethritis with metronidazole treatment in true trichomonas urethritis; in others, the parasite disappears spontaneously or after metronidazole therapy but urethritis persists and will respond to tetracycline or erythromycin in the same proportion, as does ordinary NGU.

Complications are as follows. Prostatitis is regarded by many as the commonest complication of trichomoniasis, but the diagnosis is fraught with uncertainty. Perineal discomfort is considered to be the most constant feature, together with *T. vaginalis* in prostatic secretions obtained by prostatic massage. However, one should be sceptical if the diagnosis relies on the demonstration of *T. vaginalis* in prostatic fluid obtained via the urethra, as there is no way to exclude the organism being picked up in the urethra. Trichomonal balanoposthitis has been reported by several authors, but as the organism was usually also present in the urethra, contamination may be responsible for these findings. An aetiological role for *T. vaginalis* in balanoposthitis is strengthened if the condition responds speedily to metronidazole. Trichomonal cystitis has been repeatedly described, but unless there are no other urinary pathogens and the condition responds promptly to metronidazole alone, the validity of this diagnosis remains uncertain.

In summary it can be stated that *Trichomonas* urethritis in men occurs but is probably not common, and the complications reported, mostly in the older literature, are in need of critical evaluation before they should be accepted.

VI. MICROORGANISMS ASSOCIATED WITH TRICHOMONIASIS

The best documented association is that of trichomonas vaginitis with gonorrhoea, but any infectious agent found in other STD may be present. Recently a positive association of *Gardnerella* with *T. vaginalis* has been observed (Blackwell and Barlow, 1982; Dawson and Harris, 1983), which is not surprising as the optimal pH is similar for both agents *in vivo*. Candidiasis is less often associated with trichomoniasis, possibly because the vaginal pH differs significantly in the two conditions. Lactobacilli decrease in the presence of *T. vaginalis* vaginitis and return to normal after successful treatment.

VII. PROGNOSIS

A. Untreated disease in women

It has been suggested that untreated *Trichomonas* vaginitis tends to become oligosymptomatic and eventually asymptomatic, even though the parasite may persist. Catterall (1972) found that untreated trichomonal vaginitis becomes a chronic, or recurrent, although mild, disorder.

B. Treated disease in women

Unprovoked relapses are uncommon. Sometimes the history and clinical evidence makes it fairly certain that the new attack is due to reinfection, either by the same untreated partner or by a new sexual contact. More often it is impossible to be certain whether one deals with a relapse or reinfection.

C. Sequelae

Sequelae on which there is no consensus of opinion are trichomonal pyelitis and subfertility in either sex; some authors found a low sperm count or an abnormally high proportion of deformed sperms (Bauer, 1963; Argenziano *et al.*, 1967; Gaffuri and Poggio, 1968). Davidson (1970) did not support these findings after extensive studies.

The suggestion that cervical carcinoma may follow genital trichomoniasis has been briefly mentioned. Koss and Wolinska (1959) and Teras and Kaarma

(1969) believed that there was a higher incidence of cervical carcinoma compared to controls, but Frost (1975) denied this association. However, during episodes of genital trichomoniasis cervical cells display metaplasia, which is reversible after successful treatment, and this stresses the importance of early and adequate therapy of trichomoniasis with metronidazole or its derivatives.

VIII. DIAGNOSIS

The diagnosis is essentially a laboratory one made by demonstrating and/or growing the trichomonad, as detailed earlier. Clinically, the classical features of trichomonal vaginitis should direct one's attention toward the probable diagnosis but are never a substitute for laboratory tests, which should be routinely undertaken in all women who are screened for STD and causes of vaginitis.

IX. DIFFERENTIAL DIAGNOSIS

A. Gonorrhoea; *Gardnerella*-associated vaginitis

Gonorrhoea may coexist with trichomoniasis (Fig. 9) and may be masked by it; therefore cultures for gonorrhoea are obligatory. *Gardnerella*-associated vaginitis (Fig. 10) may give rise to a fishy smelling, thin, grey discharge of low viscosity. The odour may appear immediately following intercourse. Possibly the alkaline semen reacts with the infected vaginal secretions to release volatile amines (Chen *et al.*, 1979)—a sort of amine test *in vivo*. The diagnosis can be established by microscopy, culture and the amine test (a drop of 10% KOH is mixed with a drop of vaginal secretion, when the mixture will give off the typical fishy smell, which is evanescent). As trichomoniasis may coexist, it must be sought for. A therapeutic trial with metronidazole is of no diagnostic value, as both conditions respond to this drug.

B. Other causes of vaginitis

Other causes of vaginitis such as retained foreign bodies, allergies, chemical irritants, candidiasis, threadworm infestation and "nonspecific" forms must be excluded. A number of women complain of vaginal discharge that is in fact normal. In such cases there is no evidence of infection, the pH is 4.5 or less, and the vaginal secretion show lactobacilli and large epithelial cells with large nuclei; in such individuals no specific treatment is indicated.

In men, NGU with *T. vaginalis* as a temporary passenger has to be separated from true trichomonal urethritis by the prompt response to metronidazole or its

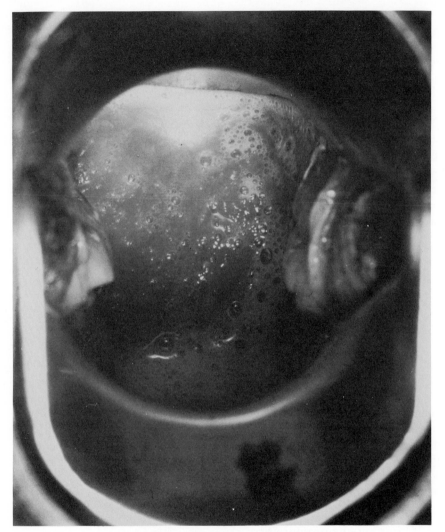

Fig. 9 Clinical signs of *Trichomonas* vaginitis.

derivatives. The difficulties in diagnosing, let alone differentiating, types of prostatitis have already been mentioned.

X. TREATMENT

Prior to 1959, the treatment of trichomoniasis was nonspecific and therefore highly unsatisfactory. Table 2 lists some of the substances that were used, which

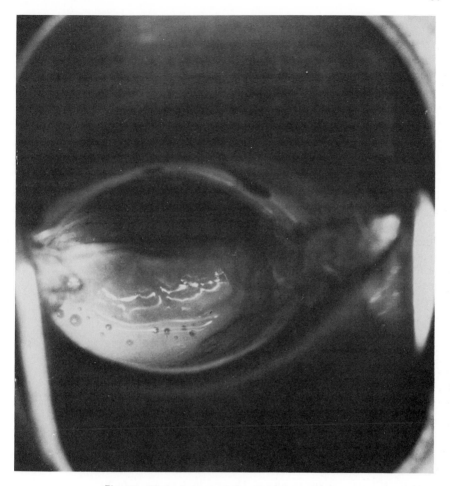

Fig. 10 Clinical signs of *Gardnerella* vaginitis.

Table 2 Compounds used for the treatment of trichomoniasis prior to the introduction of metronidazole

Acetic acid	Formalin
Acriflavine	Cocaine
Aluminium acetate	Ether in lactic acid
Alum	Iodine
Ammonium silver	Menthol
Arsenic	Mercuric chloride
Bismuth	Turpentine
Chromic acid	Silver nitrate
Picric acid	Phenol

are only of historical interest, except the locally used arsenical compound acetarsone (Stovarsol, S.V.C. pessaries) and povidone iodine (Betadine vaginal pessary), which can be of some use in cases of vaginitis not responding to the usual doses of nitroimidazole drugs.

A. Metronidazole

A number of systemic drugs were in use before the introd: iction of the nitroimidazoles and included arsenicals such as acetarsone, thiazoles, antibiotics such as ureomycin, gramicidin and trychomycin; but in spite of early enthusiastic reports, critical evaluation showed that they were of little or no value. In 1954, the French company Rhone Poulenc started a search for an effective antitrichomonal drug. From the fermentation liquors of the growth of a streptomyces, an active compound, identified as 2-nitroimidazole (I), was isolated. This 2-nitroimidazole was also shown to be identical with azomycin, an antibiotic previously isolated in Japan.

Further chemical modification of azomycin led to the preparation of metronidazole (II).

Cosar and Joulou reported on the *in vitro* and *in vivo* activity of 1-hydroxyethyl-2-methyl-5-nitroimidazole (metronidazole), both against *T. vaginalis* and *Entamoeba histolitica*. Shortly after this, Durel *et al.* (1959) used the compound clinically in human trichomoniasis. The original dosage was 200 mg t.d.s. for 7 days. The treatment has since been shortened to 800 mg b.d. for 1 day (McClean, 1971) or 2 g as a single dose (Csonka, 1971). The shorter courses are preferable because of greater acceptability and reduction of the total dose of the drug. Recently, a single dose of a 2-g rectal suppository of metronidazole, which is known to be well absorbed and to give adequate pharmacological levels, was reported to be successful in 94% of vaginal trichomoniasis (Panja, 1982). For patients having difficulty in swallowing the tablets, which have a bitter taste, benzoyl metronidazole (Flagyl-S) as a suspension containing 200 mg of the drug per 5 ml can be offered. *Trichomonas vaginalis* is sensitive to nitroimidazoles in the range of 1–10 mg/litre concentration, which is easily achieved by any current treatment schedule. The compound should be taken after food to minimise gastric upset, and alcohol must be avoided during therapy and for 24 hours following its completion, as it has an "Antabuse-like" effect. The cure rate is above 90% in both women and men and is slightly improved if the sexual partner is treated simultaneously, suggesting that some of the "treatment failures" and recurrences are due to reinfection. However, as the benefit is small, we do not insist on this if it might lead to social or marital problems.

Adverse reactions to metronidazole are rare; they include gastrointestinal disturbances, bad taste in the mouth, headaches, dizziness, rashes and peripheral neuropathy with *prolonged* treatment. Other nitroimidazoles related to metronidazole are nimorazole (Naxogin 500), which is given as a single dose of 2 g with the main meal, ornidazole (0.75–1.5 g/day for 5 days), tinidazole (Fasigyn) given as a single 2-g dose, and secnidazole, which has a long half-life of 19 hours versus 8 hours for metronidazole.

Contraindications include a history of blood dyscrasias, hypersensitivity to imidazoles and organic neurological disorders. It is not recommended during pregnancy and lactation.

1. The mechanism of metronidazole action

Müller *et al.* (1977) found that antitrichomonal action of metronidazole is mainly due to metabolites produced by the reduction of the nitrogroup. The two main compounds are the 2-hydroxymethyl and 1-acetic acid metabolite. Of these, the hydroxymethyl metabolite is the active agent against *Gardnerella*. Thus the activation of the metronidazoles depends upon the presence of a low redox potential system, which is able to reduce the nitro group of these drugs. The hydroxy metabolite is found in high concentration in the urine even after a single 2-g dose, which may be an important factor in eradicating urethral carriage of trichomonads in the male and may contribute to the therapeutic effect of metronidazole in trichomonal vaginitis (Easmon *et al.*, 1982).

2. Carcinogenicity and mutagenicity of nitroimidazoles

Rustia and Shubik (1972) reported carcinogenicity in experimental animals, but the doses given were greatly in excess to those generally used in humans.

Lindmark and Müller (1976) found nitroimidazole compounds to be weakly mutagenic in animal studies. Whilst there is no evidence of harmful effects on the human foetus, nitroimidazoles should be used during pregnancy only after due consideration of the potential benefits and possible hazards.

XI. FAILURE OF TREATMENT

This is not common and may be due to

1. Poor absorption.
2. Inactivation of the drug locally by a variety of vaginal micro-organisms.

This can be tested *in vitro* by growing the vaginal flora of the patient in the presence of metronidazole and testing it against strains of *T. vaginalis*.
3. Resistance of trichomonads to the nitroimidazoles.

Treatment failure due to poor absorption can usually be overcome by doubling the dose and prolonging treatment with metronidazole.

Microbiological inactivation of metronidazole in the vagina can be treated by using antibiotics to eliminate these organisms prior to treatment with metronidazole.

The uncommon case of failure due to partially metronidazole-resistant trichomonads may respond to more intensive therapy with an alternate preparation in this series; in patients with marked resistance, difficulties of management may arise. Stovarsol pessaries (S.V.C.) or povidone-iodine pessaries (Betadine) may then be tried.

In our experience, in treatment failure thought to be due to resistant strains, the strains are often found *in vitro* to be fully sensitive to metronidazole and its derivatives, and failure may be due to noncompliance, reinfection, poor absorption of the drug or its inactivation in the vagina by microorganisms. Truly resistant strains exist, and small numbers have been reported from widely separated countries such as Austria (Meingassner *et al.*, 1978), Britain (Waitkins and Thomas, 1981), the United States (Müller *et al.*, 1980) and Czechoslovakia (Kulda *et al.*, 1982). The method for drug testing has been reviewed by Meingassner *et al.* (1978), who believe that the tests should be performed under aerobic conditions for optimal results. It is important to note that some of the strains reported as being resistant under aerobic conditions have shown completely sensitivity using anaerobic techniques. Furthermore, in some cases where we have been able to examine the strains that have been resistant under anaerobic conditions, resistance has been lost on passage. It is not known whether resistance is induced by inadequate treatment, as in all cases treatment preceded isolation, or whether it was intrinsic to the organism isolated. In any case, a careful study of strains isolated from treatment failure is needed to allow for conclusions on the prevalence and clinical importance of metronidazole-resistant strains, especially as at present there is no really effective alternative to the nitroimidazoles.

In a recent study (John, 1980), the addition of vaginal secretion from patients with *Trichomonas* vaginitis to cultures of *T. vaginalis* reduced growth. It was then shown that there were local antibodies of the IgG class that were believed to be responsible for this effect. Humoral antibodies of the IgG class were demonstrated in about half the patients. The local antibodies disappeared after a few weeks, but humoral antibodies persisted for up to 10 months. If chemotherapy was initiated early, antibodies did not reach detectable levels, presumably because of removal of the antigen. In male contacts of *Trichomonas* vaginitis, specific antibodies were rarely found, and when present the titer was low.

It may be that these antibodies have a moderating effect on the infection, without being preventative.

XII. SUMMARY AND CONCLUSIONS

Trichomoniasis is a common cause of vaginitis. In men it appears to be rare and is either asymptomatic or occasionally results in urethritis. There is strong circumstantial evidence that the majority of trichomonal vaginitis cases are sexually transmitted, and it is probable that all or nearly all cases of trichomonal infection in males are sexually acquired. Nonsexual transmission is a possibility, as the organism is capable of surviving outside the body for 24 hours and may be transfered by fomites such as damp flannels, towels and possibly toilet seats. Asexual infection of female neonates and children by their infected mothers is documented, although rare.

Epidemiological surveys show trichomoniasis to be distributed worldwide. It is more frequent in the lower socioeconomic classes, in young females, during pregnancy, and in promiscuous individuals. In married couples, *Trichomonas* vaginitis is sometimes clearly associated with extramarital intercourse.

The clinical manifestations are more marked and characteristic in the female than in the male. Asymptomatic carriers are found in women, especially in the older age group, and are common in men. Men exposed to infection are not necessarily infected, but the chances of escaping infection are not known. In our present state of uncertainty it is advisable to treat all male sexual contacts at the same time as the female patients to reduce the chances of reinfection.

The diagnosis must be based on demonstrating the organism in the wet-mounted specimen. Culture improves the proportion of positive results.

Trichomonas vaginitis is especially associated with gonorrhoea and *Gardnerella* vaginitis. All patients with *Trichomonas* vaginitis must be carefully screened for other STD. Concomitant *Candida* infection is less common, possibly because the optimal pH of *Trichomonas* and *Candida* vaginitis differs significantly.

The treatment of choice is oral metronidazole or one of its derivatives, which gives more than 90% of cures. The routine use of trichomonicidal intravaginal preparations is not recommended. Treatment failure in the female may be due to noncompliance, inadequate absorption of the drug from the alimentary canal, inactivation of metronidazole in the vagina by a variety of vaginal microorganisms and rarely due to treatment-resistant strains of *T. vaginalis*. Most recurrences, however, are probably due to reinfection. Metronidazole has been reported to be carcinogenic in animal experiments but the dose used was in excess of the pharmacological one. Metronidazole was also found to be a weak mutagen in an animal study. Although there is as yet no evidence of harmful effects on the human foetus, it is at present recommended that the drug use be avoided during pregnancy. Genital trichomoniasis leads to marked changes of cervical cells, including metaplasia, and this has led some observers to suggest that it may give rise to cervical malignancy later on in a proportion of patients. However, these changes revert promptly following successful treatment of the infection and there is no evidence to suggest malignancy as a late sequel. In practice these changes make it necessary to repeat cervical cytology screening if the specimen was taken before the infection was cured.

REFERENCES

Adler, S., and Pulvertaft, R. J. V. (1944). *Ann. Trop. Med.* **38**, 188–189.

Anonymous (1977). *Bull. Mem. Soc. Med. Hop. Paris* **181**, 61–196.

Argenziano, G., De Luca, M., and Rossi, A. (1967). *Minerva Dermatol.* **42**, 388–391.

Asami, K., and Nakamura, M. (1955). *Am. J. Trop. Med. Hyg.* **4**, 254–258.

Baba, H. (1958). *Nisshin Igaku* **45**, 16–19.

Bauer, H. (1963). *Z. Tropenmed. Parasitol.* **14**, 86–95.

Blackwell, A., and Barlow, D. (1982). *Br. J. Vener. Dis.* **58**, 387–393.

Block, T. A., Rees, C. W., and Reardon, L. V. (1959). *Am. J. Trop. Med. Hyg.* **8**, 312–318.

Busby, S. R. M., and Copp, F. C. (1955). *J. Pharm. Pharmacol.* **7**, 112–117.

Catterall, R. D. (1972). *Med. Clin. North Am.* **56**, 1203–1209.

Chappaz, G., and Bertrand, P. (1965). *Gynaecologia* **160**, 17–23.

Chen, K. C. S., Forsyth, P. S., Buchanan, T. M., and Holmes, K. K. (1979). *J. Clin. Invest.* **63**, 828–835.

Cosar, C., and Joulou, L. (1959). *Ann. Inst. Pasteur, Paris* **96**, 238–241.

Csonka, G. W. (1971). *Br. J. Vener. Dis.* **47**, 456–458.

Csonka, G. W. (1974). *Br. J. Dermatol.* **90**, 713–714.

Davidson, A. (1970). *Br. J. Vener. Dis.* **48**, 144–145.

Dawson, S. G., and Harris, J. R. W. (1983). *Br. J. Hosp. Med.*

Dock, G. (1896). *Am. J. Med. Sci.* **3**, 1–24.

Donne, A. (1836). *C. R. Hebd. Seances Acad. Sci.* **3**, 385–386.

Durel, P., Roiron, V., Siboulet, A., and Borel, L. J. (1959). *C. R. Soc. Fr. Gynecol.* **29**, 36–45.

Easmon, C. S. F., Ison, C. A., Kaye, C. M., Timewell, R. M., and Dawson, S. G. (1982). *Br. J. Vener. Dis.* **58**, 246–249.

Forsgren, A., and Kraus, S. J. (1980). *J. Infect Dis.* **141**, 317–343.

Fouts, A. W., and Kraus, S. J. (1980). *J. Infect. Dis.* **141**, 137–143.

Frost, J. K. (1975). *In* "Textbook of Gynaecology" (E. R. Novak, G. S. Jones, and H. W. Jones, eds.). William & Wilkins, Baltimore, Maryland.

Gaffuri, S., and Poggio, A. (1968). *Minerva Ginecol.* **14**, 1260–1268.

Gillin, F. D., and Sher, A. (1981). *Infect. Immun.* **34**, 268–273.

Grys, E. (1973). *Wiad. Parazytol.* **19**, 371–373.

Heath, J. P. (1981). *Br. J. Vener. Dis.* **57**, 106–117.

Heyworth, R., Simpson, D., McNeillage, G. J. C., and Robertson, D. H. H. (1980). *Lancet* **2**, 476–478.

Hoffman, B., and Gorcynski, M. (1964). *Wiad. Parazytol.* **10**, 132–153.

Jaakmees, H., Teras, J., Roigas, E., Nigesen, U., and Tompel, H. (1966). *Wiad. Parazytol.* **12**, 378–384.

John, J. (1980). M.D. Thesis, University of Sheffield.

John, J., and Squires, S. L. (1978). *Br. J. Vener. Dis.* **54**, 84–87.

Johnson, G., Trussell, M., and Jahn, F. (1945). *Science* **102**, 126–128.
Keighley, E. E. (1971). *Br. Med. J.* **1**, 207–210.
Kolman, J. (1973). "Trichomoniasis." Wilhelm Maudrich, Vienna.
Koss, L. G., and Wolinska, W. H. (1959). *Cancer* **12**, 1171–1193.
Krieger, J. N., and Rein, D. M. F. (1982). *Infect. Immun.* **37**, 77–81.
Kulda, J., Honigsberg, B. M., Frost, J. K., and Hollander, D. H. (1970). *Am. J. Obstet. Gynecol.* **108**, 908–918.
Kulda, J., Vojtechovska, M., Tachezy, J. *et al.* (1982). *Br. J. Vener. Dis.* **58**, 394–399.
Lancely, F., and McEntegart, M. G. (1953). *Lancet* **1**, 688–671.
Lindmark, D., and Muller, M. (1976). *Antimicrob. Agents Chemother.* **10**, 476–482.
Linstead, D. (1981). *Parasitology* **83**, 125–137.
Lynch, K. M. (1915). *Am. J. Trop. Dis.* **2**, 627–634.
McClean, A. N. (1971). *Br. J. Vener. Dis.* **47**, 36–37.
McDonald, E. M., and Tatum, A. L. (1948). *J. Immunol.* **59**, 309–317.
McEntegart, M. G., Chadwick, C. S., and Nairn, R. C. (1958). *J. Pathol. Bacteriol.* **71**, 111–115.
Mantovani, A., Polentarutti, N., Peri, G. M., Martinotti, G., and Landolfo, S. (1981). *Clin. Exp. Immunol.* **46**, 391–396.
Marchand, F. (1894). *Zentralbl. Bakteriol., Parasitenkd. Infektionskr.* **15**, 709–720.
Mason, P. R. (1979). *J. Clin. Pathol.* **32**, 1211–1215.
Meingassner, J. G., Mieth, H., Czok, R., Lindmark, D. G., and Muller, M. (1978). *Antimicrob. Agents Chemother.* **13**, 1–3.
Mekki, F., and Iviv, J. (1979). *Jugosl. Ginekol. Opstet.* **18**, 15–19.
Miura, K. (1894). *Zentralbl. Bakteriol., Parasitenkd. Infektionskr.* **15**, 705–708.
Müller, M., Lindmark, D., and McLaughlin, J. (1977). *Int. Congr. Ser.—Exerpta Med.* **438**, 12–19.
Müller, M., Meingassner, J., Miller, W. A., and Ledger, W. J. (1980). *Am. J. Obstet. Gynecol.* **138**, 808–812.
Naguib, S. M. *et al.* (1966). *Obstet. Gynecol.* **27**, 607–616.
Nakabayashi, T. (1952). *Osaka Diagaku Igaku Zasshi* **4**, 11–21.
Panja, S. A. (1982). *Br. J. Vener. Dis.* **58**, 257–258.
Pheifer, T. A. *et al.* (1978). *N. Engl. J. Med.* **298**, 1429–1434.
Pierce, A. E. (1946). *Nature (London)* **158**, 343.
Rein, M. R., Sullivan, J. A., and Manuell, G. L. (1980). *J. Infect. Dis.* **142**, 575–585.
Riedmüller, L. (1932). *Schweiz. Tierheilkd.* **74**, 343–351.
Rõigas, E. M. (1975). *Parazitologiya* **9**, 278–351.
Rustia, M., and Shubik, P. (1972). *J. Natl. Cancer Inst. (U.S.)* **48**, 721–729.
Schoenherr, K. E. (1959). *Z. Immunitaets forsch. Exp. Ther.* **113**, 83–94.
Squires, S. L., and McFadzean, J. A. (1962). *Br. J. Vener. Dis.* **38**, 218–219.
Stuart, R. D. (1946). *Glasgow Med. J.* **27**, 131–134.
Teras, J. K. (1966). *Wiad. Parazytol.* **12**, 357–363.
Teras, J. K., and Kaarma, H. (1969). *Wiad. Parazytol.* **15**, 359–361.
Trevoux, R., Fari, A., De Brux, J., and Verges, J. (1976). *Rev. Fr. Gynecol. Obstet.* **71**, 27–31.
Trussell, R. E. (1946). *J. Parasitol.* **32**, 563–568.
Verges, J. (1979). *J. Urol. Nephrol.* **85**, 357–361.
Waitkins, S., and Thomas, D. J. (1981). *Lancet* **2**, 590.
Whittington, M. J. (1957). *Br. J. Vener. Dis.* **33**, 80–91.
Winston, R. M. L. (1974). *J. Obstet. Gynaecol. Br. Commonw.* **81**, 399–404.
World Health Organization (1981). Technical Report Series; 'Nongonococcal urethritis and other selected sexually transmitted diseases of public health importance' (1981). *W.H.O. Tech. Rep. Ser.* **660**, 49–52.

5 *Campylobacter* infections of man

M. B. SKIRROW

I. INTRODUCTION

The fact that a chapter on *Campylobacter* infections is included at all in this series of reviews is, of course, due to the recent recognition of campylobacter enteritis as a common cause of acute infective diarrhoea. Specific methods for the culture of *Campylobacter jejuni* from faeces are now performed routinely in many laboratories, and clinicians are becoming increasingly familiar with the disease. (Several of my colleagues have actually suffered from it.) Advances in this field have been so rapid that it is no longer possible to describe all aspects of the disease adequately in a single review. In this chapter, emphasis is placed on the pathological and clinical aspects of the disease and on some of the less common manifestations of infection that physicians and infectious disease specialists might expect to encounter.

But campylobacter enteritis is not the whole story. Nonenteric campylobacter infections were described long before enteric ones, and although infections of this sort are still uncommon they certainly deserve consideration. They are almost always septicaemic and limited to patients who are in some way compromised; most are caused by *C. fetus* ssp. *fetus,* rather than *C. jejuni.* Systemic campylobacteriosis is the term used in this chapter to describe this type of infection.

Before going on to describe these two diseases—systemic campylobacteriosis and campylobacter enteritis—passing reference must be made to two newly described groups of spiral bacteria that probably belong to the genus *Campylobacter,* or are at least closely related to it. Both are associated with disease, though their role, if any, in the pathogenesis of disease is not yet clear.

The first group has been found colonizing the stomach mucosa of patients suffering from peptic ulceration. These remarkable and completely new bacteria are found on the surface of the mucosa beneath the mucus layer, particularly in

Medical Microbiology, 4
ISBN 0-12-228004-0

the antrum, and often in enormous numbers. They are not usually present in normal people. Since their first description from Australia (Warren and Marshall, 1983) these organisms have been found in Europe, Canada and the United States. There are two reasons why they have been missed for so long: the absence, until recent years, of fibre optic instruments that permit good biopsy material to be obtained, and the fact that special staining methods (e.g., Warthin–Starry silver stain) are required to show up the organisms in histological sections. For the present these bacteria are referred to as "pyloric campylobacters," or simply as spiral bacteria of the stomach.

The second group of *Campylobacter*-like organisms (CLOs) were first isolated from rectal biopsy specimens from homosexual men in Seattle, Washington (Fennell *et al.*, 1984). There are three subgroups. All were much slower growing than *C. jejuni*, and so far they have been isolated only from biopsy material, not from faeces. Their role has yet to be determined.

II. BACTERIOLOGY

A. Classification and nomenclature

The most distinctive feature of campylobacteria is their spiral morphology. Taxonomically they are most nearly related to the spirilla—large spiral flagellated saprophytic bacteria—and they are currently included in the family Spirillaceae. Cells grow in the form of a helix and sometimes reach a length of 8 μm, when, for all the world, they look like some sort of spirochaete. Rapidly dividing forms are short, curved, or S-shaped, and it was this feature that caused them to be classified as vibrios when they were first described some 75 years ago. It was not until 1963 that their proper taxonomic status was recognized and the genus *Campylobacter* (Greek, curved rod) was established (Sebald and Véron, 1963).

In contrast to spirilla, campylobacteria are among the smallest of bacteria, measuring only 0.2–0.4 μm in width. They possess a single long flagellum at one or both poles of the bacterial cell and move extremely rapidly by spinning in the manner of a corkscrew. The guanine-plus-cytosine content of their DNA is among the lowest of any bacterial genus (29–38 mol %). Another unusual feature is that they are strictly microaerophilic: exposure to atmospheric oxygen is progressively bactericidal, yet the presence of some oxygen is essential for growth.

Difficulties with the culture and preservation of campylobacteria have, over the years, hindered work on them, and the fact that they are biochemically inactive compared with most bacteria has made it particularly difficult to recognize and define species and subspecies within the genus. It is small wonder that confusion has arisen over classification and nomenclature, but happily there is now a measure of international agreement (Skerman *et al.*, 1980). A full account

Table 1 *Campylobacter* species found in man

Approved name	Obsolete name	Site from which usually isolated	Pathogenicity
Catalase-positive group			
C. fetus ssp. fetus	C. fetus ssp. intestinalis	Blood, various	Systemic campylobacteriosis in compromised patients
C. jejuni ⎫ C. coli ⎭	C. fetus ssp. jejuni	Faeces	Acute enterocolitis
C. lardis[a]	—	Faeces	Not known
Catalase-negative group			
C. sputorum ssp. sputorum	—	Gingival crevices of mouth	Commensal
C. concisus	—	Gingival crevices of mouth	Probably commensal

[a] Proposed name (Benjamin *et al.,* 1983) for the NARTC group of Skirrow and Benjamin (1980).

of the taxonomy of campylobacteria is given by Karmali and Skirrow (1984), but here we need only mention those species that infect man (Table 1).

1. Campylobacter fetus *ssp.* fetus

This is the type-species of the genus *Campylobacter,* and it is an important cause of infectious abortion in sheep and cattle. Strains indistinguishable from these animal strains are an uncommon cause of systemic infection in debilitated or compromised patients (see Section III). *Campylobacter fetus* ssp. *fetus,* like *C. jejuni* and *C. coli,* may occasionally cause acute enterocolitis in normal people (Devlin and McIntyre, 1983; Harvey and Greenwood, 1983).

2. Campylobacter jejuni *and* C. coli

These are the species that cause acute enterocolitis in humans. They are found in a wide variety of animals, mostly as commensals of the intestinal tract but sometimes as enteric pathogens. *Campylobacter jejuni* also causes abortion in sheep, like *C. fetus* ssp. *fetus. Campylobacter jejuni* and *C. coli* together represent King's "related vibrios" (King, 1962), which she distinguished from *C. fetus* (then called *Vibrio fetus*) by their high optimum growth temperature (42°C). In the eighth edition of *Bergey's Manual of Determinative Bacteriology,* Smibert (1974) designated King's "related vibrios" *C. fetus* ssp. *jejuni,* but this name, although extensively used until recently, is no longer valid. Recent DNA analyses and hybridization experiments have shown conclusively that *C. fetus, C. jejuni* and *C. coli* are distinct species (reviewed by Owen, 1983).

Skirrow and Benjamin (1982) recognize two biotypes of *C. jejuni,* and Hébert *et al.* (1982) have proposed a provisional system for dividing *C. jejuni* and *C. coli* into eight biotypes. Although species and strain differentiation is epidemiologically important, it is of little clinical value since there is no apparent difference in the disease produced by the two species. Thus in a purely clinical context it is common (and acceptable) practice not to make the distinction, but to refer to both species collectively as *C. jejuni* (the predominant one).

(a)   Antigenic structure

Campylobacter jejuni and *C. coli* possess several surface antigens, and it is clear that there are a great many serotypes. Several serotyping systems have been developed, but two principal ones have emerged, each detecting a different class of antigen. In the one system, heat-stable antigens are detected by passive haemagglutination after extraction (Penner and Hennessy, 1980). In the other, heat-labile antigens are detected by slide agglutination of live bacteria (Lior *et al.*, 1982). To date the Penner system recognizes 60 serotypes; the raising of antisera and interpretation of results is straightforward, but the test is time-consuming to perform. The Lior system recognizes some 68 serotypes; the raising of antisera is more difficult (high-titre sera and many cross-absorptions are required), but the actual typing technique is simple. In summary, campylobacter serotyping is adolescent and not yet generally available.

3.   Campylobacter laridis

This is the name proposed (Benjamin *et al.*, 1983) for the so-called NARTC (nalidixic acid-resistant thermophilic campylobacteria) of Skirrow and Benjamin (1980). The organism is common in the intestinal contents of seagulls, where it is presumably a commensal, but it is also regularly isolated from dogs and very occasionally from human faeces. Its pathogenicity is unknown; the few patients (all children) from whom strains have been isolated had mild recurrent diarrhoea or no symptoms.

4.   Campylobacter sputorum *ssp.* sputorum *and* C. concisus

These catalase-negative campylobacteria are found in the gingival crevices of apparently healthy people. *Campylobacter sputorum* ssp. *sputorum* is said to account for 5% of the cultivable organisms from such sites. *Campylobacter concisus* has only recently been described and is of unknown pathogenicity (Tanner *et al.*, 1981).

III.   SYSTEMIC CAMPYLOBACTERIOSIS

Systemic is probably the most appropriate word to describe a variety of generalized invasive infections affecting compromised patients and usually caused by *C. fetus* ssp. *fetus*. The term nonenteric is unsuitable because some patients with systemic campylobacteriosis have diarrhoea, and the term does not convey the bacteraemic or septicaemic element that is invariably present. It could be argued that campylobacter enteritis is systemic in that bacteraemia is thought to be a regular feature of infection, but it is usually a transient phenomenon and the principal pathology is obviously enteric. Disseminated is a term that would be appropriate for some patients, but localization of infection is the exception rather than the rule.

Virtually all patients with systemic campylobacteriosis have some sort of predisposition to infection. A wide variety of compromising conditions have been reported: malignant disease (e.g., leukaemia, lymphoma, Hodgkin's disease and other reticuloses); immunosuppressive therapy; alcoholism; cirrhosis of the liver; diabetes mellitus; hypogammaglobulinaemia; pancytopoenia; cardiopathy; chronic renal failure; gastrectomy; splenectomy. Prematurity and birth trauma in newborn infants and pregnancy are also conditions that have been associated with systemic campylobacteriosis. Apart from these latter categories, most reported infections have been in men over the age of 45 years.

A. Pathogenesis and clinical manifestations

Systemic campylobacteriosis is thought to arise from intestinal colonization (Butzler *et al.*, 1977), but it is not known whether invasion of the bloodstream is an early consequence of bowel infection or whether it may arise sporadically during a period of long-term colonization. The latter is considered to be the usual pattern in ovine abortion. Whatever the mechanism in man, infections usually appear out of the blue, without any history of significant contact with animals or consumption of suspect foods. An exception to this was a bizarre outbreak of systemic *C. fetus* ssp. *fetus* infection attributed to the consumption of raw calves' liver taken during a course of "nutritional therapy" (which included coffee enemas!) in Mexico. Ten patients, all suffering from severe underlying illness, developed infection within a week of receiving such treatment (Ginsberg *et al.*, 1981). Soonattrakul *et al.* (1971) described the case of an elderly woman with *C. fetus* ssp. *fetus* septicaemia who had also ingested raw beef liver. Parenteral transmission from a blood transfusion has also been reported (Pepersack *et al.*, 1979).

Clinically the most frequent expression of disease is a nonspecific febrile illness that has been likened to brucellosis. In such cases there are no localizing signs and the diagnosis can be made only by culturing *C. fetus* ssp. *fetus* from the blood. Characteristically the infection is subacute and relapsing, and even in compromised patients spontaneous cure has been recorded. Clearly the organism is of low virulence for man. (The higher mortality attributed to *C. fetus* ssp. *fetus* bacteraemia relative to *C. jejuni* bacteraemia—a point that has been emphasised in some reviews—merely reflects the predilection of the former organism for the compromised host, who, as often as not, dies from the underlying disease.)

In some patients infection may be established in specific organs or systems, and it has been suggested that *C. fetus* ssp. *fetus* has an affinity for endovascular surfaces on account of the relative frequency of thrombophlebitis and endocarditis, but such cases are uncommon. Other forms of focal infection that have been reported are meningitis and meningoencephalitis; septic arthritis; infection of the pleura; pericarditis; spontaneous peritonitis; cholestatic hepatitis; cellulitis; and infections of the female reproductive organs, including septic abortion. Since there are several reviews that describe these infections more fully (Guerrant *et al.*, 1978; Rettig, 1979; Schmidt *et al.*, 1980), only the more clinically important or recent ones are elaborated upon here.

1. Meningitis

There are only some 24 cases of campylobacter meningitis or meningoencephalitis on record, 9 of which were neonatal. Seven of the neonatal infections were caused by *C. fetus* ssp. *fetus*, 1 by *C. jejuni* (Thomas *et al.*, 1980), and 1 by an organism that was not fully identified. Six of the 9 infants died and another suffered permanent brain damage, so the prognosis at this age—as with other forms of neonatal meningitis—is poor.

In the nonneonatal infections the identity of the organisms is not always clear from the descriptions given, but probably most were due to *C. fetus* ssp. *fetus*. Fleurette *et al.* (1971) described *C. jejuni* meningitis, preceded by diarrhoea, in a 6-month-old hydrocephalic child, and they reviewed 10 other campylobacter meningitis cases. *Campylobacter jejuni* also caused meningitis in a 37-year-old man who had had a cerebral catheter *in situ* since childhood (Norrby *et al.*, 1980); he did not have diarrhoea. Both these patients with *C. jejuni* infections survived, as did most of the patients with campylobacter meningitis outside the neonatal period.

2. Septic abortion

It would be surprising if organisms that regularly cause abortion in sheep, namely *C. fetus* ssp. *fetus* and *C. jejuni,* did not at least occasionally do so in other animals. Both organisms have caused septic abortion in women, although on very few occasions. It so happens that the first bacteriologically proven case of human campylobacteriosis was one of septic abortion (Vinzent *et al.*, 1947). The patient was a 39-year-old woman who aborted a 6-month foetus 5 weeks after suffering an influenza-like illness associated with "*Vibrio fetus*" bacteraemia. Only 5 more gestational infections, probably due to *C. fetus* ssp. *fetus*, were reported during the subsequent 30 years (Gribble *et al.*, 1981); one resulted in a still-birth, and another in premature delivery with death of the infant.

Yet in only the last 2 years, no less than 6 cases of septic abortion have been reported, all associated with *C. jejuni* or *C. coli* (Gilbert *et al.*, 1981; Gribble *et al.*, 1981; Pearce, 1981; Kist *et al.*, 1984). It seems that familiarity with these organisms as enteric pathogens has led to their recognition, where formerly they might have been missed. The gestational age of these 6 foetuses ranged from 12 to 27 weeks, whereas in the earlier reports abortions occurred in the third trimester. Only 1 of these 6 women was known to have had diarrhoea during the few days before she aborted, but all had fever. *Campylobacter jejuni* (*C. coli* in 1 case) was isolated from the blood of 5 women and from the faeces of 1 woman. Three of 5 foetuses examined were culture-positive, and inflammation, usually with infarction and necrosis, was observed in all of 4 placentas that were examined histologically. Two of the women had suffered from recurrent miscarriages of unknown cause.

The true incidence of campylobacter abortion is unknown. Possibly many infections are missed, because the diagnosis is unlikely to be made unless the organisms are looked for deliberately. On the other hand, considering the frequency of campylobacter enteritis, the chances of an infection in pregnancy ending in abortion must be very small. Certainly I have known of several patients infected in the last few weeks of pregnancy who have proceeded to a full-term uncomplicated delivery of a normal baby. There is, however, at least one report of premature labour apparently induced by severe campylobacter diarrhoea (e.g., Mawer and Smith, 1979).

Is there any evidence that uterine sepsis arises from ascending genital-tract infections? It seems not. *Campylobacter jejuni* has not been found in the cervical or vaginal flora of several groups of women: healthy women (pregnant and nonpregnant) and women with nonspecific vaginitis or vaginal discharge (Coleart and Ursi, 1979; Blaser *et al.*, 1980b); women attending a genitourinary medicine clinic (Wright *et al.*, 1982); women attending a clinic for sexually transmitted diseases (J. P. Butzler, personal communication). Moreover, since the commonly used Thayer–Martin type of gonococcal selective medium supports the growth of both *C. fetus* ssp. *fetus* and *C. jejuni*, one would have expected at least a few isolations of these organisms to have been reported if they had been at all common in genital sites. Faecal contamination would account for the isolation of *C. jejuni* from the cervix of a woman who admitted to both rectal and vaginal intercourse after having had intermittent diarrhoea during the preceding month (Wright *et al.*, 1982). Anders *et al.* (1981) report the isolation of *C. jejuni* from the vagina, but not faeces, in a woman postpartum.

3. Other infections of the female genital tract

Rare instances of infection of the uterine adnexae have been reported. Two patients with "adnexitis," one of whom had an infected ovarian cyst, are mentioned in a review by Schmidt *et al.* (1980). Brown and Sautter (1977) described a patient with clinical acute salpingitis, and Lichtenberger and Perlino (1982) reported a patient with bilateral tuboovarian and omental abscesses; *C. fetus* ssp. *fetus* was the infecting organism in both patients. Another patient with a tuboovarian abscess, also caused by *C. fetus* subsp. *fetus*, was recorded by McGechie *et al.*, 1982).

4. Male genito-urinary infection

There is a single report of the isolation of *C. jejuni* from the urine of a 77-year-old man who had haematuria and frequency of micturition, which disappeared after a course of erythromycin (Davies and Penfold, 1979). It was thought that he might have had campylobacter prostatitis. He did not have diarrhoea.

5. Cellulitis and osteitis

Muytjens and Hoogenhout (1982) isolated *C. jejuni* from an abscess at the site of a 6-month-old mastectomy wound. The parasternal lymph nodes had been irradiated postoperatively. The patient did not have diarrhoea. Paterson (1981) described cellulitis of the thigh due to *C. fetus* ssp. *fetus* in an elderly man receiving sclerotherapy for varicose veins. Pedler and Bint (1984) described a 57-year-old man with osteitis of the foot at the site of an old operation.

6. Toxic-shock syndrome

There is one report of a possible link between *C. fetus* ssp. *fetus* and toxic-shock syndrome (Van der Zwan, 1984).

B. Treatment

Since the disease is, by definition, septicaemic, a systemic antibiotic is called for. Gentamicin, erythromycin or chloramphenicol would be favoured choices, or possibly ampicillin for *C. fetus* ssp. *fetus* infections. More details of *Campylobacter* sensitivities are given in Section IV,I.

IV.   CAMPYLOBACTER ENTERITIS

A. Epidemiology

1. Incidence

In contrast to systemic campylobacteriosis, campylobacter enteritis is a common disease that affects normal people. In technically advanced countries, *C. jejuni* and *C. coli* are, with the possible exception of rotavirus, apparently the most frequent cause of infective diarrhoea. In England and Wales, laboratory isolations of these organisms currently number about 17,000/year [Communicable Disease Surveillance Centre (CDSC), London, unpublished]. Of course, this figure represents only a small proportion of the total number of infections; the true figure could be as much as 40 times higher (Skirrow, 1982). An average attack rate of 1.1% per head of population was calculated from a survey in a general practice in the south of England (Kendall and Tanner, 1982); the incidence was highest in infancy (5.4%/year), next highest in young adults aged 15–24 years (2.0%/year) and lowest in children aged 5–14 years (0.3%/year). This rather odd distribution is difficult to explain, but the relatively high incidence in young adults correlates with the greater severity of infection that is observed at this age. According to laboratory data, 1.5 times as many boys as girls become infected, but the incidence is about equal in adult men and women. The average isolation rate from patients with gastrointestinal symptoms is in the region of 7%, with a maximum of about 15%. There is universal agreement that in technically advanced countries the isolation rate from the normal healthy population is less than 0.5%.

In Britain, *C. jejuni* biotype 1 (Skirrow and Benjamin, 1982) accounts for about 75% of infections, *C. jejuni* biotype 2 for 20%, and *C. coli* for 5%. In some parts of Europe the proportion of *C. coli* is much higher.

Seasonal variation

In England and Wales about twice as many campylobacter infections are reported in the summer and autumn than in winter and early spring. This trend, which is similar to that of salmonella enteritis, has been reported from several other European countries and North America. The reasons for the pattern are obscure. Multiplication in food because of high ambient temperatures is an unlikely explanation, since campylobacteria do not grow well, if at all, in most foods. Moreover, in South Australia (Cameron *et al.*, 1982), Israel (Shmilovitz *et al.*, 1982), and Hong Kong (McGechie *et al.*, 1982), the incidence of campylobacter enteritis is higher in the cooler months of the year.

2. Campylobacter *enteritis in developing countries*

In developing countries diarrhoea is mainly a disease of infants and young children. In some areas, for example Bangladesh (Stoll *et al.*, 1982) and Ethiopia (Thorén *et al.*, 1982), rotavirus and enterotoxigenic *Escherichia coli* are the most important causes of diarrhoea. But one cannot generalize. In Zaire, De Mol *et al.*, (1983) found that *C. jejuni* was the most frequently isolated pathogen in children in both in-patients (24%) and out-patients (13.7%). Exposure to infection is apparently intense in such areas. This is reflected in the excessive number of infections in infancy, the increasing proportion of symptomless infections during childhood, presumably as a result of increasing immunity, and the virtual absence of adult disease (Richardson *et al.*, 1983). Many children with campylobacteria in their stools have other pathogens as well.

This high prevalence of campylobacteria in the developing world is also reflected in the frequency of campylobacter enteritis in travellers from countries that enjoy high standards of hygiene. Nowhere is this more strikingly shown than

Table 2 Principal pathways of infection with *Campylobacter jejuni* and *C. coli*

Pathway	Result
Direct contact with animals or animal products	
Occupational	Farmers, stockmen, poultrymen, veterinarians Workers in poultry processing plants and abattoirs; butchers
Domestic	Family pets: almost always a puppy, or occasionally a kitten, itself suffering from diarrhea Handling of raw meats, especially poultry, in the kitchen
Consumption of contaminated milk, water and food	
Raw milk	Has caused several major outbreaks; pasteurized milk is safe
Untreated water	Major outbreaks from contaminated municipal water supplies Sporadic cases from swallowing natural water (including sea water) while engaged in outdoor activities; casual consumption of natural water; unsatisfactory campsite supplies
Raw or undercooked meats	Poultry (especially barbecue, fondue); other meats probably less often; raw clams and possibly mussels
Foods cross-contaminated from raw meats	Extent unknown, but probably main cause of sporadic infections; possible role of flies in transmission; foreign travel
Contact with infected person	Surprisingly infrequent; close contact necessary; transmission most likely from young child to mother or siblings, occasionally between husband and wife

in Sweden, where 50–75% of infections are acquired abroad (Svedhem and Kaijser, 1980; Walder, 1982). Equivalent figures for Britain range from 11 to 17%.

3. Sources and transmission of infection

Campylobacter enteritis is, first and foremost, a zoonosis. Animals constitute the main reservoir of infection, whereas man is a relatively unimportant reservoir either for direct or indirect transmission. *Campylobacter jejuni* can be found in the intestinal tracts of a wide variety of animals, particularly wild birds and domestic poultry. *Campylobacter coli* is found mainly in pigs.

The routes by which infection is transmitted from animals to humans are probably many and varied, yet few have been defined; firm evidence is hard to come by. It is likely that most sporadic infections are acquired through the consumption of foods contaminated from raw animal products, particularly poultry. There is now ample evidence that poultry throughout the world harbour campylobacteria, and that contamination of carcasses at points of sale to the public is the rule rather than the exception. Infection can be acquired by handling the raw product in the kitchen or consuming it raw or undercooked. Raw or undercooked beef hamburgers, sausages, and clams, as well as poultry, have been implicated in outbreaks of campylobacter enteritis (Table 3, p. 120) but in general foodborne outbreaks, as opposed to sporadic foodborne infections, are uncommon. As already mentioned, campylobacteria do not readily multiply in food. On the other hand massive outbreaks, some affecting several thousand people, have been caused by the distribution of raw or inadequately pasteurized milk (Robinson and Jones, 1981) or inadequately treated water (e.g., Mentzing, 1981; Vogt *et al.,* 1982).

A minority of infections are caused by direct contact with infected animals or animal products. These may be occupational (e.g., farmers, veterinarians, meat and poultry workers) or domestic (usually a newly acquired puppy or kitten ill with diarrhoea). Table 2 summarizes the principal pathways of infection.

Perhaps the most important epidemiological consideration is the possibility that a patient suffering from campylobacter enteritis is part of an outbreak. Not only do outbreaks afford unique opportunities to detect new sources and routes of infection, but there is the possibility that many more infections may be prevented by the timely application of appropriate control measures.

A more detailed account of the epidemiology and control of campylobacter enteritis can be found elsewhere (Skirrow, 1982; Blaser *et al.,* 1983).

B. Pathogenesis

1. Mode of infection and minimum infective dose

Infection is acquired by ingestion. There is no other tenable explanation for the large outbreaks of campylobacter enteritis that have been associated with the consumption of untreated water and milk. Moreover, human volunteers have become infected after drinking milk containing live organisms. In one such experiment the inoculating dose was only 500 viable bacteria. In another, 5 of 10 volunteers became infected (only 1 ill) after taking a dose of 800 bacteria, and 11 of 13 became infected (5 ill) after taking a dose of 9×10^4 bacteria (Black *et al.*, 1983). The site of primary infection is presumed to be the intestine, but it has been suggested that the upper respiratory tract may be an additional or alternative site, for in some outbreaks respiratory symptoms have been present more often than would have been expected by chance.

Clinical evidence suggests that acute campylobacter proctitis in homosexual men can be transmitted by direct venereal inoculation (Quinn *et al.*, 1980).

2. Attachment and invasion

In animal experiments, colonization of the intestines rapidly follows oral (or gastric) inoculation. In mice, scanning electron microscopy has shown that colonization is accompanied by apparent attachment of bacteria to the intestinal mucosa. The striking pictures of Field *et al.* (1981) show numerous campylobacteria lying on, in, and below the mucus gel lining the epithelium of the lower ileal mucosa of neonatal mice 2 hours after intragastric inoculation. The authors likened the appearances to those seen after inoculation with *Vibrio cholerae*. Merrell *et al.* (1981) reported large mats of bacteria on the mucosal surfaces of the colons of mice within 48 hours of intraileal inoculation, although strangely none of their mice showed overt signs of illness. Similar findings were reported in calves by Taylor (1982), who, by means of silver staining, observed campylobacteria adjacent to the mucosal epithelium and the crypts of the jejunum and ileum. He also found that campylobacteria adhered to isolated brush border preparations.

This apparent ability to adhere to gut epithelium cannot be due to fimbriae or pili, for campylobacteria have neither. Merrell *et al.* (1981) suggest that a capsule might be responsible for adherence, but experiments conducted by Newell and Pearson (1982) with *in vitro* preparations of human epithelial cell lines (HeLa and foetal small intestine) suggested that flagella play a role in the process, although attachment was observed only after impaction by centrifugation. At first, flagella could be seen lying just beneath the cell surface, but after 18 hours' incubation, whole organisms were observed in vacuoles of the cells, many of which were dead or dying. Butzler showed that *C. jejuni* invaded and destroyed chicken embryo cells *in vitro,* and he demonstrated (by electron microscopy) the presence of campylobacteria in the caecal epithelia of 8-day-old chicks 1 week after oral inoculation (Butzler and Skirrow, 1979). Interestingly, 17 of 25 inoculated chicks had positive liver cultures, and 12 had positive blood cultures, yet none showed signs of illness.

Dissemination in the blood seems to be a regular feature of the early stages of infection. Taylor (1982) isolated *C. jejuni* from the lungs, gall bladder, spleen, and mesenteric lymph nodes of calves during the first 2 days after inoculation but not thereafter. Fitzgeorge *et al.* (1981) found 4 of 6 rhesus monkeys to have bacteraemia during the first 3 days after oral inoculation with *C. jejuni,* and they noted that this preceded the appearance of the organisms in the faeces. But despite bacteraemia there was only one isolation from organs not associated with the intestinal tract (urinary bladder wall). On the other hand, organisms did localize in the liver and gall bladder.

The fact that bacteraemia is seldom reported in patients suffering from campylobacter enteritis does not mean that it does not occur regularly. Blood is seldom taken for culture from patients with diarrhoea, although this was done in the volunteer studies of Black *et al.* (1983) with negative results. The prodromal febrile illness, often with rigors, that many campylobacter enteritis patients suffer is in keeping with the concept of early bacteraemia. The brisk antibody response shown by most infected patients also indicates an invasive process. In view of the evidence of invasiveness, it is odd that *C. jejuni* has consistently been found—by at least five teams of investigators—to give negative results in the Sereny (guinea pig conjuctiva) test.

Given that dissemination of organisms occurs commonly in campylobacter enteritis, it seems to be of little consequence to normal subjects, since focal infection outside the digestive system is rare. Compromised patients, of course, are a different matter (see Section III). In fact, *C. jejuni* bacteraemia is not as uncommon as it is sometimes made out to be, and not nearly as rare as *C. fetus* ssp. *fetus* bacteraemia. Eighty-one patients with bacteraemia were reported to CDSC in the period 1977–1982; most infections were due to *C. jejuni* biotype 1, but biotype 2 and *C. coli* were also represented.

3. Toxin production

Most of the earlier studies designed to detect enterotoxin production by *C. jejuni* gave negative results in conventional test systems. Recently, however, several reports have appeared which show that 60–85% of strains of *C. jejuni* and *C. coli* produce toxins under appropriate test conditions. The first of these was by Ruiz-Palacios *et al.* (1983) working in Mexico. Johnson and Lior (1984) described two types of toxin: a heat-labile cytotoxin detected in Vero cells, and a heat-stable "cytotonic" toxin that caused elongation of Chinese hamster ovary cells. Other reports are those of Wong *et al.* (1983) and McCardell *et al.* (1984). *Campylobacter jejuni* enterotoxin can be partially neutralised by antibody to cholera toxin, but genetic probing experiments have shown that the structural differences between *C. jejuni* enterotoxin and cholera or *Escherichia coli* heat-labile enterotoxin are probably greater than the immunological studies suggest (Ølsvik *et al.,* 1984).

Endotoxin-like activity (Limulus assay and dermal Schwartzmann reaction) has been shown in *C. jejuni* and *C. coli* by Fumarola *et al.* (1982), although activity was 4 to 8 times less than that of *E. coli*. Lipopolysaccharide complexes are present in the cell wall of *C. jejuni* (Naess and Hofstad, 1982; Logan and Trust, 1982).

4. Pathological changes in the intestinal tract

(a) Macroscopic lesions

Observations of the macroscopic lesions in the bowel in humans are necessarily few, since they can be made only at autopsy or laparotomy. King (1962) described haemorrhagic inflammation and congestion of the jejunum and first half of the ileum of a chicken farmer who died from campylobacter enteritis complicating alcoholic cirrhosis; there were no lesions in the colon. Evans and Dadswell (1967) described necrosis of a 12-cm segment of ileum and congestion of the caecum in a 5-month-old girl who also died apparently from campylobacter enteritis. At laparotomy, usually performed for suspected acute appendicitis, oedema and inflammation of some part of the ileum has been reported, often with mesenteric adenitis and sometimes a little free fluid in the peritoneal cavity (Skirrow, 1977; Hay and Ganguli, 1980; Pitkänen *et al.*, 1983; Pearson *et al.*, 1982). Lambert *et al.* (1982) described a woman with terminal ileitis (diagnosed by radiography and microscopy of specimens taken by retrograde ileoscopy). In a series of patients with operative evidence of acute ileitis, the commonest associated infection was *Campylobacter* (Schofield and Mandal, 1981).

Although infection seems to start in the small intestine, extension into the colon and rectum is usual; the disease is really an acute enterocolitis. This distal progression is indicated in more severely affected patients by the appearance of frank blood in the stools after 2 or 3 days of illness. [In the mouse experiments of Merrell *et al.* (1981), colonization of the ileum was only transient—the colon was the site of more lasting colonization.] In patients with colitis, endoscopy shows acute mucosal inflammation, which is haemorrhagic in severe cases. Differentiation from acute ulcerative colitis or Crohn's disease may be difficult.

(b) Microscopic lesions

The histopathological changes of campylobacter enteritis are indistinguishable from those of salmonellosis and shigellosis. There is an acute inflammatory reaction consisting of focal collections of polymorphonuclear cells in the lamina propria and lumen of mucosal capillaries, often with crypt abscess formation. Mucosal oedema is seen as a separation of the crypts of Lieberkühn and a widening of the gap between crypts and the muscularis mucosae. The epithelium may be flattened and sometimes eroded. Late in the disease the presence of chronic inflammatory cells may give rise to appearances indistinguishable from ulcerative colitis. These bowel lesions are reflected in the inflammatory cellular exudate that is usually found in the stools of patients with campylobacter enterocolitis.

5. *Haematological and biochemical changes*

The erythrocyte sedimentation rate is usually raised, sometimes to high levels. Mean values of 25–30 mm/hour with occasional values in excess of 100 mm/hour have been reported in several surveys of hospital patients. Leucocyte counts are usually normal or only moderately raised. Mean values of 7.9 × 10^9/liter (Svedhem and Kaijser, 1980) and 8.9 × 10^9/liter (range 4.1–23.0) (Pentland, 1979) are representative (see also Pitkänen et al., 1983).

Blood urea and serum electrolytic values are usually normal unless there is obvious dehydration. No significant abnormality in liver function tests were found in a series of 16 hospital patients described by Pentland (1979), but Pitkänen et al. (1983) reported raised aminotransferases in 25 (13.6%) of 184 patients in Helsinki, Drake et al. (1981) reported slightly raised SGOT values in 24% of a series of hospital patients, and McKendrick et al. (1982) reported raised (maximum 59 I.U./liter) aminotransferases in 4 of 16 hospital patients, 15 of whom had raised serum orosomucoids.

6. *Immune response*

Most patients who suffer campylobacter enteritis develop specific antibodies to their infecting strain. Antibodies appear as early as the fifth day of illness and disappear slowly over several months. This presumably confers immunity to that particular strain [rhesus monkeys were found to be resistant to reinfection when challenged with the same strain of *C. jejuni* 15 weeks after initial infection (Fitzgeorge et al., 1981)], but it is not known how long such immunity lasts. It is known that infection with one strain does not necessarily confer immunity to another. There are several reports where patients have suffered two attacks of campylobacter enteritis several months apart in which it has been shown that the infecting strains have been different (e.g., Kendall and Tanner, 1982). Constant exposure to infection in developing countries apparently gives rise to substantial immunity, as symptomatic infection is rare after early childhood in such areas. It is not known whether such immunity is dependent upon constant reexposure to infection, nor is it known whether there is any passive transfer of immunity from mother to child. Painstaking longitudinal studies are needed to answer such questions.

C. Clinical manifestations

1. *Attack rate*

Not everyone who is exposed to infection becomes infected, and not everyone who becomes infected develops symptoms. Attack rates in two major waterborne outbreaks were estimated to have been 10–30% (Mentzing, 1981) and 14–23% (Vogt et al., 1982). Attack rates of other outbreaks have ranged from 15 to 95%

Table 3 Incubation period of campylobacter enteritis in experimental infections and point-source outbreaks

Incubation period		Number of patients included in calculations	Attack rate (%)	Circumstances of infection	Source of data
Mean (days)	Range (days)				
3	—	1	—	Experimental infection; inoculating dose 10^6 organisms	Steele and McDermott (1978)
4	—	1	—	Experimental infection; inoculating dose 500 organisms	Robinson (1981)
2.8	—	6	18	Experimental infection; inoculating dose $8 \times 10^2 - 9 \times 10^4$	Black et al. (1983)
1.5	20–60 hr	101	93.5	Restaurant meal (clam salad)	Itoh et al. (1982)
2.1	20–104 hr	4	40	Household meal (chicken)	
2	1.5–7	6	30 (approx.)	Large waterborne outbreak; 6 out-of-town residents drank suspect water only once	Vogt et al. (1982)
2.8	1–6	20	15	Restaurant meal (probably under-cooked chicken)	Skirrow et al. (1981)
3.1	2–5	13	95	Restaurant meal (chicken liver fondue)	Mouton et al. (1982)
3.1	<1–8	89	72	Consumption of undercooked chicken on military field exercise	Brouwer et al. (1979)
3.9	2–6	21	15 (approx.)	Meal at barracks (raw beef hamburgers); bacteriologically confirmed cases only	Oosterom et al. (1980)
5.2[a]	2–9[a]	148	50 (approx.)	Outbreak from single distribution of unpasteurized milk; bacteriologically confirmed cases only	Porter and Reid (1980)
4 (<15y)[a] 5 (<15y)[a]	1–13[a]	616	—	Same outbreak as above, but including unconfirmed cases	Wallace (1980)

[a] Although this was a single distribution of unpasteurized milk, allowance must be made for the possibility that some patients may not have drunk the milk until 1 or 2 days later. Moreover, one cannot be sure that some of the stragglers were not secondarily infected from other

(Table 3). In a suspected milkborne outbreak in a student hall of residence, it was estimated that at least 20–25% of infections were symptomless (D. M. Jones *et al.*, 1981), and in a community milkborne outbreak reported by Porter and Reid (1980), 40% of culture-positive patients had no symptoms. Of 33 volunteers given doses ranging from 8×10^2 to 9×10^4 bacteria, 22 became infected but only 6 developed symptoms (Black *et al.*, 1983).

2. Incubation period

Early estimates of an incubation period of 3–5 days with a range of 1.5–10 days (Butzler and Skirrow, 1979) have been largely confirmed. In human volunteer experiments, incubation periods were 4 days in one person (Robinson, 1981), 3 days in another (Steele and McDermott, 1978), and an average of 68 hours (light fever) and 88 hours (light diarrhoea) in 6 others (Black *et al.*, 1983). There are several reports of individual patients developing symptoms 2 and 3 days after single exposures to known sources of infection, and mean incubation periods ranging from 1.5 to 3.9 days have been recorded from point-source outbreaks of *Campylobacter* enteritis (Table 3). The extreme range observed in such outbreaks was 20 hours to 8 days, but it should be borne in mind that bacteriological confirmation of infection was not always obtained, so it is possible that symptoms in some patients were of spurious origin. It is also possible that some late-onset infections were secondarily acquired. In the milkborne outbreak the incubation periods were almost certainly lengthened falsely through some patients not drinking the suspect milk until 1 or 2 days after it had been delivered. Thus the 13 days recorded by Wallace (1980) is almost certainly a day or two longer than the true figure. I have been unable to find an adequately substantiated report of an incubation period shorter than the 20 hours of Itoh *et al.* (1982). The important point to remember is that the usual incubation period is longer than it is for most other intestinal pathogens.

3. Onset and prodrome

The onset is typically abrupt. In most patients the first symptoms are abdominal pain and diarrhoea, but in about one-third there is a febrile prodromal period of nonspecific ''flu-like'' symptoms, which may last anything from a few hours to a few days, although usually not much more than 1 day. Patients experiencing this prodromal illness tend to develop a more severe illness than those starting with diarrhoea. Thus the incidence of prodromal symptoms is higher in patients attending hospital—e.g. 50% (McKendrick *et al.*, 1982)—than in those seen in domiciliary practice or surveyed by questionnaire during the time of an outbreak—e.g., 30% (Wallace, 1980). Typical prodromal symptoms are malaise, headache, shivering, dizziness, and generalized myalgia. Abdominal pain is usually the first symptom referable to the gastrointestinal tract, but sometimes it is preceded by nausea or vomiting. Gastric symptoms were the presenting feature

Table 4 Frequency of symptoms and signs in patients with campylobacter enteritis (mean percentage ± SD[a])

Population	Abdominal pain	Fever[b]	Rigors[c]	Vomiting	Frank blood in stools	Headache	Myalgia
Patients seen in hospitals and clinics	74 ± 18 (16)	63 ± 14 (16)	22 ± 5 (3)[d]	28 ± 13 (11)	30 ± 19 (14)	25 ± 9 (4)	29 ± 17 (3)
Patients surveyed during outbreaks	75 ± 12 (16)	50 ± 17 (14)	8 (1)[e]	16 ± 9 (16)	10 ± 9 (14)	50 ± 15 (6)	35 ± 11 (5)

[a] Figures in parentheses are numbers of surveys from which figures are derived.
[b] Includes those with symptoms of fever as well as observed fever.
[c] Does not include patients described as having "chills."
[d] Blaser et al. (1979); Pentland (1979); Pitkänen et al. (1981).
[e] Wallace (1980).

in 10% of adults and 20% of children (<15 years) affected in the milkborne outbreak of campylobacter enteritis studied by Wallace (1980). A high fever in the region of 40°C that develops in a few patients may be associated with delirium in adults and convulsions or hallucinations in children (see next subsection). Meningism has also been reported (Wright, 1979; Williams and Deacon, 1980).

The recorded frequencies of the symptoms and signs of campylobacter enteritis show wide variation according to the population studied and the criteria used. Yet extracting and sifting data from the more important studies does provide a degree of quantitation on which to base comparisons (Table 4).

4. Diarrhoeal stage

Diarrhoea is not an inevitable consequence of infection—a few patients have only abdominal pain and perhaps fever. But most patients do have diarrhoea that ranges from the passage of a few loose stools to a severe prostrating attack of enteritis. Typically the stools become fluid, foul smelling, bile-stained, often mucoid, and, in severe cases, watery. Most samples contain leukocytes and red cells. Frank blood is commonly seen from the second day of diarrhoea onwards, especially in children.

There is good agreement among published surveys that at least half of the patients attending hospitals or clinics have 10 or more bowel actions per day at the height of the disease (Blaser *et al.*, 1979; Pentland, 1979; Price *et al.*, 1979; Svedhem and Kaijser, 1980; Pitkänen *et al.*, 1983; Walder, 1982). However, Price *et al.* (1979) found that the maximum frequency of diarrhoea was less than in patients with *Salmonella* or *Shigella* infections ($p < 0.02$), and Jewkes *et al.* (1981) observed that the duration of diarrhoea was also less than in salmonella enteritis (8 days versus 10 days; $p < 0.05$). In other studies the average duration of diarrhoea was 4–7 days (Pentland, 1979; Svedhem and Kaijser, 1980; Kendall and Tanner, 1982; Kist, 1982).

Apart from the diarrhoea, abdominal pain is unquestionably the most striking symptom at this stage of the disease. The pain is initially colicky and usually periumbilical, although it may become more continuous and sometimes move to the right iliac fossa. It is temporarily relieved by the passage of stools or flatus. The study of hospital patients by Jewkes *et al.* (1981) showed that abdominal pain in campylobacter enteritis lasted longer and was more severe than in salmonella enteritis (mean duration 3 days versus 1 day, $p < 0.05$). Moreover, 2 of the 13 campylobacter-infected patients in their series underwent laparotomy (with normal findings) because of the severity of the pain (see Section IV,D,2).

Vomiting is not a conspicuous feature of the disease, and patients seldom vomit more than once or twice (Table 4).

Skin rashes, usually of unspecified type although sometimes urticarial (Bradshaw *et al.*, 1980; Hoskins, 1982), have occasionally been reported, but they are uncommon. Erythema nodosum has been reported as a late manifestation (see Section IV,E,3).

Death is rare and virtually confined to frail or compromised subjects who became irreversibly dehydrated.

5. Stage of recovery

By the time the diarrhoea has eased, patients are generally left feeling weak and washed out, and although dehydration may not be clinically apparent, many patients will have lost weight. Moreover, abdominal pain and discomfort often persist for several days. Caution over diet should be exercised when the patient's appetite returns, because any injudicious loading of the stomach, particularly with solid food, is liable to precipitate a sharp recurrence of symptoms. A temporary relapse of illness is likely to occur anyway at this time, although the symptoms are usually milder than in the original attack. Relapses of this sort have been reported in as many as 25% of infected patients (Blaser et al., 1979; Pitkänen et al., 1983); a figure of 16% was reported by Drake et al. (1981).

The average duration of illness is less than a week in about 80% of patients. The mean duration in patients involved in two outbreaks were 5.2 days (Mentzing, 1981) and 4.2 days (Mouton et al., 1982), but these would have included patients who were not ill enough to have sought medical aid. It is unusual for patients to be ill for more than 2–3 weeks; by this time one would begin to suspect that the patient had some other disease such as ulcerative colitis. In a review of 200 patients with campylobacter diarrhoea, all patients had become symptom-free by 12 days (Schofield and Mandal, 1983).

6. Convalescent excretion

The number of patients who continue to excrete campylobacteria in their faeces after an attack of acute enteritis falls off exponentially with time. Figures based on several studies show that 50% are culture-negative after 2–3 weeks, 85% after about 5 weeks, and virtually all after 3 months. There appears to be no correlation of excretion time with age, severity of symptoms, or duration of disease. These results are based on direct culture methods; probably if more sensitive enrichment culture methods were used, these periods would be somewhat longer. No long-term carriers have been reported among normal people.

D. Early onset complications

1. Campylobacter colitis

It is now clear that infection of the colon is a regular feature of campylobacter enteritis; indeed, campylobacter enterocolitis would perhaps be a more accurate description of the disease. This form of infection deserves separate consideration, because some patients present with predominantly colitic symptoms that can mimic an acute attack of ulcerative colitis or Crohn's disease.

M. E. Lambert *et al.* (1979), working in Manchester, were the first to draw attention to the presence of colonic disease in campylobacter infections, and their report was quickly followed by others in the United Kingdom (Price *et al.*, 1979; Willoughby *et al.*, 1979; McKendrick *et al.*, 1982), in Canada (J. R. Lambert *et al.*, 1979; Colgan *et al.*, 1980), and in the United States (Longfield *et al.*, 1979; Blaser *et al.*, 1980c; Duffy *et al.*, 1980; Loss *et al.*, 1980). There is general agreement that the sigmoidoscopic and histological appearances of the bowel are indistinguishable from those of other acute bacterial infections such as salmonellosis and shigellosis, but opinions differ as to whether they are distinguishable from those of acute inflammatory bowel disease (IBD). Price *et al.* (1979) and Mee and Shield (1980) had little difficulty in distinguishing between the two, but others (e.g., M. E. Lambert *et al.*, 1979) doubted whether one could reliably do so. Much depends on the timing of the examination. Early in the disease the absence of a chronic inflammatory-cell infiltrate indicates an infective cause; later on, the appearances are similar. It is important to remember that campylobacter infection can cause an acute exacerbation of IBD (Newman and Lambert, 1980; Goodman *et al.*, 1980; Chandra *et al.*, 1982; Chessin *et al.*, 1982), because specific chemotherapy can bring about rapid resolution. It is doubtful whether campylobacter infection ever causes IBD (Blaser *et al.*, 1984).

Acute dilatation of the bowel or ''toxic megacolon'' in an 83-year-old woman with severe campylobacter colitis was reported by McKinley *et al.* (1980).

Campylobacter proctitis has been reported in practising homosexual men (Quinn *et al.*, 1980), and though it is likely that these infections represent venereal transmission, this has not been proven.

2. Appendicitis and "pseudo-appendicitis"

The occurrence of severe abdominal pain, particularly before the onset of diarrhoea, can simulate an ''acute abdomen'' and lead to the admission of a patient to a surgical unit. Several surveys of campylobacter enteritis include one or two such cases, but they represent only a small proportion of all infections. The incidence was 1 of 39 patients seen in the general practice survey of Kendall and Tanner (1982), 4 (all adults) of an estimated 3500 people affected in the milk-borne outbreak of P. H. Jones *et al.* (1981), and 6 of 114 hospital and clinic patients described by Kist (1982). Inevitably, some patients with this syndrome are subjected to laparotomy, but rarely is the appendix found to be inflamed. If there is anything abnormal to see it is usually mesenteric adenitis and inflammation of the ileum. Very occasionally, however, there is genuine appendicitis. Pearson *et al.* (1982) isolated campylobacteria from 6 of 251 children admitted to hospital complaining of acute abdominal pain, and at laparotomy 3 had mesenteric adenitis but the other 3 had acute appendicitis; campylobacteria were isolated from appendix tissue of 2 (both with mesenteric adenitis) and from a peritoneal swab of 1 with genuine acute appendicitis. Megraud *et al.* (1982) isolated *C. jejuni* from the inflamed appendix of a 16-year-old girl who had had several episodes of diarrhoea in the preceding month but none at the time of operation. Chan *et al.* (1983) reported a similar patient (11-year-old boy) who had abdominal pain and a few loose stools. If campylobacteria do cause appendicitis directly, they could well precipitate it by causing inflammation and oedema in the adjacent gut.

Clinically the distinction between uncomplicated campylobacter enteritis and acute appendicitis is not usually difficult. Although the pain can move to the right iliac fossa, true localised tenderness and guarding is not a feature of the uncomplicated disease.

3.   Haemolytic uraemic syndrome
Five patients with campylobacter enterocolitis complicated by haemolytic uraemic syndrome have been reported (Denneberg *et al.*, 1982; Chamovitz *et al.*, 1983; Dickgiesser, 1983; Shulman and Moel, 1983).

4.   Gastrointestinal haemorrhage
Severe life-threatening gastrointestinal haemorrhage from campylobacter enteritis has been reported only once (Michalak *et al.*, 1980). A 24-year-old nurse, who was previously in good health, suffered a haemorrhage from an ulcer in the terminal ileum, which necessitated emergency hemicolectomy.

5.   Ulceration of ileal stoma
Two patients with long-established ileostomies, both constructed after total colectomy for inflammatory bowel disease, suffered extensive ulceration of their ileal stomas apparently as a direct consequence of campylobacter enteritis (Meuwissen *et al.*, 1981; Skirrow, 1981). In 1 patient (Skirrow, 1981), gross oedema and congestion preceded the ulceration and the mucosal damage was thought to be due to partial strangulation. Ulceration lasted several weeks in both patients, but healing was complete.

6.   Biliary-tract infection: cholecystitis and hepatitis
There are several reports of acute or acute-on-chronic campylobacter cholecystitis (Mertens and De Smet, 1979; Darling *et al.*, 1979). Most of these patients gave a history of diarrhoea shortly before they developed symptoms of cholecystitis, but de Sa Pereira *et al.* (1981) described a 43-year-old woman with severe necrotizing cholecystitis who gave no such history.

There is some evidence that *C. jejuni* can cause hepatitis. Ampelas *et al.* (1982) described bacteraemic hepatitis, with necrosis and polymorphonuclear cell infiltration in liver biopsy material, in a previously healthy 48-year-old woman with diarrhoea, and Reddy and Thomas (1982) described a 52-year-old man with campylobacter enteritis and sharply deranged liver-function tests. An alcoholic man with cholestatic hepatitis, diarrhoea and *C. jejuni* bacteraemia was reported by Nahum *et al.* (1982). Slightly raised aminotransferases have been reported in up to 25% of hospital patients (see Section IV,B,5), and occasional reports of jaundice in patients with campylobacter enteritis have been received at CDSC, London (unpublished).

It is interesting that in monkeys experimentally infected with *C. jejuni*, the liver and gall bladder were the most consistently colonized sites outside of the intestinal tract, and colonization persisted in the gall bladder of one monkey even after its faeces had become culture-negative (Fitzgeorge *et al.*, 1981). It has long been known that sheep may harbour *C. jejuni* in their gall bladders, and it has recently been shown that *C. jejuni* survives well in bile *in vitro* (Blaser *et al.*, 1980a).

7. Pancreatitis

Gallagher *et al.* (1981) reported acute pancreatitis associated with campylobacter enteritis in a 19-year-old girl. She presented with a 24-hour history of lower abdominal pain and lower right-sided backache, but at laparotomy nothing abnormal was found. Four days later she was found to have a serum amylase of 1000 I.U./litre (falling to normal within 2 weeks), and by this time she had developed diarrhoea. Pönkä and Kosunen (1981) described a 29-year-old woman with profuse watery campylobacter diarrhoea, upper abdominal pain, and raised serum amylase values. They also reported 5 other more mildly affected patients. It is not known whether these were examples of actual pancreatic infection or of secondary damage caused by infection of the adjacent biliary tract.

8. Peritonitis complicating continuous ambulatory peritoneal dialysis

Two patients on continuous ambulatory peritoneal dialysis (CAPD) who developed *C. jejuni* peritonitis within 24 hours of the onset of campylobacter enteritis have been reported (Pepersack *et al.*, 1982; CDSC, London, unpublished). Both patients were treated successfully, the former with erythromycin by mouth plus gentamicin (8 mg/litre) in the dialysis bags after co-trimoxazole (in the dialysis fluid) had failed. Vernon and Dominguez (1982) reported *C. fetus* ssp. *fetus* peritonitis in another CAPD patient who did not have diarrhoea.

9. Pneumonia

Pönkä and Kosunen (1982) described 2 elderly patients who developed mild bronchopneumonia during the acute stages of campylobacter enteritis, but there was no direct evidence that campylobacteria were infecting the lungs.

E.   Late onset complications

1.   *Reactive (aseptic) arthritis*

Since the report of Berden *et al.* (1979), reactive arthritis has become well recognized as a complication of campylobacter enteritis, just as it is a complication of salmonella, shigella or yersinia enteritis. Schaad (1982) has written a detailed review of 21 published case histories. In these patients, arthritis usually appeared within 1–2 weeks of the onset of diarrhoea, but the interval ranged from a few days to several weeks. In about one-third of patients only one joint— usually a knee—was affected, but in many the process extended to other joints such as the ankles, wrists, and small joints of the hands and feet. Arthritis affecting several joints was characteristically migratory. Four of the 21 patients and another patient not included in Schaad's review (Leung *et al.*, 1980) had Reiter's syndrome. Fever and leukocytosis were usually absent, whereas the erythrocyte sedimentation rate was raised (mean 71, range 19–130 mm/hour in 18 patients tested). Eleven of 19 patients who were tissue typed were HLA-B27 positive, as was an additional patient described by Short *et al.* (1982), i.e., 60% of those tested. The condition seems to be benign although troublesome. The mean duration of arthritic symptoms was 7.5 weeks (excluding 1 patient who had symptoms for 23 months). All patients recovered completely.

Reports of the incidence of reactive arthritis associated with campylobacter enteritis range from 1 (1.1%) of 88 patients affected in a single milkborne outbreak (Eastmond *et al.*, 1983) to 8 (24%) of 33 hospital inpatients (Gumpel *et al.*, 1981). An incidence of 2% was found in a Swedish survey (Walder, 1982). The incidence in a given community will be influenced by the prevalence of HLA-B27 in the population.

2.   *Guillain-Barré syndrome*

Four patients, 2 middle-aged men, a boy of 16 years and a woman of 34 years, were reported as developing acute peripheral polyneuritis within 9–15 days of the onset of campylobacter enteritis. All 4 had severe neurological illnesses involving the limbs, and 1 also had involvement of the sixth and tenth cranial nerves; the latter patient required positive pressure ventilation (Constant *et al.*, 1983). Two other patients were reported to have suffered severe axonal loss (Rhodes and Tattersfield, 1982; Molnar *et al.*, 1982). The authors of the fourth report (Speed, *et al.*, 1984) also presented preliminary serological evidence suggesting that *C. jejuni* enteritis may be antecedent to Guillain-Barré syndrome more often than was previously recognized (cf. Kaldor and Speed, 1984).

3.   *Erythema nodosum*

Erythema nodosum associated with campylobacter enteritis has been reported in 4 patients, all of them women (J. R. Lambert *et al.*, 1979; M. Lambert *et al.*,

1982; Ellis *et al.*, 1982; Eastmond and Reid, 1982). The lesions appeared within 1–2 weeks of the onset of diarrhoea and lasted 3–6 weeks. Terminal ileitis was present in the patient described by Lambert *et al.* (1982), and her forearms and elbows were affected as well as her shins. It is of interest that 4 patients with erythema nodosum associated with salmonella enteritis have recently been reported (Morrison *et al.*, 1983; Dobson and Hume, 1983). Again, all 4 were women (one a girl aged 10 years), and the lesions appeared 9–14 days from the diarrhoeal episode.

4. Glomerulonephritis

Menck (1981) reported mild glomerulonephritis in an 18-year-old girl following *C. jejuni* enteritis.

F. Campylobacter enteritis in children

In general, the disease in children is mild and, in contrast to rotavirus, serious dehydration is uncommon. There are several differences in the frequency of certain symptoms between children and adults, which are most apparent in children below the age of 3 years. As many as half of them vomit, but few (9%) have abdominal colic (P. A. Holt, unpublished). Under the age of 1 year, fever is much less common (20%) than in later years. None of the 5 infants under the age of 12 weeks in the series reported by Karmali and Fleming (1979) had fever, and only 1 of 8 neonates described by Anders *et al.* (1981) were febrile. Older children may develop high fever and suffer from convulsions (see below), hallucinations (Karmali and Fleming, 1979) or meningism (Wright, 1979). The passage of blood in the stools is more commonly seen in children than in adults, the highest figure (92%) being recorded by Karmali and Fleming (1979). In a German study, "pseudo-appendicitis" was almost exclusively seen in children aged 6–10 years (Kist, 1982).

In developing countries watery diarrhoea is a more prominent feature of the disease in children than is sanguinous diarrhoea. In one study (Richardson *et al.*, 1983) breast feeding did not seem to protect against colonization with *C. jejuni*.

1. Febrile convulsions

Of an estimated 2500 children affected in a milkborne outbreak of campylobacter enteritis (P. H. Jones *et al.*, 1981), 14 were admitted to hospital, 9 because of a generalized grand mal convulsion. Seven of these children had had a febrile convulsion on a previous occasion (Havalad *et al.*, 1980). The mean age of the 9 children was 5 years 8 months (range 3 years 3 months to 7 years 7 months), a much higher figure than the mean age of 22 months for children seen on the same unit with febrile convulsions not associated with campylobacter enteritis. However, the outbreak figures may be skewed by the fact that the milk was distributed mainly to children in the 5- to 7-year age group. Two other children with febrile convulsions (aged 14 months and 4 years) are described by Wright and Seager (1980).

2. Neonatal infections

Except for rare cases of meningitis (see Section III,A,1), neonatal campylobacter infections are remarkably benign. As mentioned previously, fever is unusual. The passage of blood per rectum is the usual presenting feature—diarrhoea is often mild or even absent. This has occasionally led to laparotomy for suspected intussusception, although such an outcome is probably rare, for only 1 of 57 infants with campylobacter enteritis collected over a 3-year period by Dr. P. A. Holt (unpublished) was referred with suspected intussusception and in that case surgery was avoided. There is little doubt that most neonatal infections are acquired from the mother at the time of delivery, although nosocomial spread in a neonatal unit has been recorded. There is usually a history of diarrhoea in the mother near the time of delivery, or a positive faecal culture, or both (Mawer and Smith, 1979; Karmali and Tan, 1980; Anders *et al.*, 1981; Buck *et al.*, 1982). One of the women in Anders's series had a positive vaginal culture but negative faeces culture. Symptoms generally appear within 3 days of delivery, but 3 of the babies in Anders's series did not show signs until the 11th day, which suggests that they may have become infected after delivery.

G. Laboratory diagnosis

It is not the purpose of this review to serve as a laboratory manual. Methods for the cultivation of campylobacteria are described elsewhere (e.g., Luechtefeld *et al.*, 1981; Skirrow *et al.*, 1982). The comments that follow are intended to show how the laboratory can assist in the diagnosis and management of patients with suspected campylobacter infection.

1. Collection of samples

Campylobacteria are fastidious organisms that are excessively sensitive to oxygen, even though some oxygen is essential for growth—i.e., they are strict microaerophiles. They are also sensitive to acid but tolerant to moderately alkaline conditions. Consequently, their survival in voided faeces is limited, and it is advisable to deliver specimens to the laboratory within a few hours of collection or, if delay is unavoidable, to put the specimens in a refrigerator. In fact "stale" specimens from acutely ill patients may still yield growth, because campylobacteria are usually present in very large numbers, but under these circumstances one should not place much significance on negative results. Rectal swabs or scanty specimens should be transported in a protective medium, e.g., Cary–Blair medium with reduced agar concentration (Luechtefeld *et al.*, 1981).

2. *Rapid diagnosis by direct microscopy of faeces*

It is possible to make a presumptive diagnosis of campylobacter enteritis by direct microscopy, owing to the characteristic morphology and motility of campylobacteria. This can be done by dark-ground or phase-contrast microscopy of wet preparations or by ordinary microscopy of fixed and stained smears. An experienced observer will be able to make a diagnosis in 50–60% of patients by these methods provided the samples are fresh (passed within 1 hour). Although this method is impracticable as a routine procedure, it can be valuable for the occasional acutely ill patient where correct management depends on a precise diagnosis.

3. *Culture*

One or other of several special selective agar media are required for the isolation of campylobacteria from faeces. Ideally, plates should be incubated at a temperature of 42–43°C in closed jars containing oxygen at a concentration of about 6%. If the various means by which this microaerobic atmosphere can be attained are not available (field laboratories in the tropics for example), there are acceptable simpler alternatives such as a candle extinction jar (De Boeck, 1982).

Under ideal conditions, overnight incubation is sufficient to obtain a positive culture, but it is the policy in many laboratories to leave jars closed for 48 hours before reading the plates. *Campylobacter* colonies can be rapidly identified by examining stained smears. Determination of species or biotype takes 2 or 3 days more (Table 5).

The value of selective enrichment culture for human stool samples is debatable. There is no doubt that it increases sensitivity, so it would be worthwhile if, for example, one were investigating symptomless carriage. However, for routine use it is questionable whether the extra costs are justifiable (Hutchinson and Bolton, 1983; Skirrow and Benjamin, 1984). It is probably more appropriate to examine multiple samples. In a Finnish study, where it was the policy to culture two or three samples from all patients, it was estimated that 16% of campylobacter infections would have been missed had reliance been placed on the first sample only (Pitkänen *et al.*, 1981). Enrichment methods are, however, essential for food and environmental specimens where the numbers of campylobacteria are likely to be low.

4. *Diagnosis by serology*

Occasions arise when a retrospective diagnosis of possible campylobacter enteritis is relevant to a patient's management—for example, in a patient with arthritis when it is too late to obtain positive faecal cultures. A test is required that will detect group-specific antibody in the patient—i.e., it should represent antigens common to all strains of *C. jejuni* and *C. coli,* but not any other organism. The complement-fixation (CF) test of Jones *et al.* (1980) goes a long way toward

Table 5 Main distinguishing features of the catalase-positive campylobacteria of man[a]

Characteristic	Campylobacter fetus ssp. fetus[b]	C. jejuni biotype 1	C. jejuni biotype 2	C. coli	C. laridis
Growth at:					
25°C	+	−	−	−	−
37°C	+	+	+	+	+
42°C	−	+	+	+	+
Coccal transformation on exposure to air	−	+	+	±	+
Nalidixic acid (30 µg disc)	R	S	S	S	R
Cephalothin (30 µg disc)	S	R	R	R	R
Hippurate hydrolysis	−	+	+	−	−
H_2S in iron/metabisulphite medium	−	−	+	−	+/±

[a] All strains produce oxidase and reduce nitrate to nitrite, but have no action on carbohydrates.
[b] +, positive; −, negative; ±, weak positive; R, resistant; S, sensitive.

fulfilling these criteria, although it is not very sensitive—a reaction at a serum dilution as low as 1 : 4 is considered to be positive. A positive test indicates recent infection, as CF antibody disappears after a few months. It has proved its value for screening specific populations for evidence of exposure to campylobacter infection (Jones and Robinson, 1981; D. M. Jones *et al.*, 1981). A CF antigen is now available commercially (Virion International, Switzerland). Other tests currently under development are the DIG-ELISA test of Svedhem *et al.* (1983), and the ELISA tests of Rautelin and Kosunen (1983) and Kaldor *et al.* (1983).

H. Other investigations

1. Haematological and biochemical tests
These have been described in the section on pathogenesis (Section IV,B).

2. Radiography
Straight abdominal radiographs of more severely affected patients may show dilated loops of intestine with fluid levels. Such changes were observed in 5 of 20 hospital patients (Bradshaw *et al.*, 1980), but in none of 14 patients in another hospital series (Pentland, 1979). Barium enema examination showed pancolitis in a 14-year-old boy described by M. E. Lambert *et al.* (1979) in Britain, and ulceration of the colon and ileum in a patient described by J. R. Lambert *et al.* (1979) in Canada. Otherwise, barium enema appearances have been reported as normal. Nodular mucosal thickening of the terminal ileum of a woman aged 48 years was shown on follow-through X-ray by M. Lambert *et al.* (1982) in Belgium. Noble *et al.* (1982) described unusual radiological appearances that mimicked carcinoma of the distal transverse colon in a 77-year-old diabetic man.

I. Management

Most patients seen in domiciliary practice require no special treatment beyond what is appropriate for any acute bout of diarrhoea. A glucose electrolyte mixture and possibly an antidiarrhoeal drug such as codeine, diphenoxylate (Lomotil), or loperamide (Imodium) used sparingly is all that is required. These opiate-like drugs should not be given to children because of the risk of respiratory depression. The question of specific antimicrobial chemotherapy seldom arises because patients are usually recovering by the time a bacteriological diagnosis has been made.

Hospital patients are a different matter. They will have been selected because of the severity or complicated nature of their illness, and chemotherapy may be indicated. In such cases a bacteriological diagnosis is especially important, so at least one sample of faeces should be sent for culture in the manner already described. For example, a patient with an apparent relapse of inflammatory bowel disease might in reality have campylobacter enteritis, and if the patient were to be given steroids without an appropriate antibiotic the consequences could be serious. In ill or problem patients there is much to be said for taking blood for culture as well as faeces.

1. Chemotherapy

Erythromycin has been advocated as the agent of choice for the treatment of campylobacter enteritis. It has excellent *in vitro* activity (MICs in the region of 0.2 mg/liter), low toxicity, a fairly narrow antibacterial spectrum, and relatively low cost. Resistant strains are, on the whole, rare and almost confined to *C. coli*. Resistance rates of less than 1% have been recorded in Britain (Telfer Brunton *et al.*, 1978), Canada (Karmali *et al.*, 1981) and Israel (Shmilovitz *et al.*, 1982), but rates of 2.3 and 2.8% have been reported from Belgium (Vanhoof *et al.*, 1980) and Sweden (Walder, 1982), respectively. (Figures in the region of 8% were previously reported by the Belgian and Swedish teams, so either there is a downward trend or more complete surveillance has given more representative results.)

It probably matters little what preparation of erythromycin is given (other than enteric-coated pills), but there are theoretical reasons for favouring the stearate, at least for adults. Apart from being acid-resistant and stable, it is incompletely absorbed, so there is the chance of a contact action in the bowel lumen as well as a systemic action in the blood. A dosage of 500 mg twice daily for 5 days has proved satisfactory in practice; higher doses of the stearate are liable to cause acute abdominal pain. Erythromycin ethyl succinate at 40 mg/kg/day in divided doses is recommended for children. [In fact, the efficacy of erythromycin has never been proven. Double-blind trials have failed to show significant clinical benefit, although campylobacter excretion ceased within 2 days of starting treatment (Anders *et al.*, 1982; Mandal and Ellis, 1983). Nevertheless there are many anecdotal reports of its worth in patients with severe or long-standing infection (e.g., Newman and Lambert, 1980).]

The tetracyclines are also active against campylobacteria—minocycline is the most active of the group—but the prevalence of resistant strains is too high (5–25%) for tetracyclines to be used without laboratory control. Resistance has been shown to be plasmid-mediated. Furazolidone is highly active against all strains tested, but its action is confined to the gut and it is therefore unsuitable for patients with complicated or septicaemic infections. It has been successfully used in Belgium.

Chloramphenicol and gentamicin each have a place in the treatment of life-threatening infections. Chloramphenicol is only moderately active, but in full dosage it might be a first choice for a patient with campylobacter meningitis (e.g., Norrby *et al.*, 1980). Until the recent report by Walder (1982) of a 2% resistance rate, all strains were thought to be sensitive. Only one gentamicin-resistant strain has been reported (MIC 12.5 mg/liter), and this fact, coupled with a good clinical record, makes gentamicin a first choice for the treatment of patients with life-threatening infections.

Ampicillin is the only penicillin (including mecillinam, mezlocillin and azlocillin) with any significant degree of activity against *C. jejuni* and *C. coli*, but MIC values are usually too high for it to be of much clinical use in infections with these organisms. From 5 to 16% of strains produce β-lactamase active against ampicillin (Wright and Knowles, 1980; Fleming *et al.*, 1982). *Campylobacter fetus* ssp. *fetus* is, however, sensitive to ampicillin.

Finally, it should be emphasized that campylobacteria are inherently resistant to trimethoprim and the cephalosporins, including the newer agents such as cefuroxime, cefoperazone and cefoxitin. The one exception is cefotaxime, which has moderate activity against some strains.

2. Should patients with campylobacter enteritis be isolated?

Campylobacter enteritis is a disease of low infectivity, probably because the organisms perish rapidly on exposure to air or desiccation. Experience has shown that infection does not spread, provided attendants wear disposable gloves and plastic aprons when handling bedpans or soiled linen (a rule that should be applied for the nursing of all hospital patients with diarrhoea of undetermined cause). This low infectivity was strikingly shown by the case of an unfortunate man who developed severe campylobacter enteritis and infectious hepatitis after falling into a tank of untreated sewage. He had profuse diarrhoea for 19 days, and 7 attendant nurses contracted hepatitis A, but there was no spread of *Campylobacter* infection (Sumathipala and Morrison, 1983). Nursing in a side ward is desirable, if for no other reason than to spare the patient's feelings—campylobacter enteritis in full spate is a distressing and embarrassing affliction.

Infants are a different matter; they should be isolated as soon as they develop obvious diarrhoea. On the few occasions when *Campylobacter* infection has spread in baby units, the sources of infection appear to have been baths that have not been adequately disinfected.

3. Do symptomless excreters matter?

There are few occasions when the continued excretion of campylobacteria matters once the stools have become formed again. There is no evidence that healthy culture-positive food handlers have ever caused infection, and there is no sound reason for excluding them from work, provided they can be trusted to observe the normal rules of hygiene.

REFERENCES

Ampelas, M., Perez, C., Jourdan, J., Nalet, B., Raynaud, A., Emberger, J. M., and Michel, H. (1982). *Nouv. Presse Med.* **11**, 593–595.

Anders, B. J., Lauer, B. A., and Paisley, J. W. (1981). *Am. J. Dis. Child.* **135**, 900–902.

Anders, B. J., Lauer, B. A., Paisley, J. W., and Reller, L. B. (1982). *Lancet* **1**, 131.

Benjamin, J., Leaper, S., Owen, R. J., and Skirrow, M. B. (1983). *Curr. Microbiol.* **8**, 231–238.

Berden, J. H. M., Muytjens, H. L., and van de Putte, L. B. A. (1979). *Br. Med. J.* **1**, 380.

Black, R. E., Levine, M. M., Blaser, M. J., Clements, M. L., and Hughes, T. P. (1983). *In* "Campylobacter II" (A. D. Pearson *et al.*, eds.), p. 13. Public Health Laboratory Service, London.

Blaser, M. J., Berkowitz, I. D., LaForce, F. M., Cravens, J., Reller, L. B., and Wang, W.-L. L. (1979). *Ann. Intern. Med.* **91**, 179–185.

Blaser, M. J., Hardesty, H. L., Powers, B., and Wang, W.-L. L. (1980a). *J. Clin. Microbiol.* **11**, 309–313.

Blaser, M. J., LaForce, F. M., Wilson, N. A., and Wang, W.-L. L. (1980b). *J. Infect. Dis.* **141**, 665–669.

Blaser, M. J., Parsons, R. B., and Wang, W.-L. L. (1980c). *Gastroenterology* **78**, 448–453.

Blaser, M. J., Taylor, D. N., and Feldman, R. A. (1983). *Epidemiol. Rev.* **5**, 157–176.

Blaser, M. J., Hoverson, D., Ely, I. G., Duncan, D. J., Wang, W.-L. L., and Brown, W. R. (1984). *Gastroenterology* **86**, 33–38.

Bradshaw, M. J., Brown, R., Swallow, J. H., and Rycroft, J. A. (1980). *Postgrad. Med. J.* **56**, 80–84.

Brouwer, R., Mertens, M. J. A., Siem, T. H., and Katchaki, J. (1979). *Antonie van Leeuwenhoek* **45**, 517–519.

Brown, W. J., and Sautter, R. (1977). *J. Clin. Microbiol.* **6**, 72–75.

Buck, G. E., Kelly, M. T., Pichanick, A. M., and Pollard, T. G. (1982). *Am. J. Dis. Child.* **136**, 744.

Butzler, J. P., and Skirrow, M. B. (1979). *Clin. Gastroenterol.* **8**, 737–765.

Butzler, J. P., Dereume, J. P., Barbier, P., Smekens, L., and Dekeyser, J. (1977). *Nouv. Presse Med.* **6**, 1033–1035.

Cameron, S., Roder, D., and White, C. (1982). *Med. J. Aust.* **2**, 175–177.

Chamovitz, B. N., Hartstein, A. I., Alexander, S. R., Terry, A. B., Short, P., and Katon, R. (1983). *Pediatrics* **71**, 253–256.

Chan, F. T. H., Stringel, G., and Mackenzie, A. M. R. (1983). *J. Clin. Microbiol.* **18**, 422–424.

Chandra, L., Barrowman, J. A., Jutty, K. P., Bowmer, I. M., and Fardy, P. (1982). *Can. Med. Assoc. J.* **126**, 389–390.

Chessin, L. N., Emilson, K. A., Degal, H. L., Sardisco, E. J., Stormont, J. N., Stowe, S. P., and Chey, W. Y. (1982). *Gastroenterology* **82**, 1032.

Colaert, J., and Ursi, J. P. (1979). *Med. Mal. Infect.* **9**, 46–47.

Colgan, T., Lambert, J. R., Newman, A., and Luk, S. C. (1980). *Arch. Pathol. Lab. Med.* **104**, 571–574.

Constant, O. C., Bentley, C. C., Denman, A. M., Lehane, J. R., and Larson, H. E. (1983). *J. Infect.* **6**, 89–91.

Darling, W. M., Peel, R. N., Skirrow, M. B., and Mulira, A. E. J. L. (1979). *Lancet* **1**, 1302.

Davies, J. S., and Penfold, J. B. (1979). *Lancet* **1**, 1091–1092.

De Boeck, M. (1982). *In* "Campylobacter: Epidemiology, Pathogenesis and Biochemistry" (D. G. Newell, ed.), pp. 71–72. MTP Press, Lancaster.

De Mol, P., Hemelhof, W., Butzler, J. P., Brasseur, D., Kalala, T., and Vis, H. L. (1983). *Lancet* **1**, 516–518.

Denneberg, T., Friedberg, M., Holmberg, L., Mathiasen, C., Nilsson, K. O., Takolander, T., and Walder, M. (1982). *Acta Paediatr. Scand.* **71**, 243.

de Sa Pereira, M., Lipton, S. D., and Kim, J. K. (1981). *Ann. Intern. Med.* **94**, 821.

Devlin, H. R., and McIntyre, L. (1983). *J. Clin. Microbiol.* **18**, 999–1000.

Dickgiesser, A. (1983). *Immun. Infekt.* **11**, 71–74.

Dobson, H. M., and Hume, R. (1983). *Br. Med. J.* **286**, 1146.

Drake, A. A., Gilchrist, M. J. R., Washington, J. A., II, Huizenga, K. A., and Van Scoy, R. E. (1981). *Mayo Clin. Proc.* **56**, 414–423.

Duffy, M. C., Benson, J. B., and Rubin, S. J. (1980). *Am. J. Clin. Pathol.* **73**, 706–708.

Eastmond, C. J., and Reid, T. M. S. (1982). *Br. Med. J.* **285**, 1421–1422.

Eastmond, C. J., Rennie, J. A. N., and Reid, T. M. S. (1983). *J. Rheumatol.* **10**, 107–108.

Ellis, M. E., Pope, J., Mokashi, A., and Dunbar, E. (1982). *Br. Med. J.* **2**, 937.

Evans, R. G., and Dadswell, J. V. (1967). *Br. Med. J.* **3**, 240.

Fennell, C. L., Totten, P. A., Quinn, T. C., Patton, D. L., Holmes, K. K., and Stamm, W. E. (1984). *J. Infect. Dis.* **149**, 58–66.

Field, L. H., Underwood, J. L., Pope, L. M., and Berry, L. J. (1981). *Infect. Immun.* **33**, 884–892.

Fitzgeorge, R. B., Baskerville, A., and Lander, K. P. (1981). *J. Hyg.* **86**, 343.

Fleming, P. C., D'Amico, A., De Grandis, S., and Karmali, M. A. (1982). *In* "Campylobacter: Epidemiology, Pathogenesis and Biochemistry" (D. G. Newell, ed.), pp. 214–217. MTP Press, Lancaster.

Fleurette, J., Flandrois, J. P., and Diday, M. (1971). *Presse Med.* **79**, 480–482.

Fumarola, D., Miragliotta, G., and Jirillo, E. (1982). *In* "Campylobacter: Epidemiology, Pathogenesis and Biochemistry" (D. G. Newell, ed.), pp. 185–187. MTP Press, Lancaster.

Gallagher, P., Chadwick, P., Jones, D. M., and Turner, L. (1981). *Br. J. Surg.* **68**, 383.

Gilbert, G. L., Davoren, R. A., Cole, M. E., and Radford, N. J. (1981). *Med. J. Aust.* **1**, 585–586.

Ginsberg, M. M., Thompson, M. A., Peter, C. R., Ramras, D. G., and Chin, J. (1981). *Morbid Mortal. Week. Rep.* **30**, 294–295.

Goodman, M. J., Pearson, K. W., McGhie, D., Dutt, S., and Deodhar, S. G. (1980). *Lancet* **2**, 1247.

Gribble, M. J., Salit, I. E., Isaac-Renton, J., and Chow, A. W. (1981). *Am. J. Obstet. Gynecol.* **140**, 423–426.

Guerrant, R. L., Lahita, R. G., Winn, W. C., Jr., and Roberts, R. B. (1978). *Am. J. Med.* **65**, 584–592.

Gumpel, J. M., Martin, C., and Sanderson, P. J. (1981). *Ann. Rheum. Dis.* **40**, 64–65.

Harvey, S. M., and Greenwood, J. R. (1983). *J. Clin. Microbiol.* **18**, 1278–1279.

Havalad, S., Chapple, M. J., Kahakachchi, M., and Hargraves, D. B. (1980). *Br. Med. J.* **280**, 984–985.

Hay, D. J., and Ganguli, L. A. (1980). *Postgrad. Med. J.* **56**, 205–206.

Hébert, G. A., Hollis, D. G., Weaver, R. E., Lambert, M. A., Blaser, M. J., and Moss, C. W. (1982). *J. Clin. Microbiol.* **15**, 1065–1073.

Hoskins, T. W. (1982). *Br. Med. J.* **285**, 1661.

Hutchinson, D. N., and Bolton, F. J. (1983). *J. Clin. Pathol.* **36**, 1350–1352.

Itoh, T., Saito, K., Yanagawa, Y., Sakai, S., and Ohashi, M. (1982). *In* "Campylobacter: Epidemiology, Pathogenesis and Biochemistry" (D. G. Newell, ed.), pp. 5–12. MTP Press, Lancaster.

Jewkes, J., Larson, H. E., Price, A. B., Sanderson, P. J., and Davies, H. A. (1981). *Gut* **22**, 388–392.

Johnson, W. M., and Lior, H. (1984). *Lancet* **1**, 229–230.

Jones, D. M., and Robinson, D. A. (1981). *Lancet* **1**, 440.

Jones, D. M., Eldridge, J., and Dale, B. (1980). *J. Clin. Pathol.* **33**, 767–769.

Jones, D. M., Robinson, D. A., and Eldridge, J. (1981). *J. Hyg.* **87**, 163–170.

Jones, P. H., Willis, A. T., Robinson, D. A., Skirrow, M. B., and Josephs, D. S. (1981). *J. Hyg.* **87**, 155–162.

Kaldor, J., and Speed, B. R. (1984). *Br. Med. J.* **288**, 1867–1870.

Kaldor, J., Pritchard, H., Serpell, A., and Metcalf, W. (1983). *J. Clin. Microbiol.* **18**, 1–4.

Karmali, M. A., and Fleming, P. C. (1979). *J. Pediatr.* **94**, 527–533.

Karmali, M. A., and Skirrow, M. B. (1984). *In* "Campylobacter Infections in Man and Animals" (J. P. Butzler, ed.), pp. 1–20. CRC Press, Boca Raton, Florida.

Karmali, M. A., and Tan, Y. C. (1980). *Can. Med. Assoc. J.* **122**, 192–193.

Karmali, M. A., De Grandis, S., and Fleming, P. C. (1981). *Antimicrob. Agents Chemother.* **19**, 593–597.

Kendall, E. J. C., and Tanner, E. I. (1982). *J. Hyg.* **88**, 155–163.

King, E. O. (1962). *Ann. N.Y. Acad. Sci.* **98**, 700–711.

Kist, M. (1982). *In* "Campylobacter: Epidemiology, Pathogenesis and Biochemistry" (D. G. Newell, ed.), pp. 138–143. MTP Press, Lancaster.

Kist, M., Keller, K.-M., Niebling, W., and Kilching, W. (1984). *Infection* **12**, 88–90.

Lambert, J. R., Tischler, M. E., Karmali, M. A., and Newman, A. (1979). *Can. Med. Assoc. J.* **121**, 1377–1379.

Lambert, M., Marion, E., Coche, E., and Butzler, J. P. (1982). *Lancet* **1**, 1409.

Lambert, M. E., Schofield, P. F., Ironside, A. G., and Mandal, B. K. (1979). *Br. Med. J.* **1**, 857–859.

Leung, F. Y.-K., Littlejohn, G. O., and Bombardier, C. (1980). *Arthritis Rheum.* **23**, 948–950.

Lichtenberger, C. J., and Perlino, C. A. (1982). *An. Intern. Med.* **97**, 147–148.

Lior, H., Woodward, D. L., Edgar, J. A., Laroche, L. J., and Gill, P. (1982). *J. Clin. Microbiol.* **15**, 761–768.

Logan, S. M., and Trust, T. J. (1982). *Infect. Immun.* **38**, 898–906.

Longfield, R., O'Donnell, J., Yudt, W., Lissner, C., and Burns, T. (1979). *Dig. Dis. Sci.* **24**, 950–953.

Loss, R. W., Jr., Mangla, J. C., and Pereira, M. (1980). *Gastroenterology* **79**, 138–140.

Luechtefeld, N. W., Wang, W.-L. L., Blaser, M. J., and Reller, L. B. (1981). *Lab. Med.* **12**, 481–487.

McCardell, B. A., Madden, J. M., and Lee, E. C. (1984). *Lancet* **1**, 448–449.

McGechie, D. B., Teoh, T. B., and Bamford, V. W. (1982). *In* "Campylobacter: Epidemiology, Pathogenesis and Biochemistry" (D. G. Newell, ed.), pp. 19–21. MTP Press, Lancaster.

McKendrick, M. W., Geddes, A. M., and Gearty, J. (1982). *Scand. J. Infect. Dis.* **14**, 35–38.

McKinley, M. J., Taylor, M., and Sangree, M. H. (1980). *Conn. Med.* **44**, 496–497.
Mandal, B. K., and Ellis, M. E. (1983). *In* "Campylobacter II" (A. D. Pearson *et al.*, eds.), p. 27. Public Health Laboratory Service, London.
Mawer, S. L., and Smith, B. A. M. (1979). *Lancet* **1**, 1041.
Mee, A. S., and Shield, M. (1980). *Gut* **21**, A465.
Megraud, F., Tachoire, C., Latrille, J., and Bondonny, J. M. (1982). *Br. Med. J.* **285**, 1165–1166.
Menck, H. (1981). *Ugeskr. Laeg.* **143**, 1020.
Mentzing, L. O. (1981). *Lancet* **2**, 352.
Merrell, B. R., Walker, R. I., and Coolbaugh, J. C. (1981). *Scanning Electron Microsc.* **4**, 125–131.
Mertens, A., and De Smet, M. (1979). *Lancet* **1**, 1092.
Meuwissen, S. G. M., Bakkar, P. J. M., and Rietra, P. J. G. M. (1981). *Br. Med. J.* **282**, 1362.
Michalak, D. M., Perrault, J., Gilchrist, M. J., Dozois, R. R., Carney, J. A., and Sheedy, P. F., II (1980). *Gastroenterology* **79**, 742–745.
Molnar, G. K., Mertsola, J., and Erkko, M. (1982). *Br. Med. J.* **285**, 652.
Morrison, W. M., Matheson, J. A. B., Hutchison, R. B., and Mack, R. H. (1983). *Br. Med. J.* **286**, 765.
Mouton, R. P., Veltkamp, J. J., Lauwers, S., and Butzler, J. P. (1982). *In* "Campylobacter: Epidemiology, Pathogenesis and Biochemistry" (D. G. Newell, ed.), pp. 129–134. MTP Press, Lancaster.
Muytjens, J. L., and Hoogenhout, J. (1982). *Clin. Microbiol. Newsl.* p. 166.
Naess, V., and Hofstad, T. (1982). *In* "Campylobacter: Epidemiology, Pathogenesis and Biochemistry" (D. G. Newell, ed.), p. 242. MTP Press, Lancaster.
Nahum, H. D., Kaloustian, E., Baumer, P., Papaiconomou, A. F., and Lubetski, J. (1982). *Nouv. Presse Med.* **11**, 1805–1806.
Newell, D. G., and Pearson, A. D. (1982). *In* "Campylobacter: Epidemiology, Pathogenesis and Biochemistry" (D. G. Newell, ed.), pp. 196–199. MTP Press, Lancaster.
Newman, A., and Lambert, J. R. (1980). *Lancet* **2**, 919.
Noble, C. J., Hibbert, D. J., and Patel, G. J. (1982). *J. Infect.* **5**, 199–200.
Norrby, R., McCloskey, R. V., Zackrisson, G., and Falsen, E. (1980). *Br. Med. J.* **280**, 1164.
Olsvik, Ø., Wachsmut, K., Morris, G., and Feeley, J. C. (1984). *Lancet* **1**, 449.
Oosterom, J., Beckers, H. J., Van Noorle Jansen, L. M., and Van Schothorst, M. (1980). *Ned. Tijdschr. Geneeskd.* **124**, 1631–1633.
Owen, R. J. (1983). *Eur. J. Clin. Microbiol.* **2**, 367–377.
Paterson, A. (1981). *N.Z. J. Med. Lab. Technol.* **35**, 48–50.
Pearce, C. T. (1981). *Aust. J. Med. Lab. Sci.* **2**, 107–110.
Pearson, A. D., Drake, D. P., Brookfield, D., O'Connor, S., Suckling, W. G., Knill, M. J., Ware, E., and Knott, J. R. (1982). *In* "Campylobacter: Epidemiology, Pathogenesis and Biochemistry" (D. G. Newell, ed.), pp. 147–151. MTP Press, Lancaster.
Pedler, S. J., and Bint, A. J. (1984). *J. Infect.* **8**, 84–85.
Penner, J. L., and Hennessy, J. N. (1980). *J. Clin. Microbiol.* **12**, 732–737.
Pentland, B. (1979). *Scott. Med. J.* **24**, 299–301.
Pepersack, F., Prigogyne, T., Butzler, J. P., and Yourassowsky, E. (1979). *Lancet* **2**, 911.
Pepersack, F., D'Haene, M., Toussaint, C., and Schoutens, E. (1982). *J. Clin. Microbiol.* **16**, 739–741.
Pitkänen, T., Pettersson, T., Pönkä, A., and Kosunen, T. U. (1981). *Infection* **9**, 274–278.

Pitkänen, T., Pönkä, A., Pettersson, T., and Kosunen, T. U. (1983). *Arch. Intern. Med.* **143**, 215–219.

Pönkä, A., and Kosunen, T. U. (1981). *Acta Med. Scand:* **209**, 238–240.

Pönkä, A., and Kosunen, T. U. (1982). *Ann. Clin. Res.* **14**, 137–139.

Porter, I. A., and Reid, T. M. S. (1980). *J. Hyg.* **84**, 415–419.

Price, A. B., Jewkes, J., and Sanderson, P. J. (1979). *J. Clin. Pathol.* **32**, 990–997.

Quinn, T. C., Corey, L., Chaffee, R. G., Schuffler, M. D., and Holmes, K. K. (1980). *Ann. Intern. Med.* **93**, 458–459.

Rautelin, H., and Kosunen, T. U. (1983). *J. Clin. Microbiol.* **17**, 700–701.

Reddy, K. R., and Thomas, E. (1982). *Gastroenterology* **82**, 1156.

Rettig, P. J. (1979). *J. Pediatr.* **94**, 855–864.

Rhodes, K. M., and Tattersfield, A. E. (1982). *Br. Med. J.* **285**, 173–174.

Richardson, N. J., Koornhof, H. J., Bokkenheuser, V. D., Mayet, Z., and Rosen, E. U. (1983). *Arch. Dis. Child.* **58**, 616–619.

Robinson, D. A. (1981). *Br. Med. J.* **282**, 1584.

Robinson, D. A., and Jones, D. M. (1981). *Brit. Med. J.* **282**, 1374–1376.

Ruiz-Palacios, G. M., Torres, J., Torres, N. I., Escamilla, E., Ruiz-Palacios, B. R., and Tamayo, J. (1983). *Lancet* **2**, 250–252.

Schaad, U. B. (1982). *Pediatr. Infect. Dis.* **1**, 328–332.

Schmidt, U., Chmel, H., Kaminski, Z., and Sen, P. (1980). *Q. J. Med.* [N. S.] **49**, 431–442.

Schofield, P. F., and Mandal, B. K. (1981). *Br. Med. J.* **283**, 1545.

Schofield, P. F., and Mandal, B. K. (1983). *Br. Med. J.* **286**, 646.

Sebald, M., and Véron, M. (1963). *Ann. Inst. Pasteur, Paris* **105**, 897–910.

Shmilovitz, M., Kretzer, B., and Rotman, N. (1982). *Isr. Med. Sci.* **18**, 935–940.

Short, C. D., Klouda, P. T., and Smith, L. (1982). *Ann. Rheum. Dis.* **41**, 287–288.

Shulman, S. T., and Moel, D. (1983). *Pediatrics* **72**, 47.

Skerman, V. B. D., McGowan, V., and Sneath, P. H. A. (1980). *Int. J. Syst. Bacteriol.* **30**, 270–271.

Skirrow, M. B. (1977). *Br. Med. J.* **2**, 9–11.

Skirrow, M. B. (1981). *Br. Med. J.* **282**, 1978.

Skirrow, M. B. (1982). *J. Hyg.* **89**, 175–184.

Skirrow, M. B., and Benjamin, J. (1980). *J. Hyg.* **85**, 427–442.

Skirrow, M. B., and Benjamin, J. (1982). *In* "Campylobacter: Epidemiology, Pathogenesis and Biochemistry" (D. G. Newell, ed.), pp. 40–44. MTP Press, Lancaster.

Skirrow, M. B., and Benjamin, J. (1984). *J. Clin. Pathol.* **37**, 478.

Skirrow, M. B., Fidoe, R. G., and Jones, D. M. (1981). *J. Infect.* **3**, 234–236.

Skirrow, M. B., Benjamin, J., Razi, M. H. H., and Waterman, S. (1982). *In* "Isolation and Identification Methods for Food Poisoning Organisms" (J. E. L. Corry, D. Roberts, and F. A. Skinner, eds.), pp. 313–328. Academic Press, London.

Smibert, R. M. (1974). *In* "Bergey's Manual of Determinative Bacteriology" (R. E. Buchanan and N. E. Gibbons, eds.), 8th ed., pp. 207–211. Williams & Wilkins, Baltimore, Maryland.

Soonattrakul, W., Andersen, B. R., and Bryner, J. H. (1971). *Am. J. Med. Sci.* **261**, 245–249.

Speed, B., Kaldor, J., Cavanagh, P. (1984). *J. Infect.* **8**, 85–86.

Steele, T. W., and McDermott, S. (1978). *Med. J. Aust.* **2**, 404–406.

Stoll, B. J., Glass, R. I., Huq, M. I., Khan, M. U., Holt, J. E., and Banu, H. (1982). *Br. Med. J.* **285**, 1185–1188.

Sumathipala, R. W., and Morrison, G. W. (1983). *Br. Med. J.* **286**, 1356.

Svedhem, Å., and Kaijser, B. (1980). *J. Infect. Dis.* **142**, 353–359.
Svedhem, Å., Gunnarsson, H., and Kaijser, B. (1983). *J. Infect. Dis.* **148**, 82–92.
Tanner, A. C. R., Badger, S., Lai, C.-H., Listgarten, M. A., Visconti, R. A., and Socransky, S. S. (1981). *Int. J. Syst. Bacteriol.* **31**, 432–445.
Taylor, D. J. (1982). *In* "Campylobacter: Epidemiology, Pathogenesis and Biochemistry" (D. G. Newell, ed.), pp. 163–167. MTP Press, Lancaster.
Telfer Brunton, W. A., Wilson, A. M. M., and Macrae, R. M. (1978). *Lancet* **2**, 1385.
Thomas, K., Chan, K. N., and Ribeiro, C. D. (1980). *Br. Med. J.* **1**, 1301–1302.
Thorén, A., Stintzing, G., Tufvesson, B., Walder, M., and Habte, D. (1982). *J. Trop. Pediatr.* **28**, 127–131.
van der Zwan, J. C. (1984). *Lancet* **1**, 449.
Vanhoof, R., Gordts, B., Dierickx, R., Coignau, H., and Butzler, J. P. (1980). *Antimicrob. Agents Chemother.* **18**, 118–121.
Vernon, S. E., and Dominguez, C. (1982). *Ann. Intern. Med.* **96**, 534.
Vinzent, R., Dumas, J., and Picard, N. (1947). *Bull. Acad. Natl. Med. (Paris)* **131**, 90.
Vogt, R. L., Sours, H. E., Barrett, T., Feldman, R. A., Dickinson, R. J., and Witherell, L. (1982). *Ann. Intern. Med.* **96**, 292–296.
Walder, M. (1982). *Scand. J. Infect. Dis.* **14**, 27–33.
Wallace, J. M. (1980). *Health Bull. (Edinb.)* **38**, 57–62.
Warren, J. R., and Marshall, B. J. (1983). *Lancet* **1**, 1273–1275.
Williams, G. V., and Deacon, G. J. (1980). *Med. J. Aust.* **2**, 268–271.
Willoughby, C. P., Piris, J., and Truelove, S. C. (1979). *J. Clin. Pathol.* **32**, 986–989.
Wong, P. Yeen, Puthucheary, S. D., and Pang, T. (1983). *J. Clin. Pathol.* **36**, 1237–1240.
Wright, E. P. (1979). *Lancet* **1**, 1092.
Wright, E. P., and Knowles, M. A. (1980). *J. Clin. Pathol.* **33**, 904–905.
Wright, E. P., and Seager, J. (1980). *Br. Med. J.* **281**, 454.
Wright, E. P., Balsdon, M. J., and Okubadejo, O. A. (1982). *Lancet* **2**, 380.

6 *Haemophilus ducreyi* and chancroid

S. HAFIZ, G. R. KINGHORN and M. G. McENTEGART

I. INTRODUCTION

The literature that has accumulated on *Haemophilus ducreyi* infections since Ducrey's original description in 1890 is much more extensive than might be expected on what was for long considered to be a "rare" and exotic infection. In retrospect it seems that the combination of low clinical expectation with laboratory pessimism about growing *H. ducreyi* ensured that the diagnosis of such infections in the United Kingdom was indeed rare.

Events since 1977 are slowly changing ideas and attitudes, so that there is now in many parts of the world a lively interest in the role of *H. ducreyi* in the pathogenesis of genital ulceration.

Several authors have reviewed the early events in the history of *H. ducreyi* infections (Himmel, 1901; Hewlett, 1929; Sullivan, 1940; McEntegart *et al.*, 1982), so that in order to provide an adequate understanding of the events leading to our present view of the infection we can confine ourselves to papers published in more recent years.

Rajan and Sng (1982) give an account of the epidemiology of the disease on a worldwide basis. These observations reflect not so much the spread of the disease as the growing interest in the possibility of *H. ducreyi* infections in patients with genital ulceration. Such reports have come from France (Morel, 1974; Morel *et al.*, 1982), Turkey (Nurat *et al.*, 1978), Holland (Nayyar *et al.*, 1979), Greenland (Lykke Olesen *et al.*, 1979), and Germany (Stüttgen, 1982). Similarly, accounts have been published of outbreaks in North America (Hammond *et al.*, 1980; Handsfield *et al.*, 1981; Centers for Disease Control, 1982).

In 1982 we reported a series of 22 cases of *H. ducreyi* infections diagnosed in

Medical Microbiology, 4
ISBN 0-12-228004-0

Sheffield (Hafiz *et al.*, 1982). These were unselected patients with genital ulceration. The findings were of special interest for two reasons. In many patients, *H. ducreyi* was not the sole nor indeed the principal pathogen, and the great majority of patients had acquired their infection from local contacts, very few having been abroad.

II. CULTURAL METHODS

Until more reliable cultural methods were established, the clinical diagnosis of soft sore was confirmed by the examination of stained films from the lesions, showing the organisms in a typical configuration. Of the many descriptions given, perhaps ''shoals of fish'' is the most well known and evocative (Fig. 1). Smears were generally prepared from the suspect lesion, but confirmation on the basis of a characteristic appearance was also made from cultures of ulcer material inoculated into defibrinated rabbit blood (Heyman *et al.*, 1945). In 1946 Beeson reported that both serum and erythrocytes would, when added to an agar base, support the growth of *H. ducreyi*. Perhaps the most significant finding stressed in this paper was the need for a high humidity if the organism was to be grown on solid media. New information about culture methods was very slow in gaining acceptance. Thus in 1970, Borchardt and Hoke recommended culture by the inoculation of serous fluid from the lesions into 10 ml of the patient's own blood (inactivated at 56°C for 30 min). The typical appearance of smears from such cultures were described as ''railroad tracks.'' In 1977, Tan *et al.* used a similar method whereby swabs from suspect lesions were inoculated into the patient's serum, again heat-inactivated.

Looking back, it seems likely that such methods, which based the final diagnosis on the microscopic morphology in a stained smear, may well have exaggerated the incidence in areas of high expectation whilst reducing it in others where the diagnosis was considered to be unlikely.

An indication of a change in approach to the clinical problem of genital ulceration can be found in the study of Barile and his colleagues, who in 1962 published the results on a detailed study of penile lesions in American forces in Japan. Their results show that *H. ducreyi* was isolated from 23% of patients and herpesvirus from 31%, from a few patients both organisms were isolated.

This study was perhaps seen as a rather specialized one and there was little change in the bacteriological support available to the clinician. Chapel *et al.* in 1978 made a detailed study of the flora of penile ulcerations and found a significant mixed flora in the majority of 100 patients studied. *Herpes simplex* was the most commonly identified cause. *Haemophilus ducreyi* was isolated from 2 patients only. In the light of recent studies it seems probable that this low

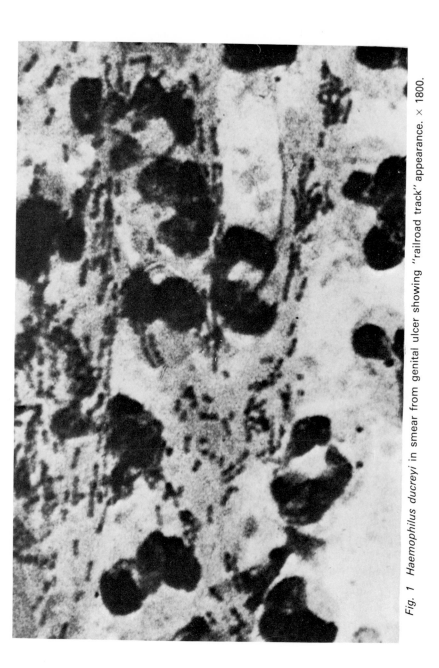

Fig. 1 *Haemophilus ducreyi* in smear from genital ulcer showing "railroad track" appearance. × 1800.

isolation rate was largely due to the absence of any adequate direct cultural method. In 1976 Kilian published a study of 426 strains of the *Haemophilus* genus, including 9 strains of *H. ducreyi*. All the strains he examined were stock strains that had originally been isolated from patients with chancroid. Of the strains he examined, he considered 7 to be unacceptable as members of the *Haemophilus* genus, although they might conform to Ducrey's original description.

A major advance in the laboratory diagnosis of *H. ducreyi* infections was the introduction by Hammond and his co-workers (1978a) of a selective chocolate blood agar medium containing 1% Isovitalex and 3 μg vancomycin/ml. The medium ensured successful isolation of *H. ducreyi* from a substantial proportion of suspected lesions. Hafiz *et al.* (1981) have subsequently reported a clear medium containing haemin to be successful in isolating the organism.

III. COLONIAL MORPHOLOGY

The most consistent observation made by workers who have grown *H. ducreyi* on solid media has been the remarkably coherent colonies produced. Although the relative hardness of the colony varies from one medium to another, colonies of *H. ducreyi* can, almost without exception, be pushed intact across the surface of the medium. They are difficult to pick up and, once removed from the medium, are difficult to emulsify and consequently difficult to quantitate as in preparing standard inocula for antibiotic sensitivity testing.

Although we have been able to improve the solid media available for *H. ducreyi* to speed up growth, and so obtain larger colonies, we have so far failed to obtain uniform turbidity in liquid medium.

In all media we have tried, the organism grows in the form of stalactites adherent to the wall of the tube and suspended in the medium. Such masses of growth are difficult to disperse and if dislodged sink to the bottom of the tube.

A. Electron microscopy of colonies

Examination of colonies under the scanning electron microscope reveals an appearance strikingly different from other organisms—for example, the gonococcus—and one that suggests that the organisms that make up the *H. ducreyi* colony are embedded in some matrix. We have failed, however, to break up this "matrix" with any enzymatic or chemical treatment we have tried. A uniform suspension can be made by sonication at amplitude of 3–6 μm for 1 minute. Clearly the reasons for the colonial character of *H. ducreyi* require further study.

IV. ULTRASTRUCTURE OF *H. DUCREYI*

The ultrastructure of *H. ducreyi* has been outlined by Kilian and Theilade (1975), Ovchinnikov *et al.* (1976) and Marsch *et al.* (1978). In tissue biopsies from chancroidal ulcers, the organism is predominantly located in the extracellular spaces and appears as a coccoid–bacillary rod, 1.25–1.40 μm long and 0.55–0.60 μm broad, with rounded ends. The cell wall has the typical trilaminar structure of Gram-negative organisms, a thickness of 115–125 Å, and is composed of two electron-dense layers separated by an electron-translucent layer. The cytoplasm is rich in ribosomes, and includes a fibrillar nucleoid; mesothomes and cross-wall formation are scanty.

V. BIOCHEMICAL ACTIVITIES OF *H. DUCREYI*

The justification for the inclusion of Ducrey's bacillus in the genus *Haemophilus* is that it is haemin-dependent, as demonstrated by the porphyrin test (Kilian, 1974). In the latter test, haemin-independent organisms, when provided with δ-aminolevulinic acid (δALA), produce porphobilinogen and porphyrins. By this test, all strains of *H. ducreyi* tested are haemin-dependent.

One of the problems in attempting to characterise *H. ducreyi* is that it is relatively inert biochemically. There is general agreement that the organism is alkaline-phosphatase-positive and reduces nitrates; the oxidase reaction is positive when tested with 1% N,N,N',N'-tetramethyl-p-phenylenediamine dihydrochloride (Nobre, 1982), but all other standard biochemical tests are negative. Most if not all strains have very little action against the normal range of bacteriological sugars, although some exceptions have been reported.

In view of this very limited carbohydrate utilization, it is interesting to record the results of work carried out in Paris by Casin and his co-workers (1982), who tested 2 reference strains and 30 other strains isolated from clinical chancroid. Of their isolates, 93% were β-lactamase producers. This group tested their strains not only by conventional biochemical methods but also by various API/ZYM systems using some 97 substrates. Their study confirmed the absence of activity in the porphyrin test and absence of any glycosidase activity. All strains showed a wide range of aminopeptidase activities, the only variation being in three strains which showed, in addition, activity against proline and hydroproline. It is surprising that this should be an uncommon activity in view of the stimulating effect on growth of gelatin, which we had thought was probably due to the presence of proline. The authors conclude that the extended knowledge of the enzymatic profile of *H. ducreyi* could lead to a better understanding of its precise growth requirements.

We have repeated this work in Sheffield and tested 12 local, 4 foreign and 2 reference strains of *H. ducreyi*. We found no strains with activity against proline or hydroxyproline; otherwise there was complete accord in the results of testing strains from different geographical areas and clinical isolates from patients with and without genital ulcers. Our results were virtually identical with those of the Parisian workers.

VI. ANTIMICROBIAL SENSITIVITY AND RESISTANCE

Although there were a number of papers published in the late 1940s recording studies on the antimicrobial susceptibility of *H. ducreyi* (Mortara *et al.*, 1944; Mortara and Saito, 1946; Beeson, 1946; Reymann, 1949; Wetherbee *et al.*, 1949; Thayer *et al.*, 1955), the major advances have been made since 1977.

As interest in the subject increased there was a need to explore the effects of a whole range of antimicrobial substances, not only to find the best drug for treatment but also to identify the most useful substances for inclusion in selective media for the isolation of *H. ducreyi*.

Understandably, in studies on the mechanisms of resistance most attention has been paid to the coding of strains for β-lactamase production and we now know a great deal about the plasmids present in ampicillin-resistant strains.

In 1978 Hammond and his co-workers published the results of their studies on 19 strains of *H. ducreyi* isolated during a circumscribed outbreak of chancroid in Canada (Hammond *et al.*, 1978c). They tested these strains against 13 antimicrobial agents. Three of their 19 isolates were resistant to β-lactam antibiotics and were β-lactamase producers. This finding fits in well with the report by Kuhlwein *et al.* (1980) of 3 patients, infected in West Africa, whose lesions were diagnosed as due to syphilis and who received 12 days penicillin treatment without benefit. These lesions responded in Hamburg to doxycycline treatment.

Plasmid-mediated ampicillin resistance in *H. ducreyi* was reported by Brunton *et al.* in 1979 when they described a 6 MDa plasmid which coded for β-lactamase production. This work was extended the following year when Mac-Lean *et al.* (1980) reported that the plasmid they had isolated coded for a TEM.1 type of β-lactamase originating from the transposon Tn 2. Handsfield *et al.* (1981) isolated six strains of *H. ducreyi* from seven clinical cases of chancroid. The first patient, infected in the Philippines infected two others in the United States, one of whom infected a further patient. Three remaining patients had been infected outside the United States. Only six strains were available for study, but their ampicillin resistance plasmids were identified and found to be of three sizes: 7.3, 5.7 and 3.2 MDa. Both plasmid size and antibiotic resistance patterns of the epidemiologically linked strains were the same, thus providing a possible marker. All the six strains isolated were resistant to ampicillin and to tetracycline (MIC greater than 16 μg/ml). Four were chloramphenicol-resistant (16 μg/ml) and one was resistant to streptomycin (16 μg/ml). All were sensitive to erythromycin and cefotaxime.

Girouard and his co-workers (1981) found that 33 of 47 strains they tested were β-lactamase producers. Using an agar dilution method, they reported the synergistic effect of clavulanic acid and ampicillin on the β-lactamase-producing strains. The combination gave MICs for ampicillin equal to those of sensitive strains. A clinical trial of this combined therapy was reported by Fast *et al.* (1982). All strains isolated from 100 patients in Nairobi were β-lactamase producers, and, although ampicillin alone failed to produce a cure, combined therapy was successful.

Sulphonamide resistance due to the presence in some strains of *H. ducreyi* of one or more plasmids of 4.9, 5.7, or 7.0 MDa was reported by Albritton *et al.* (1982). In a very detailed study, they suggest that one plasmid appeared to be closely related to the enteric plasmid pool. They comment that the demonstration of plasmid-mediated sulphonamide resistance does not exclude the possibility of chromosomal resistance in other strains of the organism.

Sanson-Le Pors *et al.* (1982) found 1 isolate amongst 29 strains of *H. ducreyi* they examined, which was resistant to chloramphenicol (MIC 16 μg/ml) and inactivated the drug. They showed that this strain produced a chloramphenicol acetyltransferase (CAT). This strain was a tetracycline-resistant β-lactamase producer, and it was thought possible that the chloramphenicol resistance was also plasmid-mediated.

W. L. Albritton (personal communication) has also described a 30-MDa plasmid encoding for tetracycline resistance and a 34.0-MDa plasmid encoding for chloramphenicol resistance.

An account of the antibiotic resistance of South African strains of the organism was given by Bilgeri and her colleagues (1982). This showed that 96 of 103 isolates of *H. ducreyi* tested in Johannesberg were β-lactamase producers. Most of these were also resistant to tetracycline and sulphonamide. All their isolates were sensitive to rifampin, erythromycin and cefoxitin. Plasmids from 7 of these strains were found to have masses of 3.95, 5.2, 5.8 and 6.4 MDa. Of these, all but the 5.8-MDa one encoded for β-lactamase production. The 5.2- and 6.4-MDa ones could be conjugally transferred to a streptomycin-resistant strain of *H. ducreyi*. They thought that this transfer occurred owing to the presence of a large plasmid in the recipient strain. Further evidence for the transfer of resistance plasmids of *H. ducreyi* was provided by Deneer *et al.* (1982), who showed that an isolate they studied had three plasmids, a cryptic one of 23.5 MDa, a 7.0-MDa ampicillin resistance one and a 4.9-MDa sulphonamide resistance one. Both the small plasmids were transferable, providing the recipient strain also harboured the 23.5-MDa plasmid, which appears, therefore, to have mobilizing capabilities. Transfer of R plasmids was also possible to *Escherichia coli* recipients and to *H. influenzae*.

McNichol *et al.* (1983) have found that the ampicillin resistance plasmids of *H. ducreyi* and *Neisseria gonorrhoeae* are similar, and it now seems clear that β-lactamase production by the two species is closely linked microbiologically and geographically.

Sng *et al.* (1982) record further observations on antibiotic sensitivity patterns of *H. ducreyi* isolates in Singapore. All 17 of the strains they studied were resistant to vancomycin (MIC > 16 μg/ml), 13 were tetracycline-resistant, 11 were sulphonamide-resistant, and 12 were β-lactamase producers. All strains were sensitive to erythromycin, co-trimoxazole and streptomycin.

It is difficult to reconcile these findings with those of Rajan and Sng (1982), who reported that 51.7% of culture-proven cases of chancroid failed to respond to streptomycin, a finding supported by a high percentage of *in vitro* streptomycin and kanamycin resistance. The authors wonder if this finding is related to the widespread use of aminoglycosides in the treatment of gonorrhoea due to penicillinase producing strains of *N. gonorrhoeae*.

Sturm and Zanen (1983), in an article entitled ''The drug of choice for chancroid,'' reported on their sensitivity patterns in a study of 19 strains of *H. ducreyi* isolated in Amsterdam. Of these, 13 were β-lactamase producers and 13 were also tetracycline-resistant. Eleven were resistant to aminoglycosides and 11 also to chloramphenicol. All were sensitive to trimethoprim and erythromycin. The resistance patterns occurred in the following combinations:

1. Fully sensitive, β-lactamase-negative
2. Fully resistant, β-lactamase-positive
3. Tetracycline-resistant, streptomycin- and chloramphenicol-sensitive, β-lactamase-positive

Our findings in Sheffield, based on the study of some 150 strains, are as follows. Only 4 were β-lactamase producers, of which 2 were known to have been acquired abroad and 2 apparently from local contacts. The majority of our strains are sensitive to ampicillin and tetracycline, erythromycin and sulphonamides. In this respect the indigenous European strains appear to differ from the very much more resistant imported strains.

A difficulty which arises when attempting to compare the findings of different groups of workers is the lack of any standard method for testing antibiotic sensitivity. This problem is aggravated by the peculiarities of the cells of *H. ducreyi*, which are coherent and very difficult to emulsify, thus making accurate quantitation of inocula difficult. Unfortunately the organism also shows a remarkable reluctance to grow in liquid media.

At present the most reliable method is the use of agar dilutions making use of inocula, standardized as well as possible, from cultures on solid media.

VII.   INFECTIVITY AND PATHOGENICITY

Clinical evidence suggests that *H. ducreyi* is an organism of low infectivity, a view supported by the results of autoinoculation and animal experiments. Thus the application of *H. ducreyi* to the intact skin does not produce a lesion— indeed, even scarification followed by the application of the organism may fail to produce a lesion in experimental animals. Only direct intradermal injection is consistently successful in producing a skin lesion in the rabbit.

The natural history of the disease in man suggests that the characteristic ulcers of chancroid result from the infection by *H. ducreyi* of minor traumatic lesions of the genital skin or mucosa or occasionally from the infection due to some other infecting agent such as *Herpes simplex* virus.

So far as we know, no specific bacterial toxin or other product has been identified to explain the tissue damage produced by the organism. Nevertheless, it is said that old laboratory strains, such as type cultures of *H. ducreyi,* may lose their pathogenicity as demonstrated by the ability to produce a typical skin lesion (Dienst, 1948).

Experimental lesions in the skin of rabbits have been studied histologically but are without any very specific features to distinguish them from any of the non-specific ulcers. Lesions produced on the chorioallantoic membrane of chick embryos are equally nonspecific. As the growing interest in *H. ducreyi* infections provides more strains than ever before, derived from many parts of the world and demonstrably different at least in antibiotic patterns and plasmid content, it should be possible to see if any differences in pathogenicity or infectivity can be detected.

Certainly the way in which chancroid can from time to time show an almost epidemic spread, as in Greenland in 1978, suggests that the infectivity of strains may vary considerably.

Likewise, the demonstration by several workers that the organism may be isolated from asymptomatic consorts or other contacts of clinical cases implies a very low infectivity in some individuals.

A.   Marker characteristics

Reference has been made to the value of plasmid molecular weights, especially in conjunction with antibiograms of organisms, as epidemiological markers to trace the spread of *H. ducreyi.* However, the study of plasmids is a costly and time-consuming one and not a realistic method for smaller clinical laboratories, which may, nonetheless, be providing diagnostic services to the local clinic.

Odumeru *et al.* (1983) examined the whole-cell proteins of 105 clinical iso-lates of *H. ducreyi* from several geographic sources by sodium dodecylsulfate–polyacrylamide gel electrophoresis (SDS-PAGE). They found heterogeneity in the protein composition of *H. ducreyi,* and at least 7 different subtypes were determined by proteins of the outer cell membrane, in the molecular weight range 24,000–50,000. Most of the isolates obtained from the Winnipeg outbreak had identical protein profiles, indicating a common origin. This method of sub-typing *H. ducreyi* could be of value in future epidemiologic studies of chancroid.

There is scope, therefore, for further study in an attempt to find some rela-tively cheap, simple and reliable typing method so that we can more accurately study the source and spread of strains of *H. ducreyi* in the community, both in the West and in Third World countries.

VIII. EPIDEMIOLOGY AND CLINICAL ASPECTS

It seems profitable before proceeding to a detailed account of the laboratory aspects of the subject to look in some detail at what we have learned about the clinical and epidemiological features of chancroidal ulceration.

Although experimental lesions have been induced in primates, rabbits and on the chorioallantoic membrane of chick embryos, man is the only natural host for *H. ducreyi* infection.

The role of *H. ducreyi* in the pathogenesis of chancroidal ulcers is supported, if not confirmed, by its isolation from ulcers as part of a mixed bacterial flora; it has been isolated in pure culture more often from inguinal bubos, although in many studies bubo fluid has been found bacteriologically sterile. It is clear that other bacteria, both anaerobic and aerobic, may cause ulcers indistinguishable from classical chancroid. Recent studies show that a polymicrobial pathogenic flora is common in such lesions (Chapel *et al.,* 1978; Kinghorn *et al.,* 1982b).

Until recently, epidemiological and clinical studies of chancroid were based on presumptive diagnoses made of typical clinical lesions, in the absence of other pathogens. Confirmation by the isolation of *H. ducreyi* was either unsuccessful or not attempted. The recent development of reliable methods for the cultivation of *H. ducreyi* has allowed a clearer view of the true incidence of bacteriologically confirmed chancroid. Such culture based studies may in time challenge tradi-tional concepts of its epidemiology.

A. Incidence

Today the worldwide incidence of chancroid exceeds that of syphilis. In recent studies, the frequency with which *H. ducreyi* has been isolated from non-treponemal genital ulcers has shown considerable geographical variation.

The conventional view of chancroid is that the disease is endemic in many tropical and subtropical countries, but rare in temperate ones. In the latter, sporadic imported cases are seen in merchant seamen and other persons returning from the tropics, and these may give rise to small localised epidemics. During the past decade, however, chancroid outbreaks have been reported in many nontropical countries both in North America and Europe, which suggests that endemic foci of infection are now occurring in these areas.

Like all sexually transmitted diseases, the incidence of chancroid rises dramatically during wartime. The higher incidence in Black compared to Causcasian servicemen has suggested a differing racial susceptibility to the infection. This may, in part, relate to the frequency of circumcision in different ethnic groups, chancroid being uncommon in circumcised men. The disease has long been associated with poor personal hygiene and low socioeconomic conditions; nevertheless, anyone coming into contact with the organism may acquire an infection, so long as there is some minor skin lesion to provide a portal of entry for the organism.

Chancroid is now most frequent in young sexually active men and women. Earlier studies showed a high male-to-female ratio of incidence. Trivial self-limiting lesions, for which medical advice is not sought, occur more often in women. Prostitutes, especially in Eastern societies, are thus an important source of the infection, as each may infect many men. In contrast, recent studies in more "liberal" Western countries have shown an equal sex incidence.

B.   Asymptomatic carriers

There are conflicting views on the role of asymptomatic carriers in the epidemiology of chancroid. Their existence particularly amongst prostitutes was suggested by the high male–female case ratio. The earliest account was that of Bruck (1916), who traced the asymptomatic female contact of two soldiers with soft sore. Further evidence was provided by the demonstration of *H. ducreyi*-like organisms in the genital tract of asymptomatic prostitutes in Singapore (Khoo *et al.*, 1977). In the 1920s, Brams (1924) and Saelhof (1925) demonstrated *H. ducreyi*-like organisms in asymptomatic men, particularly those with long-phimotic prepuces where smegma had collected. Recent African and Canadian studies have failed to demonstrate carriage of *H. ducreyi* in women without genital ulcers, although the organism could be isolated from women with asymptomatic ulcers (Ronald, 1980; Nsanze *et al.*, 1982).

Bacteriologically confirmed *H. ducreyi* has been found in the absence of genital ulcers in both men and women in Sheffield (Kinghorn *et al.*, 1983a) and in California (Centers for Disease Control, 1982), positive isolations being most likely in those harbouring other sexually transmitted pathogens. We have also found asymptomatic oropharyngeal *H. ducreyi* infections (Kinghorn *et al.*, 1983).

C. Mode of transmission

Infection is predominantly (1) sexually transmitted, but (2) accidental inoculation has resulted in extragenital lesions especially in doctors, nurses and laboratory workers; (3) autoinoculation of material from primary genital chancroid lesions may result in secondary lesions elsewhere, and (4) in asymptomatic carriers autoinfection of lesions caused by trauma or other microbial pathogens may result in secondary chancroidal ulcers.

D. Incubation period

The incubation period of sexually acquired chancroid and also of experimentally induced skin lesions is short, usually 1–5 days. In some patients, especially women, the appearance of lesions may be delayed for up to 14 days after infection. Longer incubation periods may occur in autoinfection, for we have observed a patient, without any sexual contact for 4 years, who developed secondary *H. ducreyi* infection in an area of excoriated penile psoriasis.

E. Immunity

There are very few recent studies on the immunology of *H. ducreyi*. It appears that an immune response, both humoral and cell-mediated, occurs in clinical cases, but these do not have any practical diagnostic application nor appear to provide any useful protection against autoinoculation or subsequent reinfection.

Many immunological questions arise. Is it possible that strains that are known to differ in plasmid content and antibiotic sensitivity might also differ serologically? If so, then serology of strains could contribute to epidemiology.

Could more sensitive techniques such as immunofluorescence (Denys *et al.*, 1978) or ELISA methods provide practical help in the diagnosis of cases, or even of asymptomatic carriers, especially if they were healed cases?

IX. CLINICAL FEATURES

A. Symptoms and signs

Patients usually present with painful genital ulcers and inguinal adenitis with or without suppuration. Constitutional symptoms are rare.

Any abrasion, excoriation or ulceration caused by trauma, irritation due to lack of personal hygiene, or other sexually transmitted pathogens allows *H. ducreyi* a portal of entry to infect the skin or mucosa. After 1–5 days, an initial macule or papule appears at the site of inoculation and rapidly passes through vesicular and pustular stages to form a sharply circumscribed ulcer. In classical form the chancroidal ulcer varies in diameter from 1 mm to 2 cm. The edges are irregular, often scalloped, and undermined with a surrounding erythematous halo. The ulcer crater is usually filled with a greyish or purulent exudate, which on removal reveals a base of irregular framboesiform granulation tissue which bleeds easily. Chancroidal ulcers, in contrast to the syphilitic chancre, are usually nonindurated and extremely painful.

Multiple ulcers are commoner than single lesions, especially where there is secondary *H. ducreyi* infection of genital herpes (Figs. 2 and 3). The typical appearance of lesions may be modified in some anatomical sites and by association with other genital pathogens. Follicular, dwarf, transient, papular, giant and phagadenic chancroid variants have been described. Recently a variety of the papular chancroid in the absence of lymphadenopathy, mimicking granuloma inguinale, was described by Kraus *et al.* (1982a).

B.   Location

Primary lesions usually occur in and around the genital region and are rare on the upper half of the body. In men, the preputial orifice and its internal surface, the frenulum, and the coronal sulcus are the most commonly affected sites (Fig. 4). Lesions on the glans and penile shaft are less often seen. These affected areas are often moist and macerated and particularly subject to minor trauma during intercourse. The lower temperature of these sites may also favour *H. ducreyi* growth.

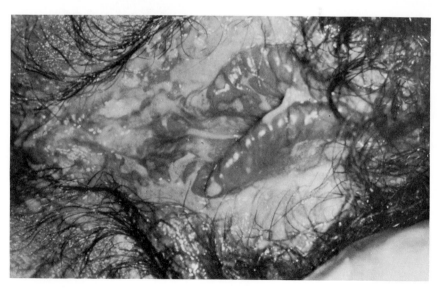

Fig. 2   Haemophilus ducreyi associated with primary herpes simplex type 2 infection in a 20-year-old woman.

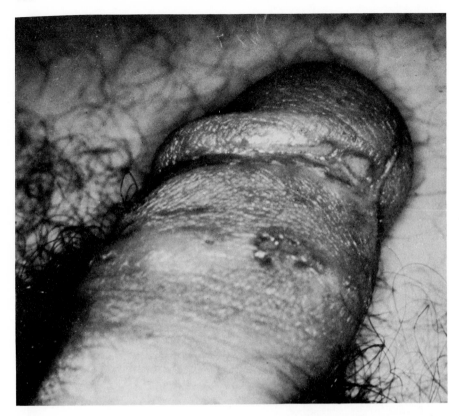

Fig. 3 Haemophilus ducreyi associated with multiple lesions of primary herpes simplex type 2.

Rarely, chancroidal urethritis has been reported. In women, the labia, clitoris and fourchette are the favoured sites, although lesions can also occur on the cervix. Lesions on the perineum and anus may occur in women and passive homosexuals.

Extragenital lesions are rare, although they have been reported in the oropharynx, breast, fingers and bulbar conjunctiva (Sullivan, 1940). In Sheffield we have described several cases of oropharyngeal ulceration from which *H. ducreyi* has been isolated (Kinghorn *et al.*, 1983).

Autoinoculation lesions may occur in the inguinal region after bubo rupture, and also on the thigh and scrotum.

C. Course and complications

Spontaneous resolution without complications occurs in up to half of untreated cases, especially in women, although the organism may persist for long periods thereafter (Kinghorn *et al.*, 1982b).

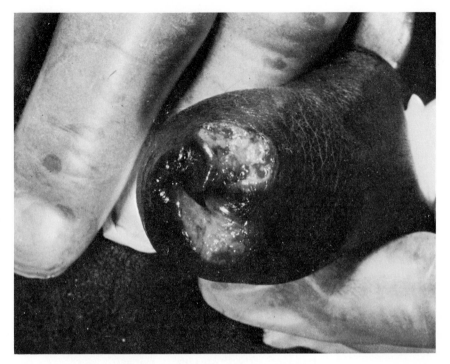

Fig. 4 Chancroid preputal ulceration.

Inguinal bubo occurs in one-third to one-half of untreated cases and is more likely the longer presentation and treatment is delayed. It is commoner with small inaccessible primary lesions, especially those associated with phimosis and poor external drainage. In two-thirds of cases the bubos are unilateral. Initially there is lymphadenitis when the glands become enlarged and tender, and subsequently matted and fused with inflammation and tenderness of the overlying skin. Unilocular suppuration may then ensue. Although spontaneous healing occurs in some cases, the resulting ulceration may develop into a giant chancroid, which extends peripherally by continuous autoinoculation (Fig. 5).

Small bubonuli may develop anywhere along the lymphatic drainage of the primary ulcer.

Autoinoculation from primary lesions may occur on the thigh, scrotum or adjacent genital skin and less frequently on the fingers and other extragenital sites.

Phimosis and paraphimosis may occur in the acute stage of infection, or as a result of the scarring of the prepuce which often follows healing of the lesion.

Phagadenic ulcers as a result of secondary anaerobic infections are most common, with ulcers on the inner aspect of the prepuce and coronal sulcus.

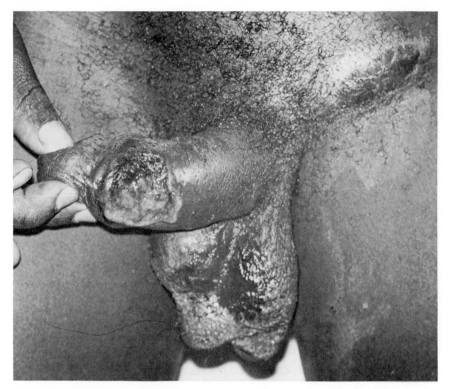

Fig. 5 Giant chancroid with left inguinal bubo (courtesy of Dr. R. S. Morton).

Concurrent infection with *Treponema pallidum, Herpes simplex,* and *Chlamydia trachomatis* strains causing lymphogranuloma venereum may be followed by complications of these infections as well as modifying the clinical appearances of the chancroidal lesions.

X.   DIAGNOSIS

A.   Isolation

Diagnosis of chancroid by the exclusion of other pathogens, and on the basis of typical clinical appearances, can no longer be accepted. A definitive diagnosis today can only be made when *H. ducreyi* is isolated from the ulcer exudate or bubo aspirate. Ideally, specimens should be inoculated directly onto plates of suitable culture media when the patient is first seen in the clinic. If this is not possible, swabs may be sent to the laboratory in Amies transport medium within 4 hours.

B. Smear examination

Gram-stained smears of ulcer exudate or bubo aspirate may show organisms in coccobacillary chains in a mucous matrix in the typical "railroad tracks" or "shoals of fish" pattern characteristic of *H. ducreyi* (Fig. 1). Although this may give a rapid presumptive diagnosis, it lacks sensitivity and specificity and should not be regarded as diagnostic. Alternatives include using Giemsa, Wright's and fluorescent staining methods.

C. Biopsy

Biopsy cannot be justified unless there is a strong suspicion of granuloma inguinale or malignancy. Heyman *et al.* (1945) have described the typical histological appearances of chancroid.

D. Skin testing

Autoinoculation of ulcer exudate intradermally into the forearm or thigh, in an attempt to produce secondary lesions from which *H. ducreyi* could be identified more easily, was used as a standard diagnostic method for many years but can rarely be justified now.

Intradermal injection of heat-killed *H. ducreyi* antigen to demonstrate delayed skin hypersensitivity by the Ito–Reenstierna test was another previously fashionable diagnostic method. This has also gone out of use, partly because of the disappearance of commercial antigen. Its usefulness was limited due to the delayed development of positivity in primary infections and also because the subsequent positive reaction was lifelong, which precluded its use in the diagnosis of reinfections.

E. Serological testing

There is no routine serological method available for diagnosis. Research into the development of sensitive serological methods is continuing.

F. Differential diagnosis

Although syphilis must be excluded in any genital ulcer, *Herpes simplex* virus and secondary pyogenic infection of traumatic lesions are the most common causes of such lesions in the United Kingdom. Lymphogranuloma venereum (LGV) and granuloma inguinale must also be considered in lesions acquired in the tropics. Excoriated scabies, allergic conditions—e.g., fixed drug eruption, genital dermatoses, and Behcet's syndrome—and neoplasms also feature in the differential diagnosis of genital ulceration.

It should be remembered not only that chancroidal ulcers may be caused by other infectious agents, but also that *H. ducreyi* may coexist in the same lesion with other pathogens, especially *Herpes simplex* and *Treponema pallidum*. It is therefore essential that all genital ulcers be thoroughly investigated for a poly-microbial aetiology.

G. Investigation of genital ulcers

Serum from abraded ulcers should be examined on three consecutive days under dark-field microscopy for the presence of *T. pallidum*. Appropriate specimens should be taken for the attempted cultural isolation of (a) *H. ducreyi*, (b) other aerobic and anaerobic bacteria, (c) *Herpes simplex* virus and (d) *Chlamydia trachomatis* (if LGV is suspected). Serum should be taken for syphilis serology, herpes antibodies, and where indicated to diagnose LGV by complement fixation or microimmunofluorescence tests. Biopsy is indicated only when malignancy or granuloma inguinale are suspected.

All serological tests should be repeated after 14–21 days, and for syphilis alone again at 5 weeks and 3 months.

XI.   MANAGEMENT

Specific treatment should not be started until all investigations of genital ulcers and other sexually transmitted diseases elsewhere in the genital tract have been undertaken.

A.   Local therapy

Saline bathes or irrigations are a useful adjunct to systemic therapy.

B.   Systemic therapy

Treponemicidal antibiotics should be avoided until syphilis has been excluded.

The antibiotic sensitivity of *H. ducreyi* isolates shows considerable geographic variation and should be taken into account in choice of therapy. Recommended treatment schedules no longer include sulphonamides or tetracyclines alone or in combination in many parts of the world.

Co-trimoxazole, 2 tablets twice daily, or erythromycin, 500 mg four times daily, are the drugs of choice. They should be given for 14 days, or until ulcers and adenopathy have healed.

Amoxycillin (500 mg), with clavulanate (250 mg) (a potent β-lactamase inhib-itor), given three times daily for 7 days, have proven successful in recent clinical trials (Fast *et al.*, 1982).

Streptomycin or kanamycin, 0.5 g i.m. twice daily for 7 days, necessitates inpatient therapy, has risks of ototoxicity and nephrotoxicity, and is rarely successful in treating bubos.

Chloramphenicol, 750 mg b.d. for 7 days, can also be used but has risks of serious haematological complications. Recently, resistance to the aminoglycosides and to chloramphenicol has become more widespread in *H. ducreyi* isolates in the Far East, and they should only be used as second-line drugs.

Single-dose therapy, which eliminates the problems of patient compliance, is increasingly being advocated. Use of co-trimoxazole (8 tablets stat.) or ceftriaxone (1 g i.m. stat.) is probably the most reliable, but doxycycline (300 mg stat.) and thiamphenicol (1.5 g stat.) have also been successfully used.

C. Bubo management

Systemic therapy of the primary lesions will abort lymphadenitis without suppuration. Small abscesses, less than 5 cm in diameter, require aspiration. The needle should be introduced through an area of healthy skin to prevent sinus formation. Larger abscesses may require a formal surgical drainage procedure to prevent scarring and subsequent deformity.

D. Other surgical procedures

Circumcision, once advocated to improve accessibility of subpreputial lesions to local treatment, or to relieve phimosis and paraphimosis and so improve drainage thereby preventing bubo formation, is now contraindicated until systemic antibiotic therapy has eradicated active infection.

E. Other management

Coexisting genital infections should receive appropriate treatment and follow-up.

F. Sexual contacts

Both primary and secondary contacts should be investigated. *Haemophilus ducreyi* may be found in swabs from the vulva or cervix in women, the subpreputial sac or terminal urethra in men, or from the oropharynx in either sex, and may occur in the absence of ulcers. Such ''carriers'' should receive systemic antibiotic therapy in full dosage. Epidemiological treatment should also be given to these contacts whose compliance with follow-up cannot be ensured, or if there are inadequate laboratory facilities for cultural diagnosis of *H. ducreyi.*

XII. PREVENTION

Chancroid is not prevented by washing with soap and water. Although topical application of sulphonamides, chloramphenicol and erythromycin and the systemic administration of sulphonamides and streptomycin have prevented infection in experimental inoculation studies, such treatment cannot be advocated. The condom, correctly used, will prevent transmission of infection in most cases.

Control of chancroid can only be achieved by thorough treatment of affected patients and by tracing and eradicating symptomatic or asymptomatic infection in consorts, thus reducing the local pool of infection.

XIII. LABORATORY ASPECTS OF DIAGNOSIS

A. Introduction

We believe that the cultivation of *H. ducreyi* should be a facility offered by any laboratory providing the diagnostic culture service for a sexually transmitted disease clinic. It is now generally accepted that successful growth of the organisms requires 5% carbon dioxide, a high humidity and a low temperature (30–34°C). Given these essentials, there are several media on which isolation will be successful. Many employ a blood or chocolate base, in keeping with the concept of a haemophilic organism. It is, however, possible to grow the organism on clear media using haemin as a source of iron. Such media have special advantages in that they permit observations around the colonies of any changes which are not seen on opaque media. In keeping with the concept of polymicrobial aetiology of genital ulcers, it is valuable to make the *H. ducreyi* medium selective by the addition of appropriate concentrations of antimicrobials, for example, vancomycin 3 µg/ml.

B. Media

In recent years a number of media have been devised for the isolation of *H. ducreyi,* including the following:

1. *Enriched chocolate agar* (Hammond *et al.,* 1978a)

GC base (Difco)		36 g
Distilled water		1000 ml
Supplements:	Haemoglobin	1%
	IsoVitalex	1%

2. *Modified enriched chocolate agar* (Handsfield *et al.,* 1981)

GC agar base		36 g
Distilled water		900 ml
Supplements:	Sheep blood (chocolatized)	5%
	IsoVitalex	1%
	Foetal calf serum	10%

3. *Foetal bovine serum agar* (Sottnek *et al.,* 1980)

Heart infusion agar (Difco)		40.0 g
Distilled water		900.0 ml
Supplements:	Agar	5.0 g
	Foetal bovine serum	100.0 cc

4. *Mueller Hinton chocolate agar* (Oberhofer and Back, 1982)

Mueller Hinton agar base		38.0 g
Distilled water		1000 ml
Supplements:	Sheep blood	5%
	IsoVitalex	1%

5. *Blood agar* (Sng *et al.,* 1982)

Bacto proteose peptone no. 3 agar (Difco)		45.5 g
Distilled water		1000 ml
Supplements:	Soluble starch	0.1%
	IsoVitalex	1.0%
	Human blood	15%

6. *Sheffield medium*

(a) Part 1

Proteose peptone	30.0 g
Rice starch	1.0 g
Potassium phosphate (dibasic)	4.0 g
Postassium phosphate (monobasic)	1.0 g
Sodium chloride	5.0 g
Gelatin	4.0 g
Glutamine	0.1 g
Glucose	0.50 g
Ferric nitrate [$Fe(NO_3)_3 \cdot 9H_2O$]	0.005 g
Agar	10 g
Distilled water	1000 ml
pH	7.2

The weighed constituents are soaked in distilled water for 30 minutes, mixed and sterilised by autoclaving at 115°C and 10 psi pressure for 15 minutes, and then cooled to 56°C in a water bath.

(b)   Part 2
Equine Haemin Type III (Sigma) (1 g) is dissolved in 25 ml of 0.2 *M* potassium hydroxide in 47.5% ethanol, then made up to 100 ml by adding distilled water, sterilized by Seitz filtration or autoclaving at 115°C and 10 psi pressure for 15 minutes and distributed in 20 ml amounts which are added to a litre of basic medium. The resulting medium contains 200 μg/ml haemin.

(c)   Alternatives

1. The Base Medium (Part 1) can be replaced by DIFCO GC Base, to each litre of which is added 15.0 g proteose peptone, 1.0 g rice starch and 4.0 gelatin.
2. 1% defined supplement (Kellogg *et al.,* 1963) or IsoVitalex (BBL).

(d)   Options

1. Add 3 μg/ml vancomycin to the final medium to give a selective medium for the isolation of *H. ducreyi* from clinical specimens (SMV).
2. Add 5–7% horse blood to the final medium to study the haemolytic effect of *H. ducreyi* (SMB).

C.   Isolation procedure

For the attempted isolation of *H. ducreyi* from suspected chancroidal ulcers proceed as follows:

1. The ulcers are sampled with a moistened cotton swab, which is inoculated immediately onto one plate of SMV and one plate of SMB.
2. The plates are incubated at 33–34°C in 5% carbon dioxide and increased humidity (or in a candle extinction jar).
3. Cultures are examined after 48 hours, and then every subsequent 24 hours for up to 7 days.

D.   Identification of *H. ducreyi* colonies

Typical *H. ducreyi* colonies appear as greenish-brown (or greyish-brown on blood-containing media), coherent, convex colonies which will push across the medium and are extremely difficult to emulsify. Colonies older than 48 hours

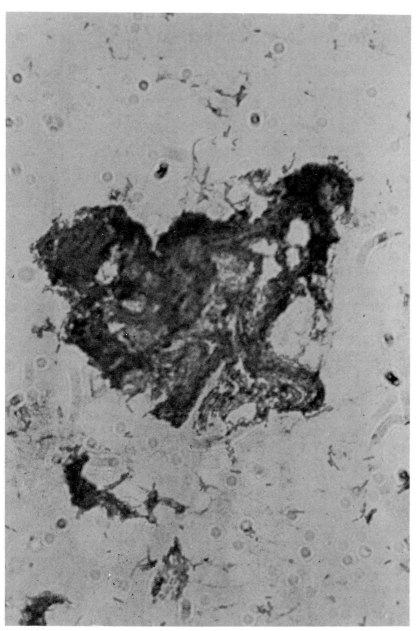

Fig. 6 Haemophilus ducreyi in Gram stain. Small Gram-negative bacilli in matrix. × 1800.

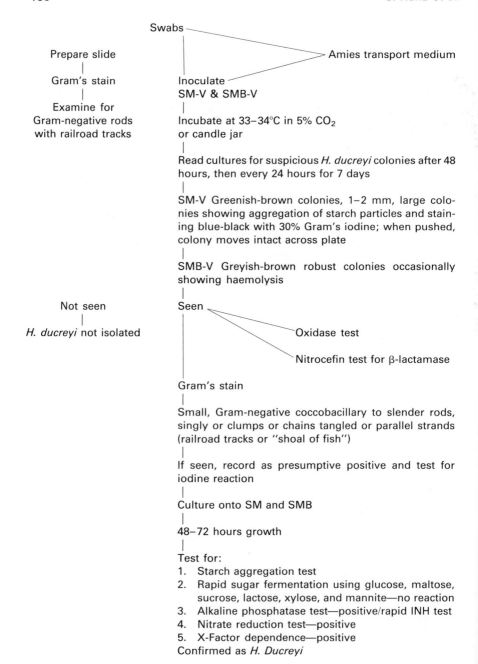

Swabs

Prepare slide → Amies transport medium

Gram's stain

Examine for
Gram-negative rods
with railroad tracks

Inoculate
SM-V & SMB-V

Incubate at 33–34°C in 5% CO_2
or candle jar

Read cultures for suspicious *H. ducreyi* colonies after 48
hours, then every 24 hours for 7 days

SM-V Greenish-brown colonies, 1–2 mm, large colonies showing aggregation of starch particles and staining blue-black with 30% Gram's iodine; when pushed,
colony moves intact across plate

SMB-V Greyish-brown robust colonies occasionally
showing haemolysis

Not seen   Seen

H. ducreyi not isolated   Oxidase test

Nitrocefin test for β-lactamase

Gram's stain

Small, Gram-negative coccobacillary to slender rods,
singly or clumps or chains tangled or parallel strands
(railroad tracks or "shoal of fish")

If seen, record as presumptive positive and test for
iodine reaction

Culture onto SM and SMB

48–72 hours growth

Test for:
1. Starch aggregation test
2. Rapid sugar fermentation using glucose, maltose,
    sucrose, lactose, xylose, and mannite—no reaction
3. Alkaline phosphatase test—positive/rapid INH test
4. Nitrate reduction test—positive
5. X-Factor dependence—positive
Confirmed as *H. Ducreyi*

Fig. 7 Procedure for *Haemophilus ducreyi*. SM = Sheffield media; SMB = with 5%
horse blood; SMV = plus vancomycin at 3 μg/ml.

also show aggregation of starch particles around them, forming a halo which will stain blue-black with 30% Gram's iodine. As the treated colonies are no longer viable and hence cannot be subcultured, the iodine should only be used as an indicator on part of the plate. When Gram-stained, the organisms appear as small pleomorphic, Gram-negative, coccobacillary to slender rods, occurring singly, in large clumps, or in tangled chains (Fig. 6). Occasionally preparations from culture give the appearance of railroad tracks ("shoal of fish") similar to those seen in ulcer smears. On these criteria, a report of "*H. ducreyi* presumptive positive" is made.

E. Confirmatory testing of isolates

Suspect colonies are subcultured onto Sheffield medium with (SMB) and without blood (SM) and incubated for 48 hours. The growth is harvested and emulsified in phosphate-buffered saline, mixing on a rotor mixer, allowing the larger clumps to settle and using the supernatant for further studies (Fig. 7).

1. X-Factor dependence

The supernatant is used to inoculate a non-haemin-containing medium, e.g., GIBCO GC base with IsoVitalex, or DIFCO GC base with added proteose peptone or defined supplement, on which a disc containing 250 μg haemin is placed, then incubated for 48 hours.

Other biochemical tests, including rapid carbohydrate fermentation, can be carried out on the supernatant.

The antibiotic sensitivity can be tested by inoculating the supernatant on SM plates, applying antibiotic discs, and reading the results after 24 hours and 48 hours of incubation in optimum conditions of temperature and humidity.

F. Viability of strains

Strains of *H. ducreyi* grown under optimum conditions will remain viable on moist slopes of SMB for about 4 weeks at 4°C. Well-grown 48-hour plates sealed to prevent drying will remain viable for about 2 weeks. To date we have been able to recover strains stored in liquid nitrogen for up to 2 years.

In our hands, freeze-drying has been less successful than freezing in liquid nitrogen. For best results we freeze-dry a suspension of the organism in foetal calf serum.

XIV. GENERAL DISCUSSION AND CONCLUSION

In little more than 5 years, chancroid has come from being a rare and, in the United Kingdom at least, insignificant infection to being one that now merits consideration in any patient with genital ulceration (Editorial, 1982).

With reports coming in and strains becoming available from many parts of the world, we may reasonably hope to find some answers to the many questions the infection poses today. We need to know more about the pathogenicity of the organism and about its infectivity. Are there really avirulent varients, or are the organisms which persist after some lesions have healed still fully virulent?

Although we have some markers in plasmids and antibiograms, is it possible that simpler ones could be developed within the scope of the general hospital laboratory?

Can we give a clear answer to the clinician who asks us if chancroid is really a specific entity rather than a laboratory-induced focus on one aspect of a poly-microbial infection? How do we explain the irregular geographical distribution? Are there truly endemic areas or is this merely a measure of laboratory enthusi-asm and success?

As laboratory media and methods for the specific diagnosis of *H. ducreyi* infections are now readily available, we hope that there will be a growing interest amongst bacteriologists in looking for an organism which is after all a much more common cause of genital ulceration today than the spirochaete of syphilis.

ACKNOWLEDGMENT

Our thanks go to Mrs. Hazel Bland for typing this chapter.

REFERENCES

Albritton, W. L., Brunton, J. L., Slaney, L., and MacLean, I. W. (1982). *Antimicrob. Agents Chemother.* **21**, 159–165.

Barile, M. F., Blumberg, J. M., Kraus, C. W., and Yaguchi, R. (1962). *Arch. Dermatol.* **86**, 273–281.

Beeson, P. B. (1946). *Proc. Soc. Exp. Biol. Med.* **61**, 81–85.

Bilgeri, Y. R., Ballard, R. C., Duncan, M. O., Mauff, A. C., and Koornhof, H. J. (1982). *Antimicrob. Agents Chemother.* **22**, 686–688.

Borchardt, K. A., and Hoke, A. W. (1970). *Arch. Dermatol.* **102**, 188–192.

Brams, J. (1924). *JAMA, J. Am. Med. Assoc.* **82**, 1166.

Bruck, C. (1915). *Müch. Med. Wschr. syp.* **129**, 170–171.

Brunton, J. L., MacLean, I. W., Ronald, A. R., and Albritton, W. L. (1979). *Antimicrob. Agents Chemother.* **15**, 294–299.

Casin, I. M., Sanson le-pors, M. J., Gorce, M. F., Ortenberg, M., and Perol, Y. (1982). *Ann. Microbiol. (Inst. Pasteur)* **133B**, 379–388.

Centers for Disease Control (1982).

Chapel, T., Brown, W. J., Jefferies, C., and Stewart, J. A. (1978). *J. Infect. Dis.* **137**, 50–56.

Deneer, H. G., Slaney, L., MacLean, I. W., and Albritton, W. L. (1982). *J. Bacteriol.* **149**, 726–732.

Denys, G. A., Chapel, T. A., and Jeffries, C. D. (1978). *Health Lab. Sci.* **15**, 128–132.

Dienst, R. B. (1948). *Am. J. Syph., Gonorrhea, Vener. Dis.* **32**, 289–291.
Ducrey, A. (1890). *Ann. Dermatol. Syphiligr. Zeser* **1**, 56.
Editorial (1982). *Lancet* **2**, 747–748.
Fast, M. V., D'Costa, L. J., Karasira, P., Nsanze, H., Plummer, F. A., MacLean, I. W., and Ronald, A. R. (1982). *Lancet* **2**, 509–510.
Girouard, Y. C., MacLean, I. W., Ronald, A. R., and Albritton, W. L. (1981). *Antimicrob. Agents Chemother.* **20**, 144–145.
Hafiz, S., Kinghorn, G. R., and McEntegart, M. G. (1981). *Br. J. Vener. Dis.* **57**, 382–386.
Hafiz, S., Kinghorn, G. R., and McEntegart, M. G. (1982). *Lancet* **2**, 872.
Hammond, G. W., Lian, C. J., Wilt, J. C., and Ronald, A. R. (1978a). *J. Clin. Microbiol.* **7**, 39–43.
Hammond, G. W., Lian, C. J., Wilt, J. C., Albritton, W. L., and Ronald, A. R. (1978b). *J. Clin. Microbiol.* **7**, 243–248.
Hammond, G. W., Lian, C. J., Wilt, J. C., and Ronald, A. R. (1978c). *Antimicrob. Agents Chemother.* **13**, 608–612.
Hammond, G. W., Slutchuk, M., Scatliff, J., Sherman, E., Wilt, J. C., and Ronald, A. R. (1980). *Rev. Infect. Dis.* **2**, 867–879.
Handsfield, H. H., Totten, P. A., Fennel, C. L., Falkow, S., and Holmes, K. K. (1981). *Ann. Intern. Med.* **95**, 315–318.
Hewlett, R. T. (1929). *In* "MRC System of Bacteriology," Chapter VII, pp. 394–419.
Heyman, A., Beeson, P. B., and Sheldon, W. H. (1945). *JAMA, J. Am. Med. Assoc.* **129**, 935–938.
Himmel, J. (1901). *Ann. Inst. Pasteur, Paris* **15**, 928–940.
Kellogg, D. S., Peacock, W. C., Deacon, W., Brown, L., and Pirkle, C. I. (1963). *J. Bacteriol.* **85**, 1273–1279.
Khoo, R., Sng, E. H., and Goh, A. J. (1977). *Asian J. Infect. Dis.* **1**, 77–79.
Killian, M. (1974). *Acta. Path. Microbiol. Scand.* **B82**, 835–842.
Kilian, M. (1976). *J. Gen. Microbiol.* **93**, 9–62.
Kilian, M., and Theilade, J. (1975). *Int. J. Syst. Bacteriol.* **25**, 351–356.
Kinghorn, G. R., Hafiz, S., and McEntegart, M. G. (1982a). *Lancet* **1**, 383.
Kinghorn, G. R., Hafiz, S., and McEntegart, M. G. (1982b). *Br. J. Vener. Dis.* **58**, 377–380.
Kinghorn, G. R., Hafiz, S., and McEntegart, M. G. (1983a). *Eur. J. Sex. Transm. Dis.* **I**, 89–90.
Kinghorn, G. R., Hafiz, S., and McEntegart, M. G. (1983b). *Br. Med. J.* **287**, 650.
Kraus, S. J., Werman, B. S., Biddle, J. W., Sottnek, F. O., and Ewing, E. P. (1982a). *Arch. Dermatol.* **118**, 494–497.
Kuhlwein, A., Konietzko, D., Reinel, D., and Rohde, B. T. (1980). *Z. Hautkr.* **55**, 661–666.
Lykke-Olesen, L., Pedersen, T. G., Larson, L., and Gaarslev, K. (1979). *Lancet* **1**, 654–655.
McEntegart, M. G., Hafiz, S., and Kinghorn, G. R. (1982). *J. Hyg.* **89**, 467–478.
MacLean, I. W., Bowden, G. H., and Albritton, W. L. (1980). *Antimicrob. Agents Chemother.* **17**, 897–900.
McNichol, P. J., Albritton, W. L., and Ronald, A. R. (1983). *J. Bacteriol.* **156**, 437–440.
Marsch, W. C., Haas, N., and Stüttgen, G. (1978). *Arch. Dermatol. Res.* **263**, 153–157.
Morel, P. (1974). *Nouv. Presse Med.* **3**, 2104–2106.
Morel, P., Casin, I., Gandiol, C., Vallet, C., and Civatte, J. (1982). *Nouv. Presse. Med.* **11**, 655–656.

Mortara, F., and Saito, M. T. (1946). *Am. J. Syph., Gonorrhea, Vener. Dis.* **30,** 352–360.

Mortara, F., Feiner, R. R., and Levenkron, E. (1944). *Proc. Soc. Exp. Biol. Med.* **56,** 163–166.

Nayyar, K. C., Stolz, E., and Michel, M. F. (1979). *Br. J. Vener. Dis.* **55,** 439–441.

Nobre, G. N. (1982). *J. Med. Microbiol.* **15,** 243–246.

Nsanze, H. (1982). *Abstr. Int. Congr. Infect. Parasit. Dis., 8th, 1982.*

Nsanze, H., Dylewski, J., Magwa, N., and D'Costa, L. J. (1982). *Abstr. Int. Congr. Infect. Parasit. Dis., 8th, 1982.*

Nurat, A., Neuzat, O., and Baransu, O. (1978). *Hautarzt* **29,** 583–585.

Oberhofer, T. R., and Back, A. E. (1982). *J. Clin. Microbiol.* **15,** 625–629.

Odumeru, J. A., Ronald, A. R., and Albritton, W. L. (1983). *J. Infect. Dis.* **148** (4), 710–714.

Ovchinnikov, N. M., Delektorskij, V. V., Tischenko, L. D., and Omjelchenko, O. G. (1976). *Vestn. Dermatol. Venerol.* **11,** 37–38.

Rajan, V. S., and Sng, E. H. (1982). *Lancet* **2,** 1043.

Reymann, F. (1949). *Acta Pathol. Microbiol. Scand.* **26,** 345–352.

Sanson Le-Pors, M. J., Casin, I., Ortenburg, M., and Perol, Y. (1982). *Ann. Microbiol. (Paris)* **133,** 311–315.

Sottnek, F. O., Biddle, J. W., Kraus, S. J., and Weaver, R. E. (1980). *J. Clin. Microbiol.* **12,** 170–174.

Sturm, A. W., and Zanen, H. C. (1983). *Lancet* **1,** 125.

Stüttgen, G. (1982). "Ulcus Molle." Grosse Verlag, Berlin.

Sullivan, M. (1940). *Am. J. Syph., Gonorrhea, Vener. Dis.* **24,** 482–521.

Tan, T., Rajan, V. S., Roe, S. L., Tan, N. K., Tab, B. H., and Goh, A. J. (1977). *Asian J. Infect. Dis.* **1,** 27–28.

Thayer, J. D., Field, F. W., and Perry, M. I. (1955). *Antibiot. Chemother. (Washington, D.C.)* **5,** 132–134.

Wetherbee, D. C., Henke, A., Anderson, R. I., Pylaski, E. J., and Kuhos, D. M. (1949). *Am. J. Syph., Gonorrhea, Vener. Dis.* **33,** 462–472.

7   The monobactams

D. P. BONNER and R. B. SYKES

I.   INTRODUCTION

The term monobactam was coined by Sykes *et al.* (1981) to describe a novel group of *mono*cyclic, *bact*erially produced β-lac*tam* antibiotics. The discovery of the monobactams was made 50 years after the momentous discovery by Fleming in 1928 and the beginning of the β-lactam era.

The realization that a fungal metabolite, penicillin, held promise for the successful treatment of infectious diseases provided the stimulus for one of the great searches in the history of medicine: antibiotics from the soil. The ensuing 15–20 years saw the discovery of almost all classes of microbially produced antibiotics in present-day usage and has rightly been referred to as the "golden era of antibiotic discovery." In contrast, the golden era of β-lactam research followed the classical period.

Until 1970, penicillins and cephalosporins were the sole representatives of the naturally occurring β-lactam antibiotics. However, with a greater commitment to selective screening and major advances in isolation technology, a variety of novel β-lactam–containing molecules have made their appearance over the last decade. During the 1970s, molecules represented by the cephamycins (Nagarajan *et al.*, 1971), clavulanic acid (Brown *et al.*, 1976), nocardicins (Aoki *et al.*, 1976), and carbapenems (Butterworth *et al.*, 1979; Okamura *et al.*, 1978; Cassidy *et al.*, 1981; Nakayama *et al.*, 1980) were described. In contrast to the fungal-produced penicillins and the cephalosporins, these novel molecules are produced by members of the actinomycetes. The discovery of bacterially produced β-lactam antibiotics was reported in 1981 by groups at Takeda (Imada *et al.*, 1981) and Squibb (Sykes *et al.*, 1981). Subsequently it has been shown that in addition to monobactams, bacteria are capable of producing carbapenems and cephalosporins (Sykes *et al.*, 1982a). Naturally occurring monobactam antibiotics and their producing organisms are shown in Table 1.

Medical Microbiology, 4
ISBN 0-12-228004-0

Table 1 Structure and source of naturally occurring monobactams

Compound	Structure	Producing organism	Culture reference	Reference
SQ 26,180		Chromobacterium violaceum	SC 11,378	Sykes et al., 1981 Wells et al., 1982a Parker et al., 1982
SQ 26,445 (Sulfazecin)		Gluconobacter sp.	SC 11,435 (ATCC 31,581)	Sykes et al., 1981
		Acetobacter pasteurianus subsp. pasteurianus	ATCC 6,033	
		Acetobacter aceti. subsp. aceti	ATCC 15,973	Liu et al., 1982
		Acetobacter peroxydans	ATCC 12,874	
		Acetobacter aceti. subsp. liquefaciens	ATCC 23,751	
		Acetobacter sp.	ATCC 21,760	
		Gluconobacter oxydans	ATCC 19,357	
		Gluconobacter oxydans subsp. oxydans	ATCC 15,178	

172

Compound	Organism	Strain	Reference
Isosulfazecin	Gluconobacter oxydans subsp. suboxydans	ATCC 19,441 ATCC 23,773	Imada et al., 1981
EM 5400	Gluconobacter oxydans subsp. industrialis	ATCC 11,894	Sykes et al., 1981
	Pseudomonas mesoacidophila	SB 72,310	Wells et al., 1982b
	Agrobacterium radiobacter	SC 11,742	Parker and Rathnum, 1982
SQ 28,332			
EM 5229-1	Flexibacter sp.	SC 11,401	Singh et al., 1983
EM 5229-2	Flexibacter sp.	ATCC 35,103	Cooper et al., 1983

	X	Y	Z	M
SQ 26,823	OCH_3	H	H	Na
SQ 26,875	OCH_3	H	OH	K
SQ 26,700	H	H	OH	K
SQ 26,970	OCH_3	OH	$OSO_3^- Na^+$	Na
SQ 26,812	OCH_3	$OSO_3^- Na^+$	$OSO_3^- Na^+$	Na

Oligopeptides

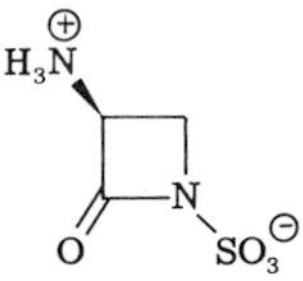

$$H_3\overset{\oplus}{N}$$

Fig. 1 3-Aminomonobactamic acid.

In addition to their scientific fascination, the monobactams provided insight into a new area of β-lactam research, the development of activated monocyclic β-lactam antibiotics. Utilizing the synthetic monobactam nucleus (3-amino-monobactamic acid) (Fig. 1), a large synthetic program was initiated similar to the semisynthetic programs carried out with the penicillins and cephalosporins. From the thousands of molecules produced to date, aztreonam has made its way from the laboratory bench into the clinic.

The concept of activating a monocyclic β-lactam nucleus to produce molecules with potent antibacterial activity has stimulated the search for additional novel activating groups. As expected, activating groups other than sulfate have been discovered, and each has made its imprint on the biological activity of the monocyclic nucleus.

This review is divided into two parts: the naturally occurring monobactams and the synthetic monocyclic compounds.

II. NATURALLY OCCURRING MONOBACTAMS

To date, 11 monobactams have been identified that differ with respect to the acylamino group at position 3 (Fig. 2). Both methoxylated and nonmethoxylated compounds are naturally produced.

The simplest monobactam isolated to date is SQ 26,180 (Wells *et al.*, 1982a) (Table 1), whose production appears to be restricted to certain strains of *Chromobacterium violaceum*. The majority of producing strains has been isolated from soil and water samples collected in the New Jersey Pine Barrens. Both pigmented and nonpigmented strains of *C. violaceum* produce SQ 26,180 (Wells *et al.*, 1982c). Although strains of *C. violaceum* are frequently isolated from natural sources, monobactam-producing strains are rare. Unlike the naturally occurring penicillins and cephalosporins, SQ 26,180 possesses weak antibac-

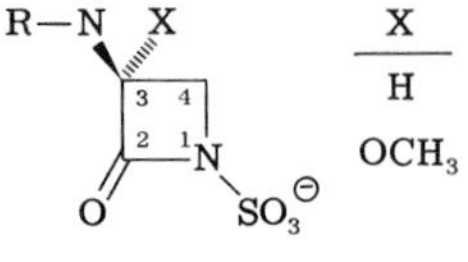

X	
H	
OCH$_3$	

Fig. 2 Structure of naturally occurring monobactams.

Table 2 Antimicrobial activity of SQ 26,180[a]

Organism	SC number	MIC[b] (µg/ml)	Organism	SC number	MIC[b] (µg/ml)
Staphylococcus aureus	1,276	50	Proteus mirabilis	3,855	>100
Staphylococcus aureus	2,399	50	Proteus rettgeri	8,479	>100
Staphylococcus aureus	2,400	100	Proteus vulgaris	9,416	>100
Staphylococcus aureus	10,165	100	Salmonella typhosa	1,195	>100
Streptococcus faecalis	9,011	>100	Shigella sonnei	8,449	>100
Streptococcus agalactiae	9,287	12.5	Enterobacter cloacae	8,236	>100
Micrococcus luteus	2,495	25	Enterobacter aerogenes	10,078	>100
Escherichia coli	8,294	>100	Citrobacter freundii	9,518	>100
Escherichia coli	10,857	>100	Serratia marcescens	9,783	25
Escherichia coli	10,896	25	Pseudomonas aeruginosa	9,545	3.1
Escherichia coli	10,909	50	Pseudomonas aeruginosa	8,329	50
Klebsiella aerogenes	10,440	>100	Acinetobacter calcoace-	8,333	25
Klebsiella pneumoniae	9,527	>100	ticus		

[a] Data from Wells et al., 1982a.
[b] Minimum inhibitory concentrations were determined by a twofold agar dilution method on DST agar (Oxoid). Final inoculum level was 10^4 colony-forming units.

Table 3 Binding of SQ 26,180 to PBPs of *Escherichia coli* and *Staphylococcus aureus*[a]

Organism	Amount (µg/ml) to inhibit penicillin binding completely						MIC (µg/ml)
Escherichia coli SC 8294	PBP1a 91K: 10	PBP1b 91K: >100	PBP2 66K: >100	PBP3 60K: >100	PBP4 49K: 10	PBP5/6 40K: 10	>100
Staphylococcus aureus SC 2399	PBP1 87K: 100		PBP2 80K: >100	PBP3 75K: >100	PBP4 41K: 2.0		100

[a] Data from Wells et al., 1982a.

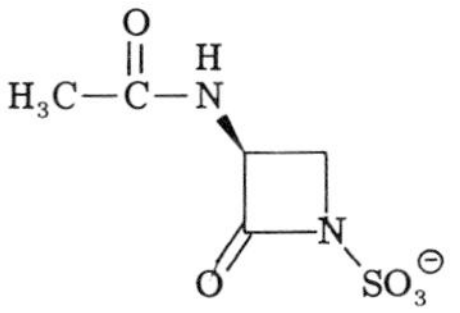

Fig. 3   SQ 26,396 (desmethoxy SQ 26,180).

terial activity (Table 2). Interestingly, it shows its greatest effect against a strain of *Pseudomonas aeruginosa*. The weak antibacterial activity of this compound can be explained by its inability to bind effectively to essential penicillin binding proteins (PBPs) of *Escherichia coli* and *Staphylococcus aureus* (Table 3).

The 3-methoxy group on the β-lactam ring of SQ 26,180 is reminiscent of that same grouping at the 7 position of the cephamycin nucleus, where it affects the compound with a high degree of stability to β-lactamases. Correspondingly, SQ 26,180 is resistant to hydrolysis by β-lactamases (Table 4). Implication of the methoxyl group in this regard can be seen from the data obtained with SQ 26,396 (Fig. 3), a synthetic derivative of SQ 26,180 that lacks the 3-methoxyl group (Table 4). SQ 26,180 shows no significant inhibition of the enzymes from *S. aureus*, *E. coli*, or *Klebsiella*. However, against the P99 β-lactamase from *Enterobacter cloacae*, it appears to act as a reversible competitive inhibitor (Wells *et al.*, 1982a).

SQ 26,445 (Table 1) as described by Squibb workers, from strains of *Gluconobacter* and *Acetobacter* species (Liu *et al.*, 1982), is identical with sulfazecin, described by workers from Takeda (Imada *et al.*, 1981) as being produced by strains of *Pseudomonas acidophila*. In terms of overall frequency of detection, SQ 26,445 is the most commonly produced monobactam. Producing

Table 4   Susceptibility to and inhibition of β-lactamases by SQ 26,180

β-Lactamase	Compound	Relative V_{max}	I_{50} (mM)
Staphylococcus aureus	Benzylpenicillin	100	—
	SQ 26,180	<0.02	>2.0
TEM-2	Benzylpenicillin	100	—
	SQ 26,180	<0.01	>2.0
K1	Benzylpenicillin	100	—
	SQ 26,180	<0.02	>2.0
P99	Cephaloridine	100	—
	SQ 26,180	<0.05	0.22
Chromobacterium violaceum	Cephaloridine	100	—
	SQ 26,180	N.D.	>0.5

Data from Wells *et al.*, 1982a.

Table 5 Activity of sulfazecin and isosulfazecin

	MIC (μg/ml)	
Organism	Sulfazecin	Isosulfazecin
Pseudomonas aeruginosa IFO 3080	800	1,600
Pseudomonas aeruginosa (sensitive mutant of IFO 3080)	0.78	0.78
Escherichia coli NIHJ JC2	12.5	100
Escherichia coli LD$_2$	6.25	50
Escherichia coli PG8 (sensitive mutant of LD$_2$)	0.39	0.78
Proteus vulgaris IFO 3988	6.25	100
Staphylococcus aureus FDA 209P	200	200

Data from Imada *et al.*, 1981.

Table 6 Interactions of β-lactamases with compounds isolated from *Agrobacterium radiobacter* SC 11,742

β-Lactamase	Compound	Relative V_{max}	K_m (mM)	I_{50} (mM)
Staphylococcus aureus	Penicillin G	100	0.03	—
	SQ 26,823	2	0.47	>0.5
	SQ 26,700	12	0.98	—
	SQ 26,875	<0.02	—	>0.4
	SQ 26,970	<0.05	—	>0.4
	SQ 26,812	N.D.	N.D.	N.D.
TEM-2	Penicillin G	100	0.08	—
	SQ 26,823	<0.01	—	>0.05
	SQ 26,700	7.1	0.28	—
	SQ 26,875	<0.01	—	>0.4
	SQ 26,970	<0.01	—	>0.4
	SQ 26,812	<0.02	—	>0.8
K1	Penicillin G	100	0.17	—
	SQ 26,823	<0.02	—	>0.5
	SQ 26,700	57	1.28	—
	SQ 26,875	<0.01	—	>0.04
	SQ 26,970	<0.01	—	>0.04
	SQ 26,812	<0.03	—	>0.08
P99	Cephaloridine	100	0.58	—
	SQ 26,823	<0.01	—	0.0008
	SQ 26,700	0.15	0.19	—
	SQ 26,875	<0.01	—	0.002
	SQ 26,970	<0.01	—	0.0007
	SQ 26,812	<0.02	—	0.002

Data from Wells *et al.*, 1982b.

strains have been isolated from many geographical areas (Wells *et al.*, 1982c). In terms of antibacterial activity, the more complex sidechain of SQ 26,445 (DGlu-DAla), is superior to the simple sidechain of SQ 26,180 (Table 5). SQ 26,445 like SQ 26,180 bears a methoxyl group at the 3 position and as such is extremely stable to hydrolysis by β-lactamases.

The Takeda group reported an epimer of sulfazecin that they referred to as isosulfazecin (Table 1). This compound was reportedly produced by a strain of *Pseudomonas mesoacidophila* (Imada *et al.*, 1981). In data reported from the Takeda group, sulfazecin shows antibacterial activity superior to isosulfazecin (Table 5).

The first bacterial strain indicated to be producing more than one monobactam was an organism identified as *Agrobacterium radiobacter* (Wells *et al.*, 1982b). This organism produces five related monobactams having N-acetylated phenylalanyl or tyrosine residues in the sidechain (Table 1). The naturally occurring nonmethoxylated monobactam SQ 26,700 was isolated from this organism. Unlike the methoxylated monobactam species produced by *A. radiobacter*, SQ 26,700 is susceptible to hydrolysis by a range of β-lactamases (Table 6). These compounds are weak antibacterial agents (Table 7).

Recently we have isolated strains of *Flexibacter* (gliding bacteria) that produce nonmethoxylated monobactams with complex acyl sidechains (Table 1) and that have molecular weights greater than 1000 (Cooper *et al.*, 1983; Singh *et al.*, 1983). Although these molecules lack the grouping that provides a high degree of stability to β-lactamases in other naturally occurring monobactams, they exhibit a high degree of stability to these enzymes. They also differ from previously isolated monobactams in being irreversible inactivators of certain β-lactamases (Cooper *et al.*, 1983).

There is little doubt that bacteria are capable of producing a whole range of monocyclic β-lactam antibiotics, in addition to the carbapenems and cephems that have also been detected in these organisms.

III. SYNTHETIC MONOCYCLIC β-LACTAMS

A. Monobactams

The successful development of penicillin and cephalosporin antibiotics has been due in a large part to modification of the acylamino sidechains leading to new entities possessing improved antibacterial activity, β-lactamase stability, and pharmacokinetic properties. Substitution programs initiated with the penicillin nucleus were later repeated with the cephalosporin nucleus, resulting in a broad array of compounds exhibiting diverse properties. Within the penicillins are compounds showing primarily anti-Gram-positive activity (penicillin G) to

Table 7 Antibacterial activity of monobactams produced by *Agrobacterium radiobacter* SC 11,742

Organism	SC number	SQ 26,823	SQ 26,875	SQ 26,700	SQ 26,970	SQ 26,812
Staphylococcus aureus	1,276	12.5	25	25	>100	>100
Staphylococcus aureus	2,399	12.5	50	25	>100	>100
Staphylococcus aureus	2,400	25	100	25	>100	>100
Staphylococcus aureus	10,165	>50	>100	>100	>100	>100
Streptococcus faecalis	9,011	>50	>100	100	>100	>100
Streptococcus agalactiae	9,287	25	50	12.5	>100	>100
Micrococcus luteus	2,495	12.5	100	12.5	>100	>100
Escherichia coli	8,294	>50	>100	>100	>100	>100
Escherichia coli	10,857	>50	100	>100	>100	>100
Escherichia coli	10,896	25	6.3	>100	25	>100
Escherichia coli	10,909	>50	100	>100	>100	>100
Klebsiella aerogenes	10,440	>50	>100	>100	>100	>100
Klebsiella pneumoniae	9,527	>50	>100	>100	>100	>100
Proteus mirabilis	3,855	>50	>100	>100	>100	>100
Proteus rettgeri	8,479	>50	>100	>100	>100	>100
Proteus vulgaris	9,416	>50	>100	>100	>100	>100
Salmonella typhosa	1,195	>50	>100	>100	>100	>100
Shigella sonnei	8,449	>50	>100	>100	>100	>100
Enterobacter cloaecae	8,236	>50	>100	>100	>100	>100
Enterobacter aerogenes	10,078	>50	>100	>100	>100	>100
Citrobacter freundii	9,518	>50	>100	>100	>100	>100
Serratia marcescens	9,783	>50	>100	>100	>100	>100
Pseudomonas aeruginosa	9,545	50	50	100	>100	>100
Pseudomonas aeruginosa	8,329	>50	>100	>100	>100	>100
Acinetobacter calcoaceticus	8,333	>50	>100	>100	>100	>100

Minimum inhibitory concentrations were determined by a twofold agar dilution method on DST agar (Oxoid). Final inoculum level was 10^4 colony-forming units. Data from Wells *et al.*, 1982b.

broad-spectrum activity such as now observed with the ureidopenicillins. A similar range is seen within the cephalosporins. Of additional interest has been the comparison between penicillins and cephalosporins containing the same or very similar sidechains. In terms of breadth of spectrum and level of antibacterial potency, piperacillin and cefoperazone, different nuclei containing a similar sidechain, exhibit similar activities. On the other hand, there are numerous examples where identical sidechains function on one type of β-lactam nucleus, either a cephalosporin or penicillin, and not on the other.

With this historical perspective in mind, an extensive program was initiated leading to alteration of the sidechain on the monobactam nucleus. Initially, a series of monobactams was synthesized bearing sidechains gleaned from the most successful of the penicillins and cephalosporins (Breuer et al., 1981; Cimarusti et al., 1982; Koster et al., 1982a).

The same problems encountered in translating the activity of a penicillin to a cephalosporin are also met when one takes the additional step to the monobactams. In general, the monobactams are like the classical β-lactams in being open to sidechain substitution, and depending on the sidechain, compounds may exhibit primarily anti-Gram-positive, anti-Gram-negative, or broad-spectrum activity. However, in terms of extremes of spectrum that can be achieved, the monobactams probably surpass their classical counterparts. Some comparisons to homologous penicillins are shown in Table 8. The penicillin G monobactam exhibits an anti-Gram-positive spectrum, but it is less active than penicillin G. Monobactams homologous to carbenicillin and mezlocillin are also less active than their penicillin counterparts, while the piperacillin monobactam is equal both in breadth of spectrum and level of activity to piperacillin. A similar situation is seen in Table 9, where monobactams are compared to their cephalosporin counterparts. The cephalothin homolog reflects the spectrum of activity but is less potent than cephalothin. The cefsulodin homolog is substantially less active than its corresponding cephalosporin, yet the monobactam based on cefoperazone reflects very well the activity of cefoperazone. A final pattern emerges when the ceftazidime comparison is considered. The innate anti-Gram-negative activity translates well between the two compounds; however, the monobactam is devoid of anti-Gram-positive activity and is demonstrably less stable to β-lactamase.

These studies underscore the unique nature of β-lactam nuclei. Although they all share a common target, inhibition of bacterial cell-wall synthesis, structural modification may subtly or drastically affect the ability of a molecule to interact with receptor sites, gain access to the receptor sites, or withstand the onslaught of β-lactamase. The monobactam nucleus is novel. While the penicillin and cephalosporin sidechains provided a general overview of the range of possible activities, they were only a start in the systematic investigations on this nucleus.

Table 8 Antibacterial relationships of penicillins to their homologous monobactams: minimum inhibitory concentrations (μg/ml) in agar dilution assays

Organism		SC number	Penicillin: benzyl penicillin CFU = 10⁴	Monobactam: SQ 26,324 CFU = 10⁴	Penicillin: carbenicillin CFU = 10⁴	Monobactam: SQ 81,393 CFU = 10⁴	Penicillin: azlocillin CFU = 10⁴	Monobactam: SQ 81,398 CFU = 10⁴
Staphylococcus aureus	PENase−	2,399	<0.05	3.1	0.2	100	0.4	1.6
Staphylococcus aureus	PENase+	2,400	3.1	6.3	6.3	100	3.1	3.1
Escherichia coli		8,294	50	25	25	>100	12.5	6.3
Klebsiella aerogenes		10,440	25	50	25	>100	25	6.3
Proteus rettgeri		8,479	3.1	25	0.4	>100	0.8	0.4
Enterobacter cloacae		8,236	>100	25	12.5	100	12.5	6.3
Pseudomonas aeruginosa		8,329	>100	>100	50	50	3.1	12.5

Organism		SC number	benzyl penicillin CFU = 10⁴	benzyl penicillin CFU = 10⁶	SQ 26,324 CFU = 10⁴	SQ 26,324 CFU = 10⁶	carbenicillin CFU = 10⁴	carbenicillin CFU = 10⁶	SQ 81,393 CFU = 10⁴	SQ 81,393 CFU = 10⁶	azlocillin CFU = 10⁴	azlocillin CFU = 10⁶	SQ 81,398 CFU = 10⁴	SQ 81,398 CFU = 10⁶
Escherichia coli	TEM+	10,404	>100	>100	50	>100	>100	>100	>100	>100	>100	>100	100	>100
Escherichia coli	TEM−	10,439	12.5	25	12.5	25	6.3	12.5	>100	>100	12.5	12.5	6.3	12.5
Enterobacter cloacae	P99+	10,435	>100	>100	>100	>100	>100	>100	>100	>100	>100	>100	>100	>100
Enterobacter cloacae	P99−	10,441	25	100	>100	>100	6.3	12.5	>100	>100	6.3	6.3	6.3	25
Klebsiella aerogenes	K1+	10,436	>100	>100	>100	>100	>100	>100	>100	>100	>100	>100	>100	>100
Klebsiella aerogenes	K1−	10,440	12.5	12.5	.50	100	6.3	12.5	>100	>100	12.5	25	6.3	6.3

(continued)

182

Table 8 (Continued)

Monobactam

Penicillin

H_3C-SO_2-N ... $-NH-CH-C-NH- = R$ (mezlocillin side structure)

H_5C_2-N ... $-NH-CH-C-NH- = R$ (piperacillin side structure)

$N-CH=N- = R$ (mecillinam side structure)

Organism		SC number	Penicillin: mezlocillin CFU = 10⁴	Monobactam: SQ 81,419 CFU = 10⁴	Penicillin: piperacillin CFU = 10⁴	Monobactam: SQ 81,427 CFU = 10⁴	Penicillin: mecillinam CFU = 10⁴	Monobactam: SQ 81,384 CFU = 10⁴
Staphylococcus aureus	PENase−	2,399	0.4	1.6	0.4	1.6	25	>100
Staphylococcus aureus	PENase+	2,400	1.6	3.1	3.1	1.6	>100	>100
Escherichia coli		8,294	3.1	6.3	3.1	0.8	<0.05	12.5
Klebsiella aerogenes		10,440	6.3	12.5	12.5	1.6	<0.05	25
Proteus rettgeri		8,479	0.4	0.8	0.1	0.1	0.1	12.5
Enterobacter cloacae		8,236	1.6	6.3	1.6	0.8	0.1	25
Pseudomonas aeruginosa		8,329	12.5	100	3.1	3.1	>100	>100

Organism		SC number	Penicillin: mezlocillin		Monobactam: SQ 81,419		Penicillin: piperacillin		Monobactam: SQ 81,427		Penicillin: mecillinam		Monobactam: SQ 81,384	
			CFU = 10⁴	CFU = 10⁶	CFU = 10⁴	CFU = 10⁶	CFU = 10⁴	CFU = 10⁶	CFU = 10⁴	CFU = 10⁶	CFU = 10⁴	CFU = 10⁶	CFU = 10⁴	CFU = 10⁶
Escherichia coli	TEM+	10,404	>100	>100	25	>100	>100	>100	25	>100	50	>100	>100	>100
Escherichia coli	TEM−	10,439	1.6	3.1	3.1	6.3	1.6	3.1	1.6	6.3	0.2	0.4	50	50
Enterobacter cloacae	P99+	10,435	50	>100	>100	>100	100	>100	>100	>100	0.8	3.1	>100	>100
Enterobacter cloacae	P99−	10,441	3.1	6.3	12.5	12.5	1.6	3.1	0.4	1.6	0.2	0.4	50	50
Klebsiella aerogenes	K1+	10,436	>100	>100	>100	>100	>100	>100	>100	>100	>100	>100	100	100
Klebsiella aerogenes	K1−	10,440	3.1	6.3	6.3	12.5	1.6	3.1	0.8	3.1	3.1	100	>100	>100

[a] Minimum inhibitory concentrations were determined by a twofold agar dilution method on DST agar.

183

Table 9 Antibacterial relationships of cephalosporins to their homologous monobactams: minimum inhibitory concentrations (µg/ml) in agar dilution assays

Monobactam general structure: R—(β-lactam ring with N—SO₃⁻)

Cephalosporin general structure: R—(cephem nucleus with N, X, COO⁻)

R groups:
- cephalothin / SQ 81,387: $S-CH_2-C(=O)-NH- = R$
- cefuroxime / SQ 81,532: $H_3C-O-N=C-C(=O)-NH- = R$ (furyl)
- cefsulodin / SQ 81,491: $^-O_3S-CH-C(=O)-NH- = R$ (phenyl)

Organism		SC number	Cephalosporin: cephalothin CFU = 10⁴	Monobactam: SQ 81,387 CFU = 10⁴	Cephalosporin: cefuroxime CFU = 10⁴	Monobactam: SQ 81,532 CFU = 10⁴	Cephalosporin: cefsulodin CFU = 10⁴	Monobactam: SQ 81,491 CFU = 10⁴
Staphylococcus aureus	PENase−	2,399	0.1	3.1	0.8	3.1	3.1	>100
Staphylococcus aureus	PENase+	2,400	0.2	3.1	0.8	6.3	3.1	>100
Escherichia coli		8,294	12.5	25	6.3	25	50	>100
Klebsiella aerogenes		10,440	6.3	50	6.3	50	100	>100
Proteus rettgeri		8,479	0.1	12.5	<0.05	12.5	12.5	100
Enterobacter cloacae		8,236	>100	100	6.3	12.5	100	>100
Pseudomonas aeruginosa		8,329	>100	>100	>100	100	1.6	>100

Organism		SC number	Cephalosporin: cephalothin CFU = 10⁴	CFU = 10⁶	Monobactam: SQ 81,387 CFU = 10⁴	CFU = 10⁶	Cephalosporin: cefuroxime CFU = 10⁴	CFU = 10⁶	Monobactam: SQ 81,532 CFU = 10⁴	CFU = 10⁶	Cephalosporin: cefsulodin CFU = 10⁴	CFU = 10⁶	Monobactam: SQ 81,491 CFU = 10⁴	CFU = 10⁶
Escherichia coli	TEM+	10,404	6.3	>100	50	>100	3.1	6.3	>100	>100	50	>100	>100	>100
Escherichia coli	TEM−	10,439	1.6	25	50	50	3.1	6.3	25	25	50	50	>100	>100
Enterobacter cloacae	P99+	10,435	>100	>100	>100	>100	>100	>100	>100	>100	>100	>100	>100	>100
Enterobacter cloacae	P99−	10,441	6.3	12.5	25	50	25	12.5	50	50	100	100	>100	>100
Klebsiella aerogenes	K1+	10,436	>100	>100	>100	>100	>100	>100	>100	>100	>100	100	>100	>100
Klebsiella aerogenes	K1−	10,440	3.1	3.1	100	100	1.6	3.1	25	50	100	100	>100	>100

(continued)

184

Table 9 (Continued)

Monobactam (generic structure)

Cephalosporin (generic structure)

	SC number	Cephalosporin: cefoperazone CFU = 10^4		Monobactam: SQ 81,491 CFU = 10^4		Cephalosporin: cefotaxime CFU = 10^4		Monobactam: SQ 81,377 CFU = 10^4		Cephalosporin: ceftazidime CFU = 10^4		Monobactam: SQ 81,402 CFU = 10^4	
Organism													
Staphylococcus aureus PENase−	2,399	0.8		3.1		0.8		6.3		12.5		>100	
Staphylococcus aureus PENase+	2,400	1.6		3.1		0.8		6.3		12.5		>100	
Escherichia coli	8,294	0.8		0.4		0.1		0.8		0.4		0.4	
Klebsiella aerogenes	10,440	0.8		0.4		0.1		0.8		0.4		0.4	
Proteus rettgeri	8,479	0.1		<0.05		<0.05		<0.05		<0.05		<0.05	
Enterobacter cloacae	8,236	0.8		0.8		0.4		0.8		0.4		0.4	
Pseudomonas aeruginosa	8,329	3.1		3.1		12.5		12.5		1.6		3.1	

	SC number	cefoperazone CFU = 10^4	CFU = 10^6	SQ 81,491 CFU = 10^4	CFU = 10^6	cefotaxime CFU = 10^4	CFU = 10^6	SQ 81,377 CFU = 10^4	CFU = 10^6	ceftazidime CFU = 10^4	CFU = 10^6	SQ 81,402 CFU = 10^4	CFU = 10^6
Organism													
Escherichia coli TEM+	10,404	3.1	>100	12.5	>100	<0.05	0.1	6.3	>100	0.4	0.4	3.1	25
Escherichia coli TEM−	10,439	0.2	0.4	0.4	0.4	<0.05	0.1	0.8	1.6	0.2	0.4	0.4	0.4
Enterobacter cloacae P99+	10,435	50	>100	>100	>100	50	>100	>100	>100	50	100	>100	>100
Enterobacter cloacae P99−	10,441	0.2	0.4	0.2	0.8	0.2	0.2	1.6	3.1	0.2	0.4	0.1	0.4
Klebsiella aerogenes K1+	10,436	>100	>100	>100	>100	1.6	100	>100	>100	0.4	1.6	>100	>100
Klebsiella aerogenes K1−	10,440	0.1	0.2	0.4	6.3	<0.05	<0.05	0.8	0.8	0.1	0.1	0.1	0.2

Minimum inhibitory concentrations were determined by a twofold agar dilution method on DST agar.

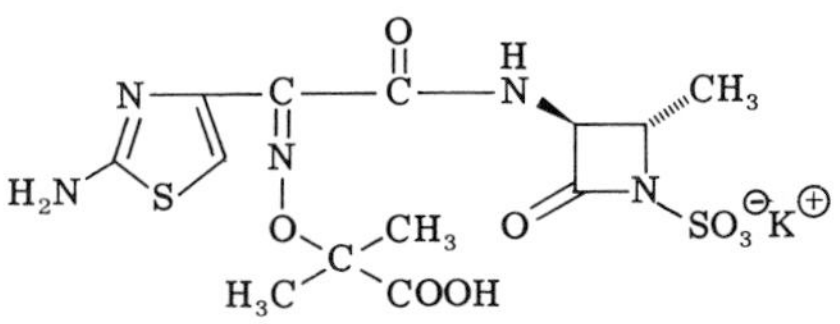

Fig. 4   Aztreonam.

B. Development of aztreonam

After examination of a wide range of penicillin and cephalosporin surrogates, attention focused on a particular class of sidechains, the aminothiazoleoximes, a sidechain class common to many of the third-generation cephalosporins. As seen in Table 11, SQ 81,402, the monobactam analog of ceftazidime, shows a similar spectrum of anti-Gram-negative activity but is unstable to many of the β-lactamases elaborated by these organisms. In addition, it is almost completely devoid of activity against Gram-positive bacteria. The unacceptable defect of instability to Gram-negative β-lactamases was overcome by derivatization at the 4 position of the monobactam nucleus. While modification at the 3 position established the range and level of intrinsic antibacterial activity, substitution of a methyl at the 4 position established β-lactamase stability. The unique property of potent activity against a wide range of Gram-negative bacteria, including *Pseudomonas aeruginosa,* allied with limited potency against Gram-positive bacteria and anaerobes, introduced a new spectrum of activity among the β-lactam antibiotics. The resulting monobactam, aztreonam (Fig. 4), on detailed study typifies a new direction in antibacterial therapy (Sykes *et al.,* 1982b).

Table 10   Antibacterial activity of aztreonam

Organism (number of isolates)	MIC_{90} (μg/ml)
Staphylococcus aureus (20)	>100
Streptococcus pyogenes (20)	12.5
Streptococcus faecalis (20)	>100
Bacteroides fragilis (10)	>100
Escherichia coli (80)	0.2
Klebsiella pneumoniae (70)	0.3
Enterobacter cloacae (30)	12.5
Serratia marcescens (120)	1.6
Proteus mirabilis (25)	<0.1
Indole-positive *Proteus* (50)	<0.1
Providencia stuartii (15)	<0.1
Citrobacter freundii (50)	0.7
Pseudomonas aeruginosa (60)	12.0
Hemophilus influenzae (50)	0.2
Neisseria gonorrhoeae (20)	0.2

Inoculum 5 × 10⁵ CFU.
Data from Sykes *et al.,* 1982b.

Table 11 Stability to chromosomally mediated β-lactamases[a]

Compound	Klebsiella K1	Proteus P1	Serratia S1	Enterobacter P99	Enterobacter E1	Providencia PD1	Bacteroides B1
			Relative efficiency of hydrolysis by β-lactamase type				
Cephaloridine	100	100	100	100	100	100	100
Aztreonam	10	0.8	<0.2	<0.01	<0.01	0.03	1.1
Ceftazidime	0.01	<0.1	<0.2	0.2	0.04	1.3	4
Cefotaxime	5	0.6	5	5	0.02	3	30
Cefoperazone	30	>1[b]	30	7	5	5	40

[a] Data from Sykes et al., 1982b.
[b] Nonlinear kinetics.

Table 12   Stability to plasmid-mediated β-lactamases[a]

Compound	Relative efficiency of hydrolysis by β-lactamase type							
	TEM-1	TEM-2	OXA-2	SHV-1	PSE-1	PSE-2	PSE-3	PSE-4
Cephaloridine	100	100	100	100	100	100	100	100
Aztreonam	0.04	0.03	1	0.10	0.02	5.5	0.8	0.01
Ceftazidime	<0.01	<0.01	<0.5	0.04	0.02	<3	0.4	<0.01
Cefotaxime	0.1	0.07	6	0.14	0.03	40	0.3	0.03
Cefoperazone	70	60	250	150	260	1900	6	280

[a] Data from Sykes et al., 1982b.

Aztreonam is specifically and solely directed against aerobic Gram-negative bacteria. Spectrum of activity and stability to chromosomal and plasmid-mediated β-lactamases is seen in Tables 10–12. Although structurally novel, the mode of action of aztreonam is very much in keeping with the present understanding of how β-lactam antibiotics effect their antibacterial activity. Binding to essential PBPs disrupts the orderly growth and proliferation of the organism, ultimately resulting in death. Aztreonam is exceptional in its high and almost exclusive predilection for PBP3 of Gram-negative bacteria (Table 13). Binding to PBP3 results in filamentation and cellular dissolution. Lack of activity against Gram-positive bacteria is similarly reflected in an absence of affinity for the essential PBPs of these organisms.

C. Monosynthams

Discovery of the monobactams established that a bicyclic ring structure was not an absolute necessity for high activity in a β-lactam antibiotic. Activation of the azetidinone ring could be accomplished otherwise, as in the case of the monobactams, by appending a sulfonic acid residue. The natural extension of this observation was to search for alternate means of activating the azetidinone. Once again, an extensive program of synthesis and study was initiated, resulting in a variety of novel monobactam subclasses.

1. Monophosphams

Preparation of 2-oxoazetidine-1-phosphonates (monophosphams) by total synthesis and confirmation of their antibacterial activities provided the first evidence that a degree of latitude existed in the chemical constraints on activation (Koster et al., 1982b). The aminothiazoleoxime sidechains proved optimal in providing compounds with noteworthy antibacterial properties. Monophosphams with arylacetyl, acylamino, or ureido sidechains are poor antibacterial agents. Distinct from their monobactam counterparts, the monophosphams are totally devoid of

Table 13 Binding of aztreonam and cephalothin to PBPs of different bacteria[a]

Organism	Compound	Concn. (µg/ml) for complete inhibition of benzylpenicillin binding									MIC (µg/ml)
		PBP1	PBP1a	PBP1b	PBP1c	PBP2	PBP3	PBP4	PBP5	PBP5/6	
Escherichia coli, SC 8,294	Aztreonam		10	≥100		>100	0.1	100		100	0.1
	Cephalothin		0.5	100		100	2.0	100		>100	0.6[b]
Proteus mirabilis, SC 3,855	Aztreonam		2.0	100		>100	0.1	100		>100	<0.05
	Cephalothin		0.1	10		100	2.0	10		>100	0.8
Proteus vulgaris, SC 9,416	Aztreonam		10	≥100		ND	0.1	ND		>100	<0.5
	Cephalothin		0.5	10		ND	2.0	ND		>100	12.5
Enterobacter cloacae, SC 8,236	Aztreonam		10	>100		>100	0.1	>100		0.1	0.1
	Cephalothin		0.1	100		>100	0.5	100		>100	>100
Klebsiella pneumoniae, SC 9,527	Aztreonam		ND[c]	>100		>100	0.1	>100		>100	0.1
	Cephalothin		ND	30		100	0.5	30		>100	<0.05
Pseudomonas aeruginosa, SC 9,545	Aztreonam		ND	100	30	>100	0.1	>100		>100	0.2
	Cephalothin		ND	10	0.5	>100	2.0	30		>100	>100
Staphylococcus aureus, SC 2,399	Aztreonam	>100				≥100	>100	>100			>100
	Cephalothin	0.5				0.5	0.5	100			0.1
Bacteroides fragilis, SC 11,085	Aztreonam	>100				100	ND	>100	>100		>100
	Cephalothin	>100				>100	ND	>100	>100		>100

[a] Data from Georgopapadakou et al., 1982.
[b] Value refers to DC2, a premeability mutant of E. coli.
[c] ND, not detected.

Table 14 Antibacterial activity of the monophosphams: MIC (μg/ml)[a]

Organism		SC number	SQ 27,023 R=—P(=O)(OCH$_3$)(O$^-$)		SQ 27,461 R=—P(=O)(OCH$_2$CH$_3$)(O$^-$)		SQ 27,498 R=—P(=O)(OCH$_2$CH$_2$F)(O$^-$)		SQ 81,377 R=SO$_3^-$	
			CFU=10^4	CFU=10^6	CFU=10^4	CFU=10^6	CFU=10^4	CFU=10^6	CFU=10^4	CFU=10^6
Staphylococcus aureus	PENase –	2,399	>100	>100	>100	>100	>100	>100	6.3	6.3
Staphylococcus aureus	PENase +	2,400	>100	>100	>100	>100	>100	>100	6.3	6.3
Escherichia coli		8,294	6.3	6.3	6.3	6.3	6.3	6.3	0.8	0.8
Klebsiella aerogenes		10,440	12.5	12.5	6.3	6.3	12.5	12.5	0.8	0.8
Proteus rettgeri		8,479	0.8	0.8	0.4	0.4	0.8	0.8	0.05	0.05
Enterobacter cloacae		8,236	3.1	3.1	3.1	3.1	6.3	6.3	0.8	0.8
Pseudomonas aeruginosa		8,329	>100	>100	>100	>100	>100	>100	12.5	12.5
Escherichia coli	TEM +	10,404	6.3	6.3	6.3	6.3	6.3	6.3	6.3	>100
Escherichia coli	TEM –	10,439	3.1	3.1	3.1	6.3	6.3	12.5	0.8	1.6
Enterobacter cloacae	P99 +	10,435	100	>100	100	>100	100	>100	>100	>100
Enterobacter cloacae	P99 –	10,441	6.3	12.5	12.5	12.5	12.5	50	1.6	3.1
Klebsiella aerogenes	K1 +	10,436	50	>100	25	100	25	100	>100	>100
Klebsiella aerogenes	K1 –	10,440	6.3	6.3	3.1	6.3	6.3	6.3	0.8	0.8

[a] Minimum inhibitory concentrations were determined by a twofold agar dilution method on DST agar.

Table 15 Antibacterial activity of monophosphams: MIC ($\mu g/ml$)[a]

Organism		SC number	SQ 27,159 $R = \overset{\overset{O}{\|}}{-P}(OCH_3)(O^-)$		SQ 27,462 $R = \overset{\overset{O}{\|}}{-P}(OCH_2CH_3)(O^-)$		SQ 81,402 $R = SO_3^-$	
			CFU = 10^4	CFU = 10^6	CFU = 10^4	CFU = 10^6	CFU = 10^4	CFU = 10^6
Staphylococcus aureus	PENase −	2,399	>100	>100	>100		>100	
Staphylococcus aureus	PENase +	2,400	>100	>100	>100		>100	
Escherichia coli		8,294	6.3	6.3	6.3		0.4	0.4
Klebsiella aerogenes		10,440	6.3	6.3	12.5		0.4	0.4
Proteus rettgeri		8,479	0.2	0.2	<0.05		<0.05	
Enterobacter cloacae		8,236	1.6	1.6	1.6		0.4	0.4
Pseudomonas aeruginosa		8,329	>100	>100	>100		3.1	3.1
Escherichia coli	TEM +	10,404	0.8	3.1	0.8	1.6	3.1	25
Escherichia coli	TEM −	10,439	1.6	1.6	1.6	1.6	0.4	0.4
Enterobacter cloacae	P99 +	10,435	>100	>100	50	>100	>100	>100
Enterobacter cloacae	P99 −	10,441	1.6	3.1	0.8	1.6	0.1	0.4
Klebsiella aerogenes	K1 +	10,436	6.3	25	6.3	25	>100	>100
Klebsiella aerogenes	K1 −	10,440	0.8	1.6	1.6	1.6	0.1	0.2

[a] Minimum inhibitory concentrations were determined by a twofold agar dilution method on DST agar.

Table 16 Antibacterial activity of the monocarbams: MIC (μg/ml)[a]

Organism		SC number	SQ 27,006 R = $-\text{CNHSO}_2\text{CH}_3$		SQ 81,823 R = $-\text{CNHSO}_2\text{NH}_2$		SQ 82,650	
			CFU = 10^4	CFU = 10^6	CFU = 10^4	CFU = 10^6	CFU = 10^4	CFU = 10^6
Staphylococcus aureus	PENase −	2,399	>100	>100	>100		>100	
Staphylococcus aureus	PENase +	2,400	>100	>100	>100		>100	
Escherichia coli		8,294	3.1		1.6		0.2	
Klebsiella aerogenes		10,440	6.3		3.1		0.4	
Proteus rettgeri		8,479	<0.05		<0.05		<0.05	
Enterobacter cloacae		8,236	3.1		1.6		0.2	
Pseudomonas aeruginosa		8,329	>100		>100		100	
Escherichia coli	TEM +	10,404	6.3	12.5	3.1	6.3	0.4	0.8
Escherichia coli	TEM −	10,439	1.6	1.6	1.6	1.6	0.2	0.2
Enterobacter cloacae	P99 +	10,435	>100	>100	100	>100	100	>100
Enterobacter cloacae	P99 −	10,441	6.3	12.5	3.1	3.1	0.8	0.8
Klebsiella aerogenes	K1 +	10,436	100	>100	25	>100	25	>100
Klebsiella aerogenes	K1 −	10,440	1.6	1.6	1.6	1.6	0.2	0.2

[a] Minimum inhibitory concentrations were determined by a twofold agar dilution method on DST agar.

Table 17 Antibacterial activity of the monocarbams: MIC (μg/ml)[a]

Structures:
$R = -\overset{O}{\underset{}{C}}NHSO_2-$ (SQ 81,991)

$R = -\overset{O}{\underset{O^-}{P}}-OCH_3$ (SQ 27,159)

$R = SO_3^-$ (SQ 81,402)

Organism		SC number	SQ 81,991 CFU = 10^4	SQ 81,991 CFU = 10^6	SQ 27,159 CFU = 10^4	SQ 27,159 CFU = 10^6	SQ 81,402 CFU = 10^4	SQ 81,402 CFU = 10^6
Staphylococcus aureus	PENase −	2,399	>100		>100		>100	
Staphylococcus aureus	PENase +	2,400	>100		>100		>100	
Escherichia coli		8,294	1.6		6.3		0.4	
Klebsiella aerogenes		10,440	1.6		6.3		0.4	
Proteus rettgeri		8,479	<0.05		0.2		<0.05	
Enterobacter cloacae		8,236	0.8		1.6		0.4	
Pseudomonas aeruginosa		8,329	6.3		>100		3.1	
Escherichia coli	TEM +	10,404	0.4	0.8	0.8	3.1	3.1	25
Escherichia coli	TEM −	10,439	0.4	0.8	1.6	1.6	0.4	0.4
Enterobacter cloacae	P99 +	10,435	6.3	25	>100	>100	>100	>100
Enterobacter cloacae	P99 −	10,441	0.8	1.6	1.6	3.1	>100	0.4
Klebsiella aerogenes	K1 +	10,436	3.1	12.5	6.3	25	0.1	0.4
Klebsiella aerogenes	K1 −	10,440	0.2	0.8	0.8	1.6	>100	0.2

[a] Minimum inhibitory concentrations were determined by a twofold agar dilution method on DST agar.

193

Table 18 Antibacterial activity of the monosulfactams[a]: MIC (μg/ml)

Organism	SC number	SQ 26,608 CFU = 10⁴	SQ 26,777 CFU = 10⁴	SQ 26,699 CFU = 10⁴
Staphylococcus aureus	PENase –	1,276	0.4	0.8	1.6
Staphylococcus aureus	PENase –	2,399	0.8	0.8	1.6
Staphylococcus aureus	PENase +	2,400	0.8	0.8	1.6
Staphylococcus aureus	PENase +	10,165	1.6	0.8	6.3
Streptococcus faecalis		9,011	50	25	6.3
Streptococcus agalactiae		9,278	0.2	0.2	0.1
Micrococcus luteus		2,495	0.4	0.4	0.4
Escherichia coli		8,294	50	25	0.4
Klebsiella aerogenes		10,440	50	25	0.8
Proteus rettgeri		8,479	12.5	12.5	<0.05
Enterobacter cloacae		8,236	>100	>100	0.4
Pseudomonas aeruginosa		8,329	>100	100	3.1

[a] Data from Gordon et al., 1982.

anti-Gram-positive activity, show substantially reduced antipseudomonal activity, and are not dependent on 4-substitution for β-lactamase stability. The range of activities and stability to β-lactamases exhibited by some of the compounds is shown in Tables 14 and 15.

2. Monocarbams

A series of carbonyl-activated azetidinones has also been prepared wherein an acidic CONHSO$_2$R moiety affixed to the *N*-1 position yielded stable monocyclic β-lactams (monocarbams), displaying notable antibacterial properties (Slusarchyk *et al.*, 1982; Breuer *et al.*, 1982). As with the monophosphams, the aminothiazoleoxime sidechains were found optimal for high intrinsic activity. Substitution at the 4 position was not necessary for β-lactamase stability. Although somewhat confined to aminothiazoleoxime sidechains at the 3 position, a wide latitude was found in R-substitution on the —CONHSO$_2$R activating moiety. Like the monophosphams, the monocarbams are devoid of anti-Gram-positive activity. Not only do they differ in showing pronounced activity against members of the Enterobacteriaceae, but also some compounds exhibit a high level of activity against *Pseudomonas aeruginosa*. Representative structures and activities are seen in Tables 16 and 17.

3. Monosulfactams

Monocyclic β-lactams bearing an OSO$_3^-$ substituent at *N*-1 (monosulfactams) have also been synthesized (Gordon *et al.*, 1982) and found to be active against bacteria. In contrast to monophosphams and monocarbams, a wide range of sidechain substitutions generating molecules with diverse antibacterial properties was possible. Depending on the sidechain, compounds exhibiting a primarily anti-Gram-positive spectrum or broad spectrum can be produced. Compounds of the former type exhibit a high degree of activity and are stable to *S. aureus* penicillinase. The broad-spectrum monosulfactams, while highly active, are susceptible to Gram-negative β-lactamase. Examples of both types can be found in Table 18.

IV. DISCUSSION

The discovery that a monocyclic β-lactam could be suitably modified to produce compounds exhibiting pronounced microbiological activity has opened up another phase in the study of this versatile chemical entity. From the initial lead provided by the soil bacterium *C. violaceum,* a host of activated azetidinones has been prepared of diverse chemical structure and consequent diverse microbiological properties. From the SO$_3^-$-activated monobactams through the monophosphams, monocarbams, and monosulfactams, compounds have shown varying degrees of β-lactamase stability, levels of activity, and breadth of spectrum. The range of specifically anti-Gram-positive, specifically anti-Gram-negative, to broad spectrum is unparalleled with the traditional penicillin and cephalosporin nuclei. Furthermore, due to the structural simplicity of the monocyclic nucleus, we have the first class of β-lactam antibiotics amenable to total chemical synthesis both on the experimental and manufacturing scales.

Realizing that the monocyclic β-lactam nucleus is the basic essential structural feature very quickly led us to examine alternative activating groups. The dispatch with which these groups were found argues that a wide latitude in activation is possible and that many of the future breakthroughs in β-lactam research may very well center around a nucleus with a single ring.

REFERENCES

Aoki, H., Sakai, H. I., Kohsaka, M., Konomi, T., Hosoda, J., Kubochi, Y., Iguchi, E., and Imanaka, H. (1976). *J. Antibiot.* **29**, 492–500.
Breuer, H., Cimarusti, C. M., Denzel, T. L., Koster, W. H., Slusarchyk, W. A., and Treuner, U. D. (1981). *J. Antimicrob. Chemother.* **8E**, 21–28.
Breuer, H., Denzel, T., Straub, H., Lindner, K. R., Bonner, D. P., and Slusarchyk, W. A. (1982). *In* "Abstracts of 22nd Interscience Conference on Antimicrobial Agents and Chemotherapy," p. 184. Am. Soc. Microbiol., Washington, D.C.
Brown, A. G., Butterworth, D., Cole, M., Hanscomb, G., Hood, J. D., Reading, C., and Rolinson, G. N. (1976). *J. Antibiot.* **29**, 668–669.
Butterworth, D., Cole, M., Hanscomb, G., and Rolinson, G. N. (1979). *J. Antibiot.* **32**, 287–294.
Cassidy, P. J., Albers-Schonberg, G., Goegelman, R. T., Miller, T., Arison, B., Stapley, E. O., and Birnbaum, J. (1981). *J. Antibiot.* **34**, 637–648.
Cimarusti, C. M., Sykes, R. B., Applegate, M. A., Bonner, D. P., Breuer, H., Chang, M. W., Denzel, T. L., Floyd, D. M., Fritz, A. W., Koster, W. H., Liu, W. C., Parker, W. L., Rathnum, M. L., Slusarchyk, W. A., Treuner, U. D., and Young, M. G. (1982). *In* "New Beta-Lactam Antibiotics: A Review from Chemistry to Clinical Efficacy of the New Cephalosporins" (H. C. Neu, ed.), pp. 35–44. College of Physicians of Philadelphia, Philadelphia, Pennsylvania.
Cooper, R., Bush, K., Principe, P. A., Trejo, W. H., Wells, J. S., and Sykes, R. B. (1983). *J. Antibiot.* **36**, 1252–1257.
Georgopapadakou, N. H., Smith, S. A., and Sykes, R. B. (1982). *Antimicrob. Agents Chemother.* **21**, 950–956.
Gordon, E. M., Ondetti, M. A., Pluscec, J., Cimarusti, C. M., Bonner, D. P., and Sykes, R. B. (1982). *J. Am. Chem. Soc.* **104**, 6053–6060.
Imada, A., Kitano, K., Kintaka, K., Muroi, M., and Asai, M. (1981). *Nature (London)* **289**, 590–591.
Koster, W. H., Cimarusti, C. M., and Sykes, R. B. (1982a). *In* Chemistry and Biology of β-Lactam Antibiotics" (R. B. Morin and M. Gorman, eds.), Vol. 3, pp. 339–375. Academic Press, New York.
Koster, W. H., Zahler, R., Bonner, D. P., Chang, H. W., Cimarusti, C. M., Jacobs, G. A., and Perri, M. (1982b). *In* "Abstracts of 22nd Interscience Conference on Anti-

microbial Agents and Chemotherapy,'' p. 184. Am. Soc. Microbiol., Washington, D.C.

Liu, W. C., Parker, W. L., Wells, J. S., Principe, P. A., Trejo, W. M., Bonner, D. P., and Sykes, R. B. (1982). *In* "Current Chemotherapy and Immunotherapy" (P. Periti and G. G. Grossi, eds.), pp. 328–329. Am. Soc. Microbiol., Washington, D.C.

Nagarajan, R., Boeck, L. D., Gorman, M., Hamill, R. L., Higgins, G. E., Hoehn, M. M., Stark, W. M., and Whitney, J. G. (1971). *J. Am. Chem. Soc.* **93,** 2308–2310.

Nakayama, M., Iwasaki, A., Kimura, S., Mizoguchi, T., Tanabe, S., Murakami, A., Watanabe, I., Okuchi, M., Itoh, M., Saino, Y., Kobayashi, F., and Mori, T. (1980). *J. Antibiot.* **33,** 1388–1390.

Okamura, K., Hirata, S., Okumura, Y., Fukagawa, Y., Shimauchi, Y., Kouno, K., Ishikura, T., and Lein, J. (1978). *J. Antibiot.* **31,** 480–482.

Parker, W. L., and Rathnum, M. L. (1982b). *J. Antibiot.* **35,** 300–305.

Parker, W. L., Koster, W. H., Cimarusti, C. M., Floyd, D. M., Liu, W. C., and Rathnum, M. L. (1982a). *J. Antibiot.* **35,** 189–195.

Singh, P. D., Johnson, J. H., Ward, P. C., Wells, J. S., and Sykes, R. B. (1983). *J. Antibiot.* **36,** 1245–1251.

Slusarchyk, W. A., Applegate, H. E., Bonner, D. P., Breuer, H., Dejneka, T., and Koster, W. H. (1982). *In* "Abstracts of 22nd Interscience Conference on Antimicrobial Agents and Chemotherapy,'' p. 182. Am. Soc. Microbiol., Washington, D.C.

Sykes, R. B., Cimarusti, C. M., Bonner, D. P., Bush, K., Floyd, D. M., Georgopapadakou, N. H., Koster, W. H., Liu, W. C., Parker, W. L., Principe, P. A., Rathnum, M. L., Slusarchyk, W. A., Trejo, W. H., and Wells, J. S. (1981). *Nature (London)* **291,** 489–491.

Sykes, R. B., Parker, W. L., and Wells, J. S. (1982a). *In* "Trends in Antibiotic Research" (H. Umezawa, A. L. Demain, T. Hata, and C. R. Hutchinson, eds.), pp. 115–124. Japan Antibiotics Research Association, Tokyo.

Sykes, R.B., Bonner, D. P., Bush, K., and Georgopapadakou, N. H. (1982b). *Antimicrob. Agents Chemother.* **21,** 85–92.

Wells, J. S., Trejo, W. H., Principe, P. A., Bush, K., Georgopapadakou, N., Bonner, D. P., and Sykes, R. B. (1982a). *J. Antibiot.* **35,** 184–188.

Wells, J. S., Trejo, W. H., Principe, P. A., Bush, K., Georgopapodakou, N., and Sykes, R. B. (1982b). *J. Antibiot.* **35,** 295–299.

Wells, J. S., Hunter, J. C., Astle, G. L., Sherwood, J. C., Ricca, C. M., Trejo, W. H., Bonner, D. P., and Sykes, R. B. (1982c). *J. Antibiot.* **35,** 814–821.

8 Effect of low level of antibiotics on bacterial susceptibility to phagocytosis

CURTIS G. GEMMELL

I. INTRODUCTION

At least two qualities are needed of any pathogenic microorganism to allow it to multiply *in vivo*. Firstly, it must be able to utilize the complex chemical components present in the tissues of the host animal, allowing it to outgrow the commensal bacteria also present within that environment. Secondly, it should be able to inactivate (or fail to stimulate) the various host defence mechanisms, which would otherwise kill or remove it. In this respect the cellular elements of the body's reticuloendothelial system, namely polymorphonuclear leukocytes (PMN), monocytes (MO), and macrophages (MAC), are most important. These reticuloendothelial cells usually provide adequate protection for the host against microorganisms, but there are circumstances in which such cells protect the bacteria and disseminate them within the host. This occurs when the bacteria are able to survive and grow within wandering phagocytes, either through being endowed with structural aggressins (e.g., Vi antigen in *Salmonella typhi* and V and W antigens in *Yersinia pestis*) that impair the normal killing mechanisms or when bacteria are ingested by PMN deficient in some or all of the normal killing sequence (e.g., diminished myeloperoxidase enzyme activity in patients with chronic granulomatous disease).

It is in this arena that significant advances have been made in the study of phagocytosis *in vitro*, as reviewed recently by Horwitz (1982). Methods are now available for the isolation and purification of PMN and MO from peripheral blood, of MAC by bronchial lavage in man and of peritoneal macrophages in rodents, and the functions of the phagocytic cell are summarised in Table 1. In addition, a variety of methods exist for the accurate measurement of the kinetics

C. G. Gemmell

Table 1 Functions of phagocytic cell

Maturation and release of cells in bone marrow
Adherence to vascular endothelium
Random migration and chemotaxis
Adherence of particles
Phagocytosis
Intracellular killing and digestion
Degranulation

of uptake of various bacterial species by phagocytic cells (see Table 2). These studies have also shown that serum opsonization, either with antibody or complement or both, is an essential prerequisite for efficient phagocytosis, which progresses in various stages as outlined in Table 3.

The ingestion and subsequent destruction of microorganisms by phagocytic cells is a critical determinant of resistance to infectious diseases. The phagocytic process can be divided into two stages, attachment and ingestion. The particle to be ingested attaches to the phagocytic surface, and this attachment can be affected by a number of factors, including the surface charge of the particle, whether it is coated by opsonins, and whether the particle is attached to a surface. Bacteria can be phagocytosed if attached to surfaces, but free bacteria are less easily phagocytosed. The process is made much more efficient by the attachment to the bacterial surface of the activated third component of complement, C3b, either via the alternative pathway or by activation of the classical pathway by immune complexes containing IgG or IgM antibody. The route of complement activation followed depends to some extent on the bacterial species involved, and this association is summarised in Fig. 1. The phagocytic cell membrane carries receptors for C3b and for the Fc component of IgG. Each receptor is functionally independent, and attachment is dependent upon divalent cations such as Ca^{2+} and Mg^{2+}. Attachment of the particle can be separated from the ingestion process using inhibitors such as cytochalasin B, and attachment and phagocytosis are accompanied by subsequent lysosomal degranulation within the PMN. Microbial killing within the phagocytic cell is undertaken by two types of lysosomal

Table 2 Methods of studying phagocytosis

Cytological staining
Uptake of radioactive label
Reduction of nitro-blue tetrazolium
Chemiluminescence
Measurement of colony-forming units
Electron microscopy

Table 3 Stages of phagocytosis

Attachment
Ingestion
Mobilization of granules
Formation of phagosome
Binding of granules to phagosome
Reiease of granule enzymes
Activation of myeloperoxidase system
Generation of superoxide radicals
Destruction of bacterial cell
Release of bacterial debris from cell

granule: one, the azurophil (primary) granule, a large round neutral, dense body containing myeloperoxidase, neutral proteases, lysozyme and acid hydrolases; the other the specific (secondary) granule, being more numerous, electron-lucent, and containing lysozyme and lactoferrin. The ingestion of most bacteria is followed by fusion of both primary and secondary lysosomal granules with the phagosome, releasing a mixture of hydrolytic enzymes, which proceed to destroy any trapped bacterial cells.

The microbicidal mechanisms of phagoyctic cells comprise an oxygen-requiring one, such as the myeloperoxidase-mediated generation of hydrogen peroxide

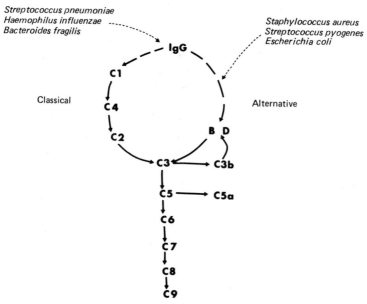

Fig. 1 Activation of complement by different bacterial pathogens.

and the production of the superoxide anions, and an oxygen-independent system. The former system requires cofactors such as iodide and thiocyanate ions and is inhibited by catalase, and organisms producing free catalase can exhibit enhanced virulence under these circumstances. The oxygen-independent process is primarily composed of acid, lysozyme, unsaturated lactoferrin, and cationic proteins. Although phagocytes have a significantly reduced microbicidal capacity under anaerobic conditions, killing still occurs. Fuller details of these intracellular biochemical pathways have been reviewed by Goren (1977) and Babior (1978a,b).

Antibiotic concentrations equal to the minimal inhibitory concentration (MIC) or greater than the MIC (minimal bactericidal concentration, MBC) for a given organism produce very different effects on the bacterial cell than those which result from concentrations below the MIC (sub-MIC). Different modes of action at these concentrations are real and not merely less pronounced. Lorian and Sabath (1972) were the first to show that exposure of *Proteus mirabilis* to sub-MIC's of penicillin and several cephalosporins presented different and distinct morphologies. Later, with the discovery that other drugs were capable of similar morphological effects on other organisms (Lorian, 1975), a term was needed to define the lowest concentration of an antibiotic that could affect bacterial structure or growth rate, or both. Lorian and de Freitas (1979) proposed the term minimum antibiotic concentration (MAC), indicating the minimum concentration of an antibiotic that could produce a structural change seen either by light or electron microscopy. These changes have been extensively reviewed (Lorian, 1980; Atkinson and Amaral, 1982).

The effects of antibiotics on bacterial cells have traditionally been demonstrated primarily *in vitro*, with clinical efficiency being deduced from experimental animal infections. Nevertheless, it is generally recognised that several host factors can exert independent effects *in vivo* as part of the host's defence against any bacterial invader, and these may well determine the outcome of an infection. The importance of host factors acting synergistically with the antibacterial action of a particular drug may modulate the speed and magnitude of the host response to a particular drug regimen. With the considerable advances now being made in the *in vitro* study of phagocytosis by white blood cells, we can now gain an understanding of how changes in the efficiency of this bacteria-scavenging system might affect the host response to particular antibiotic therapy. In particular, for individuals with defects in their immune system, acquired either congenitally or through other forms of medical treatment, antimicrobial chemotherapy remains a potent force in the treatment of any bacterial infection therein. Since host defense mechanisms and antibacterial agents may act in synergy, concentrations of the latter below those that will kill bacteria *in vitro* (i.e., sub-MIC) should be considered in the evaluation of any effect that might be achieved *in vivo*. Empha-

Table 4 Antiphagocytic substances produced by bacteria

Structural components	Organisms
Capsules	*Streptococcus pneumoniae, Escherichia coli*
M Protein	*Streptococcus pyogenes*
Pili	*Escherichia coli, Neisseria gonorrhoeae*
Protein A	*Staphylococcus aureus*
Microcapsule	*Salmonella typhi*

sis will be placed on the changes in bacterial susceptibility to phagocytosis that may arise following their exposure to antibacterial agents that fail to kill them or to inhibit their growth. Most of the studies discussed in this review concentrate on a fairly select group of microorganisms that display particular virulence determinants that, in the absence of any antibacterial agent, contribute to their resistance to the attentions of the phagocytic cell. A selection of such surface components associated with microbial pathogenicity is summarised in Table 4.

II. SOME FEATURES OF BACTERIAL RESISTANCE TO PHAGOCYTOSIS

The limiting surface layer of most Gram-positive bacteria comprises a "back-bone" of peptidoglycan in which other components such as lipoteichoic acid and proteins can be intercalated. As such, these structures resist phagocytosis through impairment of adherence of the bacteria to the phagocytic cells. However, certain proteins of the serum complement cascade can associate with these cell wall structures; factors B and C3b are particularly involved at this stage. Thereafter, C3 convertase is activated on the bacterial surface, amplifying the deposition of C3b onto the bacteria and potentiating their subsequent attachment to the C3b receptor of the phagocytic cells. In this respect, quite efficient phagocytic uptake and killing can take place in the absence of specific antibody. However, specific antibody binding to the bacterial cell provides a further attachment site on the leukocyte via the Fc receptor.

Several bacterial species carry on their surfaces a polysaccharide capsule that fails to activate the alternative complement pathway. Such "nonactivating" surfaces require the presence of specific antibody before complement activation via the classical pathway can take place. In particular, C1q is activated by the antibody–surface polysaccharide antigen complex, leading to generation of C3 convertase and C3b deposition as before. Thus there exists a fundamental difference between capsulated and noncapsulated bacteria in terms of the route by which prephagocytic opsonization occurs. In the former, the classical pathway of complement activation together with specific antibody is needed; in the latter, the alternative pathway of complement activation alone is required (Fig. 1).

Complement activation can still occur with some capsulated bacteria, although this does not allow adequate opsonization to take place. For example in *Staphylococcus aureus* M, C3 is fixed onto the bacterial surface below the capsular polysaccharide to the same extent as occurs with a noncapsulated variant of the same strain. In addition, both bacterial strains share a similar capacity for C3–C9 consumption in pooled normal human serum, C2-deficient serum, or immunoglobulin-deficient serum (Peterson *et al.*, 1978a,b). For effective opsonization of the encapsulated *S. aureus* M strain to occur before PMN phagocytosis type-specific antibodies must be present in the serum. Heat-inactivated immune rabbit serum (no active complement remaining) was found to have an increased opsonic capacity for the intact capsulated organism but not for a particle lacking capsule. In the currently accepted thinking, phagocytosis of capsulated bacteria by PMN requires specific plasma membrane receptors for the Fc portion of antibody molecules and the C3b component of complement to bind to the surface of the bacterium. The mechanism by which the capsule can mask the cell's surface from the attentions of serum opsonins is not yet clear. However, there are two possible explanations: (1) the capsule acts as a physicochemical barrier preventing access of opsonic factors to the peptidoglycan or (2) the capsule in some way interferes with the opsonic activity of serum factors, even though they may become bound to the bacterial cell surface. In either case, the capsule interferes with the normal recognition of the bacterium by leukocyte receptors. In an elegant study, Horwitz and Silverstein (1980) have shown that specific antibody and serum complement are needed to opsonize a capsulated strain of *Escherichia coli,* whereas serum complement alone was needed to opsonize a noncapsulated strain of the same organism.

III. MODIFICATION OF BACTERIA BY EXPOSURE TO ANTIBIOTICS

During the treatment of a bacterial infection with any antimicrobial agent, an important interaction must occur between the drug administered and the defenses of the host to eradicate the invading bacteria as expeditiously as possible. Much is known about the way in which antimicrobial agents attack microorganisms even at the molecular level and of the way in which the host responds to a particular microorganism. However, relatively little is known of the way in which specific antimicrobial agents might affect the encounter between the host's reticuloendothelial system and the bacteria, either by modifying the surface or other virulence properties of the organism or changing phagocytic function.

A. At levels greater than MIC

Since the discovery (Eagle and Musselman, 1949; Eagle *et al.*, 1950) that penicillin at $\geq$ MIC exerts paradoxical effects on the viability of staphylococci when incubated together, it has been discovered that the bacteria could survive under these conditions even in the presence of several times the MIC of the drug.

These studies led to the development of the concept of the postantibiotic effect (PAE) by Craig and his colleagues (Bundtzen *et al.*, 1981). They showed that antibiotics *in vitro* could retard bacterial growth and metabolism for a period beyond the period of exposure to the antibiotics. Working primarily with *Staphylococcus aureus*, but also with streptococci and *Haemophilus influenzae*, a variety of drugs were shown to induce a consistent postantibiotic effect ranging from minutes to several hours (McDonald *et al.*, 1977; Gerber and Craig, 1981). In these experiments bacterial suspensions were exposed for 2 hours to 4 × MIC of the appropriate antibiotic, followed by complete removal of the drug from the culture medium. The survival and subsequent regrowth of the drug-treated bacteria was then measured. Table 5 summarises the PAE values obtained for several antistaphylococcal drugs.

Gram-negative bacteria also exhibit an extended survival time when treated for a short time with chloramphenicol, conditions that interfere with protein synthesis by suppressing peptidyl transferase activity on the 50S subunit of the bacterial ribosome. The first of a series of studies followed (Pruul and McDonald, 1979) that examined the effect of a brief nonlethal exposure of *Escherichia coli* to chloramphenicol on subsequent *in vitro* antibacterial activity of human leukocytes and serum. *Escherichia coli*, when exposed to 5 × MIC chloramphenicol for 10 minutes, failed to resume normal growth for 1–4 hours in the presence of leukocytes and serum after removal of the drug from the reaction

Table 5 Postantibiotic effects (PAEs) of various antimicrobial agents on *Staphylococcus aureus* when exposed to 5 × MIC for 2 hours[a]

Drug	PAE (hr)
Penicillin	1.5
Ampicillin	1.7
Methicillin	1.9
Vancomycin	2.2
Erythromycin	3.1
Clindamycin	2.9
Gentamicin	0.3

[a] Taken from studies of Bundtzen *et al.* (1981).

mixture. This postantibiotic effect required white cells as well as specific antibody and complement to operate successfully. Pretreatment of leukocytes with chloramphenicol (50 μg/ml) failed to potentiate antibacterial activity, indicating that potentiation of the PAE was due entirely to an action of the drug on the bacteria within the pretreatment period. Later (Pruul *et al.*, 1981) it was shown that human leukocytes killed chloramphenicol-pretreated *E. coli* more efficiently than they did untreated control bacteria. Phagocytosis was measured by the uptake of radiolabelled bacteria and by direct microscopic counting of ingested bacteria. The decrease in bacterial viability was associated with enhanced intracellular killing of phagocytosed antibiotic-damaged bacteria. Leukocytes failed to kill chloramphenicol-pretreated *E. coli* in the presence of phenylbutazone; instead, an accumulation of intracellular bacteria occurred. This drug is an inhibitor of oxidative metabolism and causes a reduction in superoxide-dependent and myeloperoxidase-mediated bactericidal activities. Cytochalasin B also inhibited leukocidal activity against antibiotic-damaged bacteria. This drug inhibits translocation of myeloperoxidase-containing granules to the phagosomes of human neutrophils, probably by disruption of the contractile microfilament system of the cell. The inhibition of PMN killing action by these drugs may also be due to a decrease in phagocytic uptake of the antibiotic-damaged bacteria.

Bacterial opsonization via complement activation was essential, since Trypan blue, which binds to the C3 receptors of human PMN, inhibits killing of chloramphenicol-pretreated *E. coli* by leukocytes. In addition, anaerobic glycolysis was needed in the killing process, since iodoacetic acid was also inhibitory. The nonlethal damage sustained by initial contact with the drug has now been shown to render the bacteria more susceptible to intracellular killing—a good example of synergy between an antibiotic and PMN.

With *Staphylococcus aureus* and exposure to 10 × MIC of penicillin G, erythromycin, amoxycillin, or rifampicin for 10 min, McDonald *et al.* (1981) showed that pretreated bacteria proved to be more susceptible to phagocytosis by leukocytes than were the untreated control organisms. In the absence of leukocytes there occurred no significant depression of staphylococcal growth with any of the antibiotics.

With *E. coli,* only exposure to gentamicin was as effective as chloramphenicol in sensitizing the bacteria to phagocytic killing. Amoxycillin, ampicillin, and cefoxitin were rather less active in this respect. The degree to which chloramphenicol or gentamicin sensitized bacteria to phagocytosis depended to some extent on the strain of *E. coli* used, but no correlation with the presence or absence of K antigen was apparent.

Finally, it has been shown (Pruul *et al.*, 1982) that the sensitivity of several strains of *E. coli*, as well as *Klebsiella pneumoniae, Salmonella minnesota* and *Shigella sonnei*, to killing by acetate extracts of polymorphonuclear leukocyte granules could be altered by prior exposure for short periods of time to several antibiotics. For example, the quantity of granule extract needed to kill 50% of the target organism was significantly lower after prior exposure of the bacteria to chloramphenicol, tetracycline, streptomycin and gentamicin, but not after exposure to ampicillin or cefoxitin. Those results would not fit with those obtained earlier for the leukocyte activity against *E. coli,* which was particularly refractory to the bactericidal activity of the extract but was rendered susceptible after exposure to chloramphenicol and tetracycline. These findings would suggest that the enhanced phagocytic killing demonstrated earlier might be due in part to an increased fragility of the drug-treated bacterial cells to the components of the granule extract.

Preliminary evidence has also been obtained (H. Pruul, personal communication) that shows that an anaerobe, *Bacteroides fragilis,* can also be modified by exposure to chloramphenicol and clindamycin in terms of its susceptibility to phagocytic killing. Enhancement of killing was proportional to the time of exposure and to antibiotic concentration. Antibiotics such as penicillin G, amoxycillin, cefoxitin, and carbenicillin also potentiated killing, but not as markedly as seen with chloramphenicol and clindamycin. An accentuated leukocyte granule extract activity was seen following pretreatment with the latter two drugs.

The host's response to a microbial infection is determined to some extent by the relative efficiency of uptake and killing by phagocytic cells of the reticuloendothelial system, followed by the production of both specific antibodies to the pathogen and mediators of cellular immunity. The likelihood exists that antibiotics can influence this process either by potentiating bacterial cell killing or by reducing the amount of the antigenic stimulus needed to produce specific immunity. In addition, a too-rapid killing of bacteria (especially of Gram-negative bacteria such as *E. coli*) may lead to the rapid release of endotoxin, causing intravascular shock.

Clinical experience has shown that for antimicrobial therapy to be effective, a functional host defence system is required. If an antibacterial agent is prescribed at a dose well above its minimal inhibitory concentration, it becomes more difficult to take account of the host's contribution towards the final eradication of the pathogen.

B. At levels less than MIC

Several research groups have looked at the interaction of the bacterial pathogen with the host cell defence system in the presence or absence of antibiotics at very low levels. However, it must be understood that different methodologies have been used in each study.

In the early 1970s, Adam's group in West Germany looked at the effects of several antibiotics (gentamicin, polymyxin, dihydrostreptomycin, ampicillin, tetracycline, and chloramphenicol) in sub-growth-inhibitory concentrations on phagocytic and intracellular killing activity of mouse peritoneal macrophages (MAC) and human monocytes (MO) with *E. coli* and *Listeria monocytogenes* as target organisms. For example, both ampicillin and tetracycline at a concentration of 0.05 μg/ml each ($\frac{1}{20}$ × MIC) enhanced phagocytosis by human monocytes of *L. monocytogenes* by 41 and 75%, respectively (Adam *et al.*, 1974). In a similar way, dihydrostreptomycin at approximately $\frac{1}{70}$ × MIC enhanced both the phagocytic uptake and killing of *E. coli* by MAC (Adam *et al.*, 1972). Neither of these effects was due to a direct action of the drug on the isolated macrophages, since it was also shown that macrophages pretreated with the antibiotics in identical concentrations and washed free of drug prior to incubation with the test organism showed the same phagocytic activity as did control untreated MAC. However, different results have been obtained with the different methodologies used to study phagocytic function. For example, Midtvedt *et al.* (1982) looked at the effects of 13 antibiotics on the process of elimination of phagocytosed bacterial cell components from human PMN adhering to glass cover slips. Using ^{32}P-labelled *E. coli* as target organism, it was found that amphotericin B, fusidic acid, nalidixic acid, and rifampicin enhanced the degree of elimination occurring within 3 hours incubation with the drugs. On the other hand, doxycycline, metronidazole, and trimethoprim depressed the elimination of the labelled *E. coli*. However, high drug concentrations were needed to produce these effects.

Another group (Brunner and Undeutsch, 1982) has examined the effects of gentamicin and cephalothin on the phagocytic uptake and killing activity of guinea pig alveolar MAC for *Klebsiella pneumoniae*. It was shown that phagocytosis of this organism depended on adequate opsonization by specific antibodies. A 50-fold increase in uptake of bacteria occurred in the presence of specific antibody compared to that occurring in its absence. Uptake of *Klebsiella* organisms was neither enhanced nor impaired by the presence of gentamicin or cephalothin at their minimal bactericidal concentration. However, the number of viable bacteria within the macrophages was significantly reduced in the presence of the antibiotics. Of interest in this respect was the finding that sub-growth-inhibitory concentrations of the antibiotics also caused a reduction in the numbers of bacteria surviving intracellularly compared to that caused by higher concentrations of the same drugs. These data provide evidence that subinhibitory concentrations of some antibiotics might be sufficient to eradicate bacteria from the infected host, provided that the efficiency of phagocytic uptake and killing in the presence of appropriate opsonins is not impaired by the drugs.

The measured chemiluminescence (CL) by polymorphonuclear leukocytes in the presence of luminol and preopsonised target bacteria has been recognised as a function of membrane perturbation by the particles. Such a procedure has been used by Easmon and Desmond (1982) to examine the effects of sub-growth-inhibitory concentrations of a variety of antibiotics on the uptake of several bacteria by polymorphonuclear leukocytes. For group B streptococci, treatment with both penicillin G and clindamycin enhanced CL but had little effect on the observed uptake of the bacteria by the phagocytic cells. With a capsulated *Staphylococcus aureus* (M strain) a more variable effect was seen. For penicillin G, vancomycin, rifampicin, and clindamycin, negligible intracellular uptake of the organism was observed microscopically. Nevertheless, CL was enhanced by penicillin G and vancomycin but repressed by rifampicin- and clindamycin-grown bacteria. With a third target organism, *E. coli,* rifampicin and chloramphenicol treatment markedly enhanced chemiluminescence, but again no change was seen in the numbers of bacteria present within the PMN. With this study at least, little real evidence was obtained to show that changes in phagocytic uptake could be correlated with changes in luminol-enhanced chemiluminescence. However, in one experiment, the efficacy of killing of group B streptococci was improved by penicillin G or vancomycin pretreatment of the target bacteria.

Based on an earlier observation that protein exotoxins elaborated by several strains of *Streptococcus pyogenes* were not produced in the presence of sub-growth-inhibitory concentrations of various antibiotics, Gemmell and Amir (1979) examined the same bacteria for the presence of structural antigens, including the M and T proteins. These proteins are present as a surface "fuzz" associated with lipoteichoic acid of the cell wall of the bacterium (Swanson *et al.,* 1968). Using serological methods, lincomycin and clindamycin were shown to impair the expression of these antigens. A reduction in the M protein content of the treated cells was later shown to affect their susceptibility to phagocytosis by PMN. In a carefully controlled study, Gemmell *et al.* (1981) showed that the absence of M protein potentiated opsonization by normal human serum lacking specific antibodies to the surface antigens. Enhanced bacterial opsonization was reflected both in measurements of complement consumption via the alternative pathway (Table 6) and by the visual deposition of C3b on the surface of the bacterial cells by specific fluorescent antibody. Electron micrographs of thin sections of the drug-treated bacteria revealed that there remained little if any of

Table 6 Complement consumption by *Streptococcus pyogenes* after growth in the presence of clindamycin[a]

Target bacteria[b]	% Consumption of complement after	
	15 Minutes	60 Minutes
Untreated bacteria	19	54
$\frac{1}{4}$ × MIC clindamycin-grown bacteria	31	100

[a] Normal human serum was used at a concentration of 10% to treat 1 × 10^8 CFU *S. pyogenes.*
[b] Grown for 4 hours in shaken culture at 37°C.

the electron-dense "fuzz" corresponding to M protein (Figs. 2 and 3). Thus clindamycin even at $\frac{1}{10}$ × MIC impaired M protein synthesis and by so doing potentiated serum opsonization. When such opsonized bacteria were used as targets for measurement of phagocytosis by isolated human PMN and MO by the method of Verhoef *et al.* (1977), enhanced rates of phagocytosis were possible with clindamycin-grown bacteria. The results of such an experiment are shown in Table 7. Later it was shown that at least 2 hours' contact with the drug was necessary before any stimulation of phagocytic uptake occurred. The enhanced phagocytosis can also be illustrated microscopically (Fig. 4). In addition, these authors showed that drug treatment also potentiated the rate of killing of the streptococci by both PMN and MO.

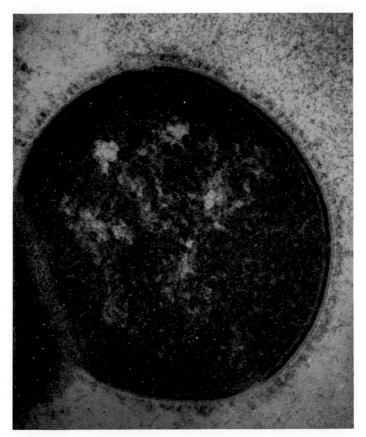

Fig. 2 Transmission electron micrograph of *Streptococcus pyogenes* S43 grown for 4 hours in the absence of any antibiotic. Note presence of an electron-dense "fuzz" around the cell, representing M protein. × 70,000.

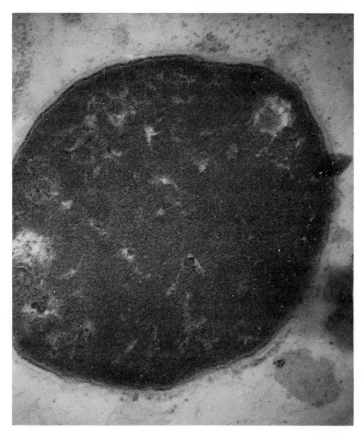

Fig. 3 Transmission electron micrograph of *Streptococcus pyogenes* S43 grown for 4 hours in the presence of ½ × MIC clindamycin. Note absence of an electron-dense "fuzz" around the cell. × 70,000.

Table 7 Phagocytosis of *Streptococcus pyogenes* by PMN after growth in clindamycin at sub-growth-inhibitory concentrations

Target bacteria	% Phagocytic uptake by PMN after	
	15 Minutes	30 Minutes
Untreated bacteria	8.2	9.0
½ × MIC clindamycin-grown[a]	30.4	38.6
¼ × MIC clindamycin-grown[a]	28.2	40.4

[a] Grown for 4 hours in shaken culture at 37°C.

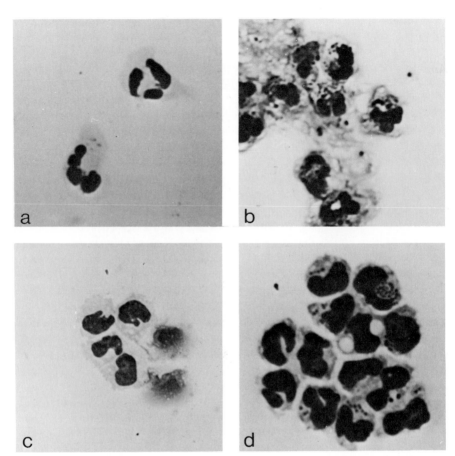

Fig. 4 Phagocytosis of *Streptococcus pyogenes* grown in the presence or absence of $\frac{1}{2}$ × MIC clindamycin. (a) PMN + normal *S. pyogenes;* (b) PMN + drug-grown *S. pyogenes;* (c) MO + normal *S. pyogenes;* (d) MO + drug-grown *S. pyogenes.*

In this context the studies of Horne and Tomasz (1980, 1981) are relevant. They showed that pretreatment of group B streptococci with benzyl penicillin, other β-lactam antibiotics or vancomycin increased the susceptibility of these bacteria to the bactericidal activity of a mixture of PMN and serum. This method contrasts with that of Gemmell *et al.* (1981), in which the drug-grown bacteria were preopsonised with normal human serum before being exposed to the leukocytes. Horne and Tomasz (1981) in their system showed that only β-lactam antibiotics at sub-MIC levels enhanced killing by leukocytes. Gentamicin and chloramphenicol, inhibitors of bacterial protein synthesis, failed to affect the susceptibility of the streptococci to phagocytosis. Penicillin treatment at $\frac{1}{8}$ ×

MIC induced the release of substantial quantities of cell surface components (lipoteichoic acid, lipid, and capsular polysaccharide). Earlier work by Amir (1980), using a somewhat simplified microscopic measurement of phagocytosis, had shown that exposure of a strain of group B streptococcus to lincomycin and clindamycin enhanced its susceptibility to phagocytosis. The percentage of PMN showing active uptake of the organism in 30 minutes increased from 38 to 62 and 66%, respectively, whereas neither erythromycin nor chloramphenicol treatment had any effect. Measurement of NBT (nitro-blue tetrazolium) reductase by histochemical staining also demonstrated increased enzymic activity when lincomycin- or clindamycin-exposed bacteria were the targets for the PMN. At this time also, preliminary experiments with capsulated *Streptococcus pneumoniae* (NCTC 9798), refractory to phagocytosis, showed that the same drugs as well as penicillin failed to potentiate phagocytosis. In this organism at least, the presence of a capsule would appear to protect the organism from drug-induced modulation.

One microorganism that has been studied in some detail in relation to its interaction with polymorphonuclear leukocytes has been *Staphylococcus aureus*. Numerous reports have been generated from laboratories in both Europe and the United States showing that phagocytosis of *Staphylococcus aureus* is dependent on adequate opsonization via activation of the alternative complement cascade (Peterson *et al.*, 1978b). However, two surface components of the cell are known to impair this process, namely protein A (Peterson *et al.*, 1977) and capsular polysaccharide (Wilkinson *et al.*, 1979).

Armed with such knowledge, several investigators have used a variety of antibiotics and several strains of *Staphylococcus aureus* to study the role of its surface structures in terms of their antiopsonic, and hence antiphagocytic, capabilities. Early work had shown that pretreatment of staphylococci with penicillin accelerated their subsequent phagocytosis by mouse macrophages (Friedman and Warren, 1974, 1976) and that the use of sub-MIC penicillin increased the susceptibility of staphylococci to killing by mixtures of lysozome and trypsin (Warren and Gray, 1966) or to lysosomal extracts (Efrati *et al.*, 1976).

The β-lactam antibiotics produce two major effects on susceptible bacteria when used at sub-MIC levels: inhibiting cross-wall formation so that unusually long filamentous cells are formed (Lorian, 1975), or causing the formation of thickened cross-walls without subsequent separation (Lorian and Atkinson, 1976).

Root *et al.* (1981) showed that *Staphylococcus aureus* 502 A pretreated with $\frac{1}{4}$ × MIC penicillin G during its logarithmic phase of growth, causing the appearance of thickened cross-walls, became more susceptible to killing by PMN as measured by their intracellular survival time. For example, a mean survival rate of $0.17 \pm 0.04\%$ was seen with drug-grown bacteria, compared to $1.5 \pm 0.38\%$ following their interaction with the PMN and normal human serum.

Again, it should be noted that no preopsonization with serum was allowed before phagocytic uptake and killing were measured. In other experiments, Root *et al.* were able to show that this enhanced susceptibility to killing by PMN occurred even when phagosome formation was inhibited by cytocholasin B. In this case, $65.6 \pm 4.6\%$ of the penicillin-treated bacteria were killed after the same period of incubation with the PMN. Pretreatment of *Staphylococcus aureus* with vancomycin similarly enhanced susceptibility to killing by cytochalasin-B–treated PMN ($51.1 \pm 2.8\%$ compared to $29.3 \pm 4.9\%$), but no effect was seen with gentamicin pretreatment. In fact, fewer staphylococci were killed in 30 minutes compared to the untreated bacteria ($12.6 \pm 5.3\%$, versus $29.3 \pm 4.9\%$). Penicillin was shown to be effective even when used at $\frac{1}{16} \times$ MIC, whereas vancomycin was active only as low as $\frac{1}{8} \times$ MIC.

Although the rate of killing was enhanced by pretreatment of the bacteria by penicillin, no change was detectable in either the rate of phagocytic uptake by the PMN or of the activity of PMN–myeloperoxidase-mediated protein iodination. By measuring inorganic iodide fixed to trichloroacetic acid–precipitated protein, no differences were seen in PMN incubated in 10% serum with normal or penicillin-treated bacteria (0.138 ± 0.09 versus 0.159 ± 0.01 nmol). In addition, little evidence was apparent from electron microscopy suggesting that penicillin-pretreatment caused earlier cell lysis within the phagolysosome.

Somewhat contradictory results were reported in a carefully controlled study by Milatovic (1982). She examined the effect of sub-MIC levels of penicillin, cefotiam, piperacillin, vancomycin, clindamycin, and doxycycline against another strain of *Staphylococcus aureus* in terms of its rate of uptake and susceptibility to killing by PMN. Of the six drugs tested, only clindamycin and doxycycline had any potentiating effect on the rate of uptake of radiolabeled bacteria. Clindamycin was active in this respect even at $\frac{1}{32} \times$ MIC, whereas doxycycline was active at $\frac{1}{64} \times$ MIC. These effects were seen under conditions in which only 1% serum was present in the reaction mixture. However, no significant difference was apparent in the efficiency of PMN killing of these drug-grown organisms within 30 minutes. In view of the fact that the experimental set-up chosen meant that the bacteria had to be opsonized as well as taken up and killed by the PMN within a short time, any differences in killing rate might be difficult to detect. Neither penicillin nor the other cell-wall active antibiotics had any action on phagocytic uptake or killing staphylococci. Against this, however, Root *et al.* (1981) did find differences with penicillin treatment within this time and under somewhat similar experimental conditions.

In another study, Lorian and Atkinson (1980) grew 14 different strains of *Staphylococcus aureus* on membrane filters placed on agar containing sub-minimal inhibitory concentrations ($\frac{1}{2}$ or $\frac{1}{4} \times$ MIC) of either oxacillin or nafcillin. Clusters of staphylococci held together by thick cross-walls resulted. Such bacteria, as well as the same strains grown without any drug present in the agar, were eluted from the membranes and incubated with human PMN and serum (concentration unknown). Phagocytosis was measured either by phase contrast microscopy or by Giemsa-stained smears, and the authors reported no difference in rate of phagocytic uptake of staphylococci, whether or not they had been exposed to oxacillin or nafcillin. However, the drug-grown organisms were less susceptible to phagocytic killing than were the control organisms (no drug present). This was statistically significant over the first 60 minutes of incubation but not thereafter. It is almost certain that the poorer efficiency of killing of the drug-grown bacteria was related to the fairly complex ultrastructure of the enlarged bacterial

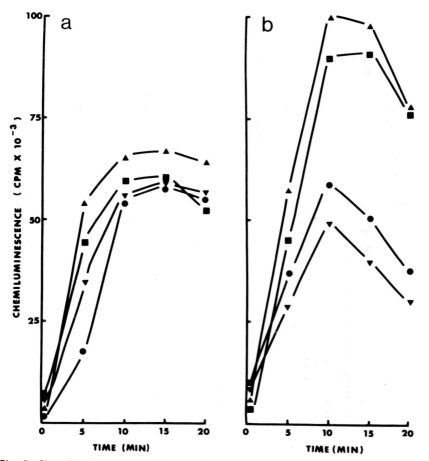

Fig. 5 Chemiluminescence of human PMN in response to *Staphylococcus aureus* grown in absence of any drug or in the presence of (a) sub-MIC clindamycin or (b) sub-MIC fusidic acid: ●———● no drug present; ▲———▲ $\frac{1}{2}$ × MIC; ■———■ $\frac{1}{4}$ × MIC; ▼———▼ $\frac{1}{8}$ × MIC.

cells having multiple cross-walls. After 30 and 60 minutes incubation with PMN, the killing rates for oxacillin-grown versus control staphylococci were 52 and 70% versus 65 and 85%, respectively.

However, in none of the studies reported to date has much attention been paid to the mechanism whereby different drugs either enhance or repress phagocytic uptake and killing. Recently experiments in this laboratory (Gemmell and O'Dowd, 1983) have measured protein A on the staphylococcal surface (*Staphylococcus aureus* Cowan 1) with and without exposure to either clindamycin or fusidic acid, both ribosomal protein synthesis inhibitors. In view of the findings of Peterson *et al.* (1977) in which the presence of protein A on the surface of the cell was recognised as an inhibitor of serum opsonization, it seemed logical to explore whether differences in opsonization might explain some of the discrepancies described earlier in staphylococcal killing rates by PMN following exposure to the drugs. Staphylococci were exposed to either clindamycin or fusidic acid for either 6 or 18 hours in drug concentrations of between $\frac{1}{2}$ and $\frac{1}{16} \times$ MIC before their opsonization in human serum. Exposure of these preopsonized bacteria to PMN allowed the discrete measurement of phagocytic uptake without any interference by concomitant opsonization. The rate of phagocytic uptake was potentiated by exposure to either drug. In the case of clindamycin, this effect was seen at $\frac{1}{4} \times$ MIC and for fusidic acid at $\frac{1}{8} \times$ MIC. By following chemiluminescence as a measure of phagocytic uptake of bacteria, the magnitude of the CL

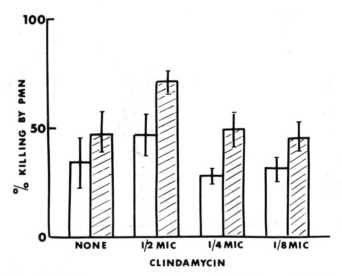

Fig. 6 Killing of *Staphylococcus aureus* by human PMN after growth in the presence or absence of low levels of clindamycin: open bars, percentage killed after 30 min; cross-hatched bars, percentage killed after 60 min.

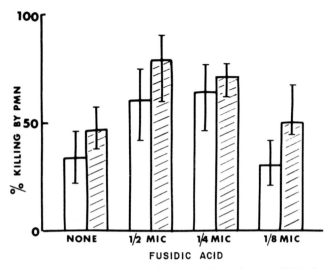

Fig. 7 Killing of *Staphylococcus aureus* Cowan strain by human PMN after growth in the presence or absence of low levels of fusidic acid: open bars, percentage killed after 30 min; cross-hatched bars, percentage killed after 60 min.

response was greater with staphylococci exposed to either drug than in their absence. A typical experiment is illustrated in Fig. 5. Finally, killing curves were obtained for both the clindamycin treated and fusidic-acid–treated bacteria, and this showed an enhanced rate of destruction of viable cells (see Figs. 6 and 7). Protein A was markedly reduced on the surface of the drug-exposed organisms. It was also apparent that this loss was due in part to an increased release of the protein from the bacterial cell surface during growth in the presence of the drugs. These studies provide some ''common ground'' between the conflicting evidence of the other groups who have investigated the effect of drug exposure on staphylococcal susceptibility to phagocytosis. Therefore some change (probably attributable to protein A or to some other structural component of the cell) occurs when *Staphylococcus aureus* is exposed to antibiotics at sub-growth-inhibitory levels. In this context it is worth noting that *S. aureus* M carrying a polysaccharide capsule is not affected by growth in either clindamycin or fusidic acid (C. G. Gemmell, unpublished observations), nor is phagocytosis potentiated or repressed under these circumstances.

1. Gram-negative bacteria

Much less is known about the effects of sub-growth-inhibitory levels of antibiotics on the susceptibility of both aerobic and anaerobic Gram-negative bacteria to host defence systems. In this respect only *Escherichia coli, Haemophilus influ-*

enzae, and *Bacteroides fragilis* have been looked at in any detail, and they will be briefly reviewed.

(a)   Escherichia coli

Early studies by Lorian and Atkinson (1979) showed that several members of the Enterobacteriaceae exposed to low concentrations of antibiotics were equally or less susceptible than control organisms to the bactericidal effect of serum. Organisms that were serum-sensitive were killed in less than 30 minutes. Filaments and rounded cells arising from exposure to sub-MICs of ampicillin or mecillinam were equally susceptible to serum killing over 30 minutes. When organisms that were resistant to serum were exposed to certain β-lactam antibiotics, the morphologically abnormal forms also remained resistant. In one case a serum-sensitive strain of *E. coli* appeared to become more serum-resistant after exposure to the antibiotic. In contrast, Taylor *et al.* (1981) showed that each of four serum-resistant strains of *E. coli* after growth in the presence of various subinhibitory concentrations of mecillinam or pivmecillinam became more serum-susceptible. Production of ovoid or rounded cells in the presence of the drugs was not a prerequisite for serum sensitization. Growth in the presence of mecillinam did not alter the serum sensitivity of a serum-susceptible *E. coli* strain. In addition, Alexander *et al.* (1980) have found that rifampicin at subinhibitory concentrations could convert an *E. coli* strain from being serum-resistant to being serum-sensitive. Such a finding may be important when one considers the studies of Bar-Shavit *et al.* (1980), who looked at the uptake of *E. coli* by mouse peritoneal MAC. They showed that the mannose-binding activity of *E. coli* determined the recognition of the organisms by the phagocytic cells. Nonseptate filamentous cells were formed by growing the organisms in the presence of cephalexin. The internalization of filamentous cells by peritoneal macrophages was much less efficient (uptake only 20%) compared to that found with normal rod-shaped single cells (90% uptake) after 30 minutes.

(b)   Haemophilus influenzae

Only one report exists that has sought to examine the ability of PMN to kill *Haemophilus influenzae* type b cells that have previously been exposed to sub-growth inhibitory concentrations of antibiotics (Cates and Caparas, 1981). Bacteria were exposed to either ampicillin or chloramphenicol at a concentration of either $\frac{1}{8}$ × MIC for 3 hours at 37°C or 25 × MIC for 10 min at 37°C. Such antibiotic-treated cells were then washed and mixed with PMN and serum before measurement of killing. After 1 hour there was significantly more killing of the *Haemophilus* exposed to either sub-MIC ampicillin or a pulsed dose of 25 × MIC ampicillin (26 and 61%) compared to ampicillin alone (no PMN) with mean killing of 1 and 38% respectively. Similar pretreatment of *Haemophilus influenzae* with chloramphenicol (from $\frac{1}{2}$ to $\frac{1}{12}$ × MIC) had no effect on killing by PMN. However, no mechanism was proposed whereby this differential effect of the two antibiotics on *Haemophilis influenzae* could be explained. It is possible that alterations occurred in the degree of encapsulation in this organism after exposure to the drugs.

(c) Bacteroides fragilis

Recognition of the role of *Bacteroides fragilis* in the aetiology of a variety of infectious processes has fostered research into the pathogenicity of this organism and its interaction with host defences. Improved methods of electron microscopy with and without ruthenium red staining for polysaccharide have demonstrated that pathogenic strains of *B. fragilis* are endowed with a polysaccharide capsule (Kasper *et al.* 1979). Others (Onderdonk *et al.*, 1977) have demonstrated a close association between encapsulation and virulence (Simon *et al.*, 1982), especially with regard to the development of an experimental model of peritoneal abscesses (Onderdonk *et al.*, 1976) and skin abscesses (Joiner *et al.*, 1980) in association

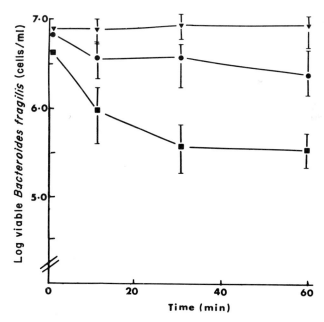

Fig. 8 Killing of *Bacteroides fragilis* UC 6428 grown in the presence or absence of $\frac{1}{2}$ × MIC clindamycin: ●——● serum-opsonized bacteria grown in absence of drug + PMN; ■——■ serum-opsonized bacteria grown in presence of drug + PMN; ▼——▼ non-opsonized bacteria grown in absence of drug + PMN.

with *E. coli*. In addition, Bjornson and her colleagues (Bjornson and Bjornson, 1978; Bjornson *et al.*, 1980) have unravelled the opsonic requirements of the organism and its susceptibility to phagocytosis. Adequate opsonisation requires both the presence of specific antibody and activation of the alternative complement pathway.

In this context, some investigations in our laboratory have sought to understand the role of the polysaccharide capsule in the pathogenicity of the organism. Since *B. fragilis* is very sensitive to clindamycin, attempts were made to modify its virulence by growing it in the presence of sub-growth-inhibitory concentrations of the drug. Under these circumstances its ability to elaborate the capsule was impaired: electron microscopy failed to detect any capsule on the cell surface, even with the use of ruthenium red staining (Gemmell *et al.*, 1983). Such cells were more rapidly phagocytosed and killed by human PMN (see Fig. 8). It would appear that loss of the capsule enhanced the host cellular response to the pathogen. It is possible that within the anaerobic abscess in circumstances where poor penetration of chemotherapeutic drugs may take place (Joiner *et al.*, 1981), the ability of a drug to act at sub-growth-inhibitory concentrations might be more important, especially where an adequate phagocytic response is necessary for the resolution of the abscess. As Joiner *et al.* (1980) have shown, the anaerobic abscess is composed of a focus of infection surrounded by a halo of phagocytic cells. Under these conditions any enhancement of phagocytic function through antibiotic-induced modification of the bacterial cell could undoubtedly alter the course of the infectious process.

IV. ANTIBIOTICS—THEIR UPTAKE AND INTERACTION WITH PHAGOCYTIC CELLS

The last 10 years have seen the emergence of interest in the effects of antibacterial agents on phagocytic function. In particular their effect on chemotaxis, phagocytic uptake and killing has been examined using a variety of experimental methods and was reviewed recently by Mandell (1982). Since this chapter is more concerned with the direct action of the antibacterial agents on the bacteria and only indirectly on phagocytic cells, attention will be directed only towards the possible action of antibiotics within the phagocytic cells which might affect their microbicidal function. A number of studies have shown that concentration of several antibiotics can take place within the phagocytic cell, whereas others fail to penetrate the cell to any extent. Johnson *et al.* (1980) have examined the uptake of numerous antibiotics by rabbit alveolar macrophages. These cells failed to concentrate penicillin G, cefazolin, cefamandole, cephalexin, gentamicin, tetracycline and isoniazid. Limited concentration intracellularly was seen with rifampicin, lincomycin and chloramphenicol, with ethambutol and erythromycin being taken up to a greater extent. By far the best uptake was shown by clindamycin, which was concentrated 40-fold within the MAC. Clindamycin uptake by PMN was rapid, saturable and temperature-dependent (Klempner and Styrt, 1981); accumulated within the host cell's lysosomes; and remained bioactive therein. These studies probably explain the early work of Mandell and Vest (1972), who studied the microbicidal activity of several antibiotics on staphylococci within human PMN. Although extracellular bacteria were killed by all the drugs tested, only rifampicin was able to eliminate completely intracellular organisms as well. A direct correlation may exist between this study and the improved therapeutic efficiency of rifampicin in lethal staphylococcal intraperitoneal infections and subcutaneous abscesses in mice (Lobo and Mandell, 1972). However, when the same drug was tried against *Mycobacterium tuberculosis* in human monocyte cultures (Clini and Grassi, 1970), it was no more capable of inactivating intracellular organisms than either cycloserine or ethambutol. In another study (Pesanti, 1980), neither rifampicin nor penicillin at up to $50 \times$ MIC enhanced the intracellular killing of *Staphylococcus aureus* within unstimulated mouse peritoneal macrophages. More recently, Elliot *et al.* (1982) incubated PMN that had already ingested *S. aureus* with $\frac{1}{10} \times$ MIC of either penicillin, cephalothin or clindamycin for up to 16 hours at 37°C. Lower survival rates within the PMN were seen with each drug, suggesting drug action intracellularly.

V. *IN VIVO* EFFECTS OF SUB-GROWTH-INHIBITORY CONCENTRATIONS OF ANTIBIOTICS

Not long after the discovery that sub-growth-inhibitory concentrations of antibiotics could affect the expression of soluble virulence factors by *Staphylococcus aureus* (Gemmell and Shibl, 1976), it was discovered that the same drugs (clindamycin, fusidic acid and lincomycin) could also impair toxinogenesis in experimental staphylococcal skin lesions in mice. At the same time, the extent and histological features of the infection were reduced whenever these drugs were administered to the animals (Gemmell, 1978). Later, Comber *et al.* (1977) achieved 50% protection of mice infected with *E. coli* by maintaining $\frac{1}{4} \times$ MIC amoxycillin in the animal's bloodstream. In contrast, ampicillin, also at $\frac{1}{4} \times$ MIC, failed to protect the animals (Zak and Kradolfer, 1979). Later these same authors showed that ampicillin and gentamicin (both at $\frac{1}{3} \times$ MIC), if maintained at these concentrations for up to 6 hours in the peritoneal fluid of rabbits experimentally infected with *E. coli,* could enhance the survival of some of the animals. Of those animals that were given therapy and subsequently died, survival time was longer than in the control animals given no drug. Additionally it was found that ampicillin ($\frac{1}{3}$ × MIC), cephaloridine ($\frac{1}{3}$ × MIC) and gentamicin ($\frac{1}{6}$ × MIC) could also protect rabbits infected with *Proteus mirabilis*.

Nevertheless, another study (Zak *et al.*, 1977) showed that drug therapy (at sub-MIC levels) failed to enhance survival of the experimentally infected animals. Animals infected with *Salmonella typhimurium* died sooner (21 hours) when ampicillin was administered to achieve $\frac{1}{3}$ × MIC in the peritoneal cavity compared to the control animals, which died in 26 hours. Enhanced endotoxin release may explain these results.

Smith and Kong (1981) reported that sub-growth-inhibitory concentrations of nafcillin enhanced the virulence of *Staphylococcus aureus* in mice. In a limited study using 10 control mice and 10 mice challenged with nafcillin-damaged bacteria, a difference in time to death was seen in the two groups: the antibiotic-damaged staphylococci brought forward mortality by 2 hours. No explanation was given for this difference.

VI. SUMMARY AND CONCLUSIONS

In such a review as this, it is immediately apparent that "the state of the art" reflects primarily on the various *in vitro* experiments that have been performed in various laboratories. Since the outset, antibacterial chemotherapy has been based upon the quantitative assay of the inhibition of bacterial growth or bacterial killing using cultural techniques. It has always been assumed that the achievement of serum levels greater than those that inhibit bacterial growth will be effective therapeutically. Since many drugs reach only up to half of their serum concentrations in some tissues, and since administration of many antibiotics is only intermittent, a knowledge of how the drug may perform at concentrations below those that inhibit bacterial growth may be of value to the clinician. However, there exist only a few reports of the use of sub-growth-inhibitory concentrations of antibiotics in humans. Reymann *et al.* (1979) reported that a group of patients with Gram-negative sepsis who were not immunosuppressed, when treated with gentamicin, showed the same rate of mortality when the serum

Table 8 Antibiotics shown to alter microbial susceptibility to phagocytic uptake

Antibiotic	Target
Ampicillin	*Haemophilus influenzae*
Clindamycin, fusidic acid, doxycycline	*Staphylococcus aureus*
Clindamycin, penicillin G	*Streptococcus pyogenes*

Table 9 Antibiotics shown to alter microbial susceptibility to phagocytic killing

Antibiotic	Target
Clindamycin	*Streptococcus pyogenes*
Penicillin, vancomycin	*Streptococcus* (group B)
Penicillin, clindamycin, fusidic acid	*Staphylococcus aureus*
Clindamycin	*Bacteroides fragilis*

levels of drug were lower than $\frac{1}{8} \times$ MIC for the infecting organism as did patients who had gentamicin levels higher than $\frac{1}{8} \times$ MIC.

In addition, Ben Redjib *et al.* (1982) reported good therapeutic results when 10 mg ampicillin and 2 litres of water were given to patients with urinary-tract infections due to *E. coli*. It was calculated that this therapy resulted in sub-MIC levels of ampicillin in the urine. Notwithstanding these reports, which perhaps do not accurately reflect the complex picture of the host–parasite relationship as it exists in most bacterial infections (namely, the phagocytic encounter between bacteria and cells of the reticuloendothelial system), it is fair to propose that at least some of the subtle effects of antibiotics on bacterial virulence factors described in this review (see Tables 8 and 9) might take place *in vivo*. Some of the animal experiments would certainly support this concept. However, the biological effects of low levels of antibiotics will continue to generate interest within the medical and scientific communities and can only lead to a greater understanding of the host–parasite relationship, especially with regard to the immune-compromised host exposed to an increasing variety of antibacterial and antiinflammatory drugs in association with more sophisticated surgical procedures and organ transplantation.

ACKNOWLEDGMENT

The excellent secretarial assistance of Ms. Alison Smith is gratefully acknowledged.

REFERENCES

Adam, D., Staber, F., Belohradsky, B. H., and Marget, W. (1972). *Infect. Immun.* **5,** 537–541.
Adam, D., Schaffert, W., and Marget, W. (1974). *Infect. Immun.* **9,** 811–814.
Alexander, W. J., Cobbs, C. G., and Curtiss, M. R. (1980). *Infect. Immun.* **28,** 923–926.
Amir, M. K. A. (1980). Ph.D. Thesis, University of Glasgow.

Atkinson, B. A., and Amaral, L. (1982). *CRC Crit. Rev. Microbiol.* **9**(2), 101–138.

Babior, B. M. (1978a). *N. Engl. J. Med.* **298**, 659–668.

Babior, B. M. (1978b). *N. Engl. J. Med.* **298**, 721–725.

Bar-Shavit, Z., Goldman, R., Ofek, I., Sharon, N., and Mirelman, D. (1980). *Infect. Immun.* **29**, 417–424.

Ben Redjib, S., Slim, A., Horchani, A., Zmerli, S., Boujnah, A., and Lorian, V. (1982). *In* "Current Chemotherapy and Immunotherapy" (P. Periti and G. G. Grassi, eds.), p. 13. Am. Soc. Microbiol., Washington, D.C.

Bjornson, A. B., and Bjornson, H. S. (1978). *J. Infect. Dis.* **138**, 351–358.

Bjornson, A. B., Bjornson, H. S., and Kitko, B. P. (1980). *Infect. Immun.* **28**, 633–637.

Brunner, H., and Undeutsch, C. (1982). *In* "The Influence of Antibiotics on the Host–Parasite Relationship" (H.-V. Eickenberg, H. Hahn, and W. Opferkuch, eds.), pp. 129–138. Springer-Verlag, Berlin and New York.

Bundtzen, R. W., Gerber, A. U., Cohn, D., and Craig, W. A. (1981). *Rev. Infect. Dis.* **3**, 28–37.

Cates, K. L., and Caparas, L. (1981). *Antimicrob. Agents Chemother.* **21** (Abstr. 658).

Clini, V., and Grassi, C. (1970). *Antibiot. Chemother. (Washington, D.C.)* **16**, 20–26.

Comber, K. R., Boon, R. T., and Sutherland, R. (1977). *Antimicrob. Agents Chemother.* **12**, 736–744.

Eagle, H., and Musselman, A. D. (1949). *J. Bacteriol.* **58**, 475–490.

Eagle, H., Fleischman, R., and Musselman, A. D. (1950). *Ann. Intern. Med.* **33**, 544–571.

Easmon, C. S. F., and Desmond, A. M. (1982). *In* "The Influence of Antibiotics on the Host–Parasite Relationship" (H. V. Eickenberg, H. Hahn, and W. Opferkuch, eds.), pp. 202–206. Springer-Verlag, Berlin and New York.

Efrati, C., Sacks, T., Ne'eman, N., Lahav, M., and Ginsburg, I. (1976). *Inflammation* **1**, 371–407.

Elliot, G. R., Peterson, P. K., Verbrugh, H. A., Freiberg, M. R., Hoidal, J. R., and Quie, P. G. (1982). *Antimicrob. Agents Chemother.* **22**, 781–784.

Friedman, H., and Warren, G. H. (1974). *Proc. Soc. Exp. Biol. Med.* **146**, 707–711.

Friedman, H., and Warren, H. G. (1976). *Proc. Soc. Exp. Biol. Med.* **153**, 301–304.

Gemmell, C. G. (1978). *In* "Current Chemotherapy," (W. Siegenthaler and R. Lüthy, eds.), pp. 512–514. Am. Soc. Microbiol., Washington, D.C.

Gemmell, C. G., and Amir, M. K. (1979). *In* "Streptococci and Streptococcal Disease" (M. T. Parker, ed.), pp. 67–68. Reedbooks, Chertsey, England.

Gemmell, C. G., and O'Dowd, A. (1983). *J. Antimicrob. Chemother.* **12**, 587–597.

Gemmell, C. G., and Shibl, A. M. (1976). *In* "Staphylococci and Staphylococcal Infections" (J. Jeljaszewicz, ed.), pp. 657–664. Fischer, Stuttgart.

Gemmell, C. G., Peterson, P. K., Schmeling, D., Kim, Y., Mathews, J., Wannamaker, L., and Quie, P. G. (1981). *J. Clin. Invest.* **67**, 1249–1256.

Gemmell, C. G., Peterson, P. K., Schmeling, D., Mathews, J., and Quie, P. G. (1983). *Eur. J. Clin. Microbiol.* **2**, 327–334.

Gerber, A. U., and Craig, W. A. (1981). *J. Antimicrob. Chemother.* **8**, Suppl. C, 81–91.

Goren, M. B. (1977). *Annu. Rev. Microbiol.* **31**, 507–533.

Horne, D., and Tomasz, A. (1980). *In* "Current Chemotherapy and Infectious Disease" (J. D. Nelson and C. Grassi, eds.), pp. 1127–1129. Am. Soc. Microbiol., Washington, D.C.

Horne, D., and Tomasz, A. (1981). *Antimicrob. Agents Chemother.* **19**, 745–753.

Horwitz, M. A. (1982). *Rev. Infect. Dis.* **4**, 104–123.

Horwitz, M. A., and Silverstein, S. C. (1980). *J. Clin. Invest.* **65**, 82–94.

Johnson, J. D., Hand, W. L., Francis, J. B., King-Thomson, N., and Corwin, R. W. (1980). *J. Lab. Clin. Med.* **95,** 429–439.

Joiner, K. A., Onderdonk, A. B., Gelfand, J. A., Bartlett, J. G., and Gorbach, S. L. (1980). *Br. J. Exp. Pathol.* **61,** 97–107.

Joiner, K. A., Lowe, B. R., Dzink, J. L., and Bartlett, J. G. (1981). *J. Infect. Dis.* **143,** 487–494.

Kasper, D. L., Onderdonk, A. B., Polk, B. F., and Bartlett, J. G. (1979). *Rev. Infect. Dis.* **1,** 278–288.

Klempner, M. S., and Styrt, B. (1981). *J. Infect. Dis.* **144,** 472–479.

Lobo, M. D., and Mandell, G. L. (1972). *Antimicrob. Agents Chemother.* **2,** 195–200.

Lorian, V. (1975). *Bull. N.Y. Acad. Sci.* [2] **51,** 1046–1055.

Lorian, V. (1980). *In* "Antibiotics in Laboratory Medicine" (V. Lorian, ed.), pp. 342–408. Williams & Wilkins, Baltimore, Maryland.

Lorian, V., and Atkinson, B. (1976). *Antimicrob. Agents Chemother.* **9,** 1043–1055.

Lorian, V., and Atkinson, B. A. (1979). *Rev. Infect. Dis.* **1,** 797–806.

Lorian, V., and Atkinson, B. (1980). *Antimicrob. Agents Chemother.* **18,** 807–813.

Lorian, V., and de Freitas, C. (1979). *J. Infect. Dis.* **139,** 599–603.

Lorian, V., and Sabath, L. D. (1972). *J. Infect. Dis.* **125,** 560–564.

McDonald, P. J., Craig, W. A., and Kunin, C. M. (1977). *J. Infect. Dis.* **135,** 217–227.

McDonald, P. J., Wetherall, B. L., and Pruul, H. (1981). *Rev. Infect. Dis.* **3,** 38–44.

Mandell, G. L., and Vest, T. K. (1972). *J. Infect. Dis.* **125,** 486–490.

Mandell, L. A. (1982). *Rev. Infect. Dis.* **4,** 683–697.

Midtvedt, T., Lingaas, E., and Melby, K. (1982). *In* "The Influence of Antibiotics on the Host–Parasite Relationship" (H.-V. Eickenberg, H. Hahn, and W. Opferkuch, eds.), pp. 118–128. Springer-Verlag, Berlin and New York.

Milatovic, D. (1982). *Eur. J. Clin. Microbiol.* **1,** 97–101.

Onderdonk, A. B., Bartlett, J. G., Louie, T., Sullivan-Seigler, N., and Gorbach, S. L. (1976). *Infect. Immun.* **13,** 22–26.

Onderdonk, A. B., Kasper, D. L., Cisneros, R. L., and Bartlett, J. G. (1977). *J. Infect. Dis.* **136,** 82–89.

Pesanti, E. L. (1980). *Antimicrob. Agents Chemother.* **18,** 208–209.

Peterson, P. K., Verhoef, J., Sabath, L. D., and Quie, P. G. (1977). *Infect. Immun.* **15,** 760–764.

Peterson, P. K., Wilkinson, B. J., Kim, Y., Schmeling, D., and Quie, P. G. (1978a). *Infect. Immun.* **19,** 943–949.

Peterson, P. K., Kim, Y., Wilkinson, B. J., Schmeling, D., Michael, A. F., and Quie, P. G. (1978b). *Infect. Immun.* **20,** 770–775.

Pruul, H., and McDonald, P. J. (1979). *Antimicrob. Agents Chemother.* **16,** 695–700.

Pruul, H., Wetherall, B. L., and McDonald, P. J. (1981). *Antimicrob. Agents Chemother.* **19,** 945–951.

Pruul, H., Wetherall, B. L., and McDonald, P. J. (1982). *In* "The Influence of Antibiotics on the Host–Parasite Relationship" (H.-V. Eickenberg, H. Hahn, and W. Opferkuch, eds.), pp. 208–218. Springer-Verlag, Berlin and New York.

Reymann, M. T., Bradac, J. A., Cobbx, C. G., and Dismukes, W. E. (1979). *Antimicrob. Agents Chemother.* **16,** 353–361.

Root, R. K., Isturiz, R., Molavi, A., Metcalfe, J. A., and Malech, H. L. (1981). *J. Clin. Invest.* **67,** 247–259.

Simon, G. L., Klempner, M. S., Kasper, D. L., and Gorbach, S. L. (1982). *J. Infect. Dis.* **145,** 72–77.

Smith, I. M., and Kong, Y. L. (1981). *In* "Staphylococci and Staphylococcal Infections" (J. Jeljaszewicz, ed.), pp. 693–698. Fischer, Stuttgart.

Swanson, J., Hsu, K. C., and Gotschlich, E. C. (1968). *J. Exp. Med.* **141,** 1329–1347.

Taylor, P. W., Gaunt, H., and Unger, F. M. (1981). *Antimicrob. Agents Chemother.* **19,** 786–788.

Verhoef, J., Peterson, P. K., and Quie, P. G. (1977). *J. Immunol. Methods* **14,** 303–311.

Warren, G. H., and Gray, J. (1966). *Can. J. Microbiol.* **13,** 321–328.

Wilkinson, B. J., Sisson, S. P., Kim, Y., and Peterson, P. K. (1979). *Infect. Immun.* **26,** 1159–1163.

Zak, O., and Kradolfer, F. (1979). *Rev. Infect. Dis.* **1,** 862–879.

Zak, O., Kradolfer, F., Tosch, W., and Vischer, W. (1977). *Antimicrob. Agents Chemother.* **17** (Abstr. 418).

9 Effect of antibiotics on colonization resistance

D. VAN DER WAAIJ

I. INTRODUCTION

Colonization resistance (CR) could be defined as the resistance encountered by a potentially pathogenic microorganism (PPMO) when it tries to colonize a "landing site" on the mucosa in one of the three tracts that have an open communication with the outside world (van der Waaij, 1982a,b, 1983). The CR of the digestive tract is a rather complex mechanism in which host factors and anaerobic microflora cooperate in limiting the colonization of the digestive tract by PPMO's (see Table 1). The strength of CR can be measured and expressed as the log of the oral dose of PPMO's such as *Escherichia coli, Klebsiella,* or *Pseudomonas* species (or intestinal pathogenic organisms) that results in colonization for a minimum of 2 weeks in 50% of a group (humans and animals) (van der Waaij *et al.,* 1971). In the respiratory and in the urinary tract, the CR-determining forces—mucus, IgA secretion, cell desquamation, and mechanical cleansing forces such as ciliary movement and bladder emptying, respectively—are entirely host related.

In the digestive tract, however, although CR-determining host factors comparable to those in both other tracts are present—saliva and mucus production, IgA secretion, cell desquamation, and swallowing, that is, peristalsis—and effectively contribute to the CR, the (anaerobic) resident microflora plays a major role. The various anaerobes that maintain intestinal CR appear to live in close association with the mucosal lining of the ileum and the colon (Costerton, 1982), forming a "living wallpaper" that is susceptible to a number of antibiotics. Colonization by PPMO's is perhaps only possible when they find open patches in the otherwise confluent "anaerobic wallpaper" of the gut wall. Adherence of large numbers of PPMO's appears to be associated with detectable penetration of

Medical Microbiology, 4
ISBN 0-12-228004-0

Table 1 Colonization resistance of the digestive tract

Host related		Flora related	
Site	Susceptible to	Organisms	Susceptible to
Mucosal lining	Chemotherapy Irradiation Starvation Disease (diabetes, uraemia, coma, etc.) Ageing	Anaerobic flora viridans strepto- cocci	Antibiotics (penicillin and its derivatives, tetracycline, chlorampheni- col, aminoglyco- sides, clindamycin, most cephalo- sporins)
Saliva and mucus secretion	Anaesthesia Morphine Disease		
Swallowing and peristalsis	(Sjögren syndrome, megacolon etc.)		
Immune system (S-IgA)	Immune suppression congenital deficiency, etc.		

the epithelial lining and PPMO migration into the lymphatic organs (translocation of bacteria) (van der Waaij *et al.*, 1972a,b; Berg, 1980).

Anaerobes shed from the adherent layer and those multiplying in the intestinal
contents compete successfully with PPMO's for nutrients, and this forms another
effective mechanism (Guiot, 1982). Thus, CR in the gut depends markedly upon
the "crowding out" effect and the nutrient depletion effect maintained by the
commensal flora.

II. CONSEQUENCES OF CR IN ANTIMICROBIAL TREATMENT

Antibiotics are perhaps among the most abused drugs of the many that have
become available in the last half century. It is understandable that this abuse has
developed and has not been stopped: In the 1940s, serious, often fatal, infections
such as pneumococcal pneumonia and typhoid were suddenly curable in several
days, as if by magic. Therefore, antibiotics were often applied to the treatment of
conditions such as viral infections, which would not respond to such therapy.
The adverse effects of many antibiotics came to be recognized. Particularly in
relation to prophylactic use of antibiotics, much controversy ensued (Johanson *et*

al., 1969; Myerowitz *et al.*, 1971; Greene *et al.*, 1973; Roberts and Douglas, 1978; LeFrock *et al.*, 1979a,b). This is understandable, because the target groups of opportunistic bacteria to be suppressed may differ from patient to patient. Furthermore, even if the endogenous PPMO flora of a particular patient is susceptible to antibiotics applied for prophylactic purposes, environmental strains of similar organisms occurring in hospitals and wards in which many similar cases have been recently treated may be resistant and may have increased virulence in terms of their invasive potential and colonizing ability.

The importance of hand washing in preventing the transfer of bacteria from patient to patient is obvious, as reported by several investigators (Seiden *et al.*,

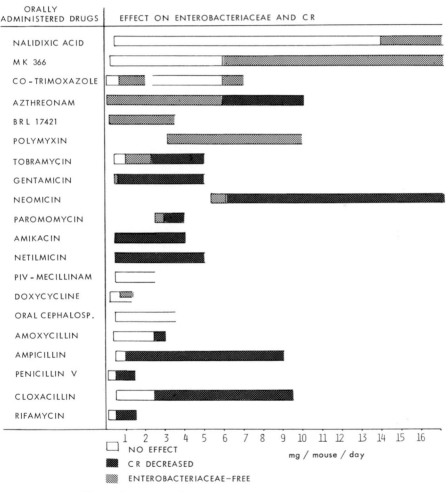

Fig. 1 Screening of antibiotics in mice, oral treatment.

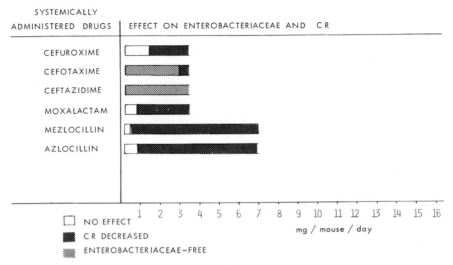

Fig. 2 Screening of antibiotics in mice, systemic treatment.

1971; Weinstein, 1982). If antibiotics are used that suppress the microflora responsible for normal CR, the resistant bacteria and yeasts of fungi, either endogenously present at admission or acquired in the ward, may take their chance and massively colonize the digestive tract, often in both the throat and the intestines. This condition is often followed by contamination and colonization of places with decreased CR in either one of the other tracts—for example, due to obstruction, like canulation—which may lead to (re-)infection.

Screening of antibiotics in mice for their effect on the CR-constituting anaerobic flora by either oral (Thijm and van der Waaij, 1979; Emmelot and van der Waaij, 1980; van der Waaij *et al.*, 1982a; Wiegersma *et al.*, 1982) or parenteral treatment (van der Waaij *et al.*, 1982b) of groups of animals with different daily doses has given some insight into the range of drugs that may influence the autochthonous flora and thus the CR (Figs. 1 and 2). Since mice and humans differ in quality and location of their gut flora, these results require confirmation in humans. There is evidence, however, that the CR-constituting flora of man is affected by the same antibiotics as that of mice (Hinton, 1970; Hirsh *et al.*, 1973; Sutter and Finegold, 1974; Hartley *et al.*, 1978; Heimdahl *et al.*, 1982; Heimdahl and Nord, 1982; Mulligan *et al.*, 1982; Arvidsson *et al.*, 1982).

III. TAILOR-MADE ANTIMICROBIAL TREATMENT AND PROPHYLAXIS

Since antibiotic prophylaxis has been repeatedly tried and modified in surgery as well as in medicines, it may be relevant to briefly review the progress and difficulties in this area.

Just as the anaesthesists have developed their discipline to take account of individual patient responses to their "standard" drugs and to recognize the importance of monitoring for individual reactions, bacteriologists should recognize general and individual adverse effects of their therapy. It is surprising that the need for individual monitoring during antimicrobial therapy has not been adequately recognized by clinical microbiologists in their approaches to prophylaxis and treatment of infections. Patients with infections caused by the same bacterial species may respond differently to a standard antibiotic regimen. This is not primarily due to pharmacokinetic differences in individual patients, and it is not invariably attributable to differences in susceptibility to toxicity. It is in most cases due to the fact that antibiotics may influence not only the patient and a particular pathogen, but also the patient's flora, which comprises an essential (functional) part of the patient and should be inventoried and monitored during antibiotic treatment.

As a result of excretion of antibiotics by the liver and/or saliva or intestinal secretions, parenterally administered antibiotics may often reach the gut in inhibitory concentrations. Many orally administered antibiotics that are not rapidly absorbed or are inactivated in the proximal section of the gastrointestinal tract may be "dumped" in active form in the distal gut.

Depending upon the spectrum of the antimicrobial drug(s) employed, there may be a marked effect on the anaerobes, with suppression of the flora and a consequent loss of CR (Table 1). During circumstances of decreased CR, ingested resistant opportunistic environmental strains may successfully colonize the gut in high concentrations. If these strains carry resistance plasmids, they may transfer their genetic information to other PPMO strains (Lacey, 1975; Rubens et al., 1981). In addition, mutation may occur more frequently among resistant strains, since they may multiply more readily when the CR is decreased. More mutations increase the risk of the development of a more pathogenic mutant. If the antibiotic(s) given have an indifferent effect on the CR, there may nevertheless be selection of resistant flora with some enrichment of these PPMO's. If the antibiotic(s) on the other hand positively decrease the CR—an aspect of antibiotic toxicity not yet fully appreciated, whereby the defensive capacity of the gut is compromised—the patient is rendered more susceptible to colonization by resistant strains acquired from the environment (e.g., from other patients, sinks, hospital food, etc.)

The possibility of this damaging effect occurring during antibiotic treatment underlines the necessity to monitor the flora-dependent part of the CR as long as antibiotics are used. Since monitoring of the CR by quantitative and qualitative culturing of aerobic and anaerobic flora is very laborious, difficult, and expensive, monitoring of the CR by biochemical means, as suggested by Welling (1979), seems indicated. A biochemical approach is certainly less expensive. It involves only the preparation of a faecal suspension, with its centrifugation and subsequent analytical high voltage electrophoresis, to estimate the concentration of a dipeptide, β-aspartylglycine. β-Aspartylglycine is an end product of protein metabolism and is normally digested by enzymes produced by CR-constituting flora (Welling, 1979).

IV. IMMUNOCOMPROMISED PATIENTS

Most defences can be severely decreased by a combination of bone marrow suppression and decrease of the host-dependent CR. The flow of saliva is inhibited and the condition of the mucosa of the digestive tract is affected by the cytotoxic chemotherapy. A decrease in one or more host-dependent CR factors can be related to the acquisition of opportunistic microorganisms and colonization of the patient by these, so one should take note of the following: (1) the PPMO's that colonize the patient at the time of a host-dependent CR-decrease, and their resistance patterns; and (2) the strains and species in the (hospital) environment and their resistance patterns. This calls for longitudinal bacteriological monitoring of the opportunistic flora of the patient's oropharynx and faeces during antimicrobial therapy. However, whilst flora monitoring is always of epidemiological interest, it is not by itself enough for the protection of severely neutropenic patients with decreased CR.

A. Selective decontamination of the digestive tract

Severely immunologically compromised patients require properly selected prophylactic antimicrobial treatment which should not reduce the anaerobic flora (should not be CR-decreasing), and this concept has become the basis of selective decontamination (SD). Selective decontamination (van der Waaij, 1982b) implies daily oral administration of a combination of antimicrobial drugs that do not affect the CR and are otherwise selected for their effectiveness on both patient-colonizing and environmental PPMO's. If such antimicrobials are administered in a sufficiently high daily dose, the endogenous PPMO flora should disappear from the digestive and other tracts, whilst environmental PPMO's are suppressed or killed after contamination by the antimicrobial concentration inside the alimentary canal (Sleijfer *et al.*, 1980; Guiot *et al.*, 1981; Jehn *et al.*, 1981; Kurrle, 1981; Dekker *et al.*, 1981). A basic rule in SD is that in this kind of prophylactic treatment it is often not sufficient to give patients a standard set of antimicrobial drugs each day. Frequent monitoring of the presence of PPMO components in the oropharyngeal and faecal flora during SD is necessary for an optimal result (De Vries-Hospers *et al.*, 1981). Ideally, both sites of the digestive tract should become free of PPMO (Gram-negative bacteria, *Staph. aureus* and yeasts) soon after the start of this prophylactic treatment, although it must be conceded that the list of PPMO's appears to be infinite. If the samples reveal well-known opportunistic organisms on culture after several days of treatment, SD treatment should be readjusted according to the sensitivity patterns of the strain(s) isolated. Again, the important point is that individual monitoring is essential.

B. Cross-infection during SD

It has been reported that in a ward in which virtually all patients receive SD treatment, the risk of cross-infection is greatly reduced (De Vries-Hospers *et al.*, 1981). In the majority of the patients, the threshold for colonization by PPMO's is maintained largely intact (flora-dependent part of the CR). This does not mean that the usual precautions such as hand washing between treatment of different patients and frequent disinfection of collectively used sinks in the ward are no longer necessary. However, the safety of the individual patient in terms of acquisition of nosocomial infections is greatly supplemented by SD.

The SD strategy reduces and may even eliminate the major source of multi-resistant Gram-negative bacteria, since the patient with ''overgrowth'' of such bacteria can be regarded as a major source.

V. PREVENTION OF INDUCTION OF RESISTANCE AND ITS TRANSFER

Induction of resistance and transfer of resistance plasmids between patients in wards in which bacteria are occasionally used should be prevented or minimised if preference is given to CR-indifferent antimicrobial drugs for therapy (Table 2). These drugs should apparently be applied either in doses that give salivary and intestinal concentrations of less than the minimal inhibitory concentration (MIC) for the commensal PPMO's that commonly colonize the digestive tract, or in concentrations that are well above the MIC of these strains. In the first situation, resistance is not induced, because the bacteria present are already (naturally) resistant to the concentrations existing in the gut; in the second situation—which implies SD—all susceptible PPMO's are eliminated from the gut microflora so that no resistance develops. Resistant strains, other than those maintaining the CR, colonizing the patient at the time of CR-indifferent antimicrobial treatment, may remain. As long as the host-related part of the CR is intact, they will not tend to overgrow in the alimentary tract during therapy.

However, if the sensitivity pattern of an infecting organism calls for CR-decreasing antibiotic(s) in therapy, additional SD of the digestive tract may be indicated. This is particularly the case when patients are treated for longer periods with CR-decreasing drugs on a ward with immunologically compromised patients. Without SD, the chances for induction of resistance and of acquisition of resistant strains from the (hospital) environment increase with time. In addi-

Table 2   Prevention of overgrowth by resistant
microorganisms during antibiotic therapy

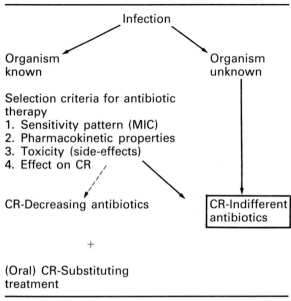

Infection

Organism   Organism
known   unknown

Selection criteria for antibiotic
therapy
1. Sensitivity pattern (MIC)
2. Pharmacokinetic properties
3. Toxicity (side-effects)
4. Effect on CR

CR-Decreasing antibiotics   CR-Indifferent
                                   antibiotics

+

(Oral) CR-Substituting
treatment

tion, transfer of resistance may occur *in vivo* under circumstances of decreased
CR and overgrowth by transferable plasmid carrying PPMO's. It is recognized
that acquisition of resistant nosocomial strains during antibiotic therapy can be
limited and possibly prevented by strict isolation of the patient (Dankert *et al.*,
1978). However, in a hospital setting, the efficiency of reverse isolation of
patients in specially designed isolators or (Dietrich *et al.*, 1975) laminar air flow
systems (van der Waaij *et al.*, 1973) may be relatively poor unless very costly
arrangements are introduced (Dietrich *et al.*, 1975).

VI.   THE "IDEAL ANTIBIOTIC"

The information presented in this review may provide a lead for an outline of
properties of the "ideal antibiotic." In addition to the classical criteria (Table 2)
such as lack of toxicity and good pharmaconkinetic properties, an ideal antibiotic
should fulfil the following criteria:

   1. As Gram-positive PPMO's often share susceptibility with many CR-in-
      stituting anaerobic bacteria, an ideal antibiotic should operate over a narrow
      spectrum limited to Gram-negative bacteria; alternatively, if it is broad-

spectrum or if it mainly affects Gram-positive bacteria, it should not be excreted into the digestive tract in concentrations that decrease the CR.

2. Safety with respect to "toxicity to the CR" as well as to the chance that resistance develops or is transmitted, preferably with drugs with high activity (low MIC), should be considered for therapy. High activity may in many cases permit lower dosing, which may help to minimize excretion by the liver and therewith the risk of resistance induction within the alimentary canal. In particular, if during systemic treatment excretion occurs by the salivary glands and with intestinal means, marginal suppressive amounts of the drug to (potentially) pathogenic bacteria may emerge inside the digestive tract.

3. Drugs designed for oral treatment (in suspensions, tablets, or capsules) should either be completely absorbed in the small intestine, resulting in virtually zero concentrations in the colon, i.e., lower than the MIC of any intestinal flora component. If "complete absorption" in the proximal gut is impossible, the drug should have a narrow spectrum limited to Gram-negative bacteria or be present in an inactive form. Active drugs with a narrow, mainly Gram-negative spectrum (CR-indifferent) should be only partially or poorly absorbed. A sufficient (CR-indifferent) amount of drug should in this case reach the colon to establish a concentration that guarantees a cidal (killing) effect on all susceptible potential "target organisms." A target organism is any PPMO that can cause an infection in the same or in any other (immunocompromised) host organism. These target organisms should disappear from the oropharynx or, perhaps more importantly, from the intestinal contents before resistance by selection and/or mutation can develop.

REFERENCES

Arvidsson, A., Alvan, G., Angelin, B., Borga, O., and Nord, C. E. (1982). *J. Antimicrob. Chemother.* **10**, 207–215.

Berg, R. D. (1980). *Infect. Immun.* **29**, 1073–1081.

Costerton, J. W. (1982). *In* "Action of Antibiotics in Patients" (L. D. Sabath, ed.), pp. 160–176. Huber, Bern.

Dankert, J., Gaus, W., Gaya, H., Krieger, D., Linzenmeier, G., and van der Waaij, D. (Gnotobiotic Project Writing Committee) (1978). *Infection* **6**, 175–191.

Dekker, A. W., Rozenberg-Arska, M., Sixma, J. J., and Verhoef, J. (1981). *Ann. Intern. Med.* **95**, 555–559.

De Vries-Hospers, H. G., Sleijfer, D. T., Mulder, N. H., van der Waaij, D., Nieweg, H. O., and Van Saene, H. K. F. (1981). *Antimicrob. Agents Chemother.* **19**, 813–820.

Dietrich, M., Abt, C., and Pflieger, H. (1975). *Med. Prog. Technol.* **3**, 85–89.

Emmelot, C. H., and van der Waaij, D. (1980). *J. Hyg.* **84**, 331–340.

Greene, W. H., Moody, M., Schimpff, S., Young, V. M., and Wiernik, P. H. (1973). *Ann. Intern. Med.* **79,** 684–689.

Guiot, H. F. L. (1982). *Infect. Immun.* **38,** 887–892.

Guiot, H. F. L., Van der Meer, J. W. M., and Van Furth, R. (1981). *J. Infect. Dis.* **143,** 644–654.

Hartley, C. L., Clements, H. M., and Linton, K. B. (1978). *J. Med. Microbiol.* **11,** 125–135.

Heimdahl, A., and Nord, C. E. (1982). *Eur. J. Clin. Microbiol.* **1,** 38–48.

Heimdahl, A., Kager, L., Malmborg, A. S., and Nord, C. E. (1982). *Infection* **10,** 120–124.

Hinton, N. (1970). *Curr. Ther. Res.* **12,** 341–352.

Hirsh, D. C., Burton, G. C., and Blenden, D. C. (1973). *Antimicrob. Agents Chemother.* **4,** 69–71.

Jehn, U., Ruckdeschell, G., Saner, H., Clemm, C., and Wilmans, W. (1981). *Klin. Wochenschr.* **59,** 1093–1099.

Johanson, W. G., Pierce, A. K., and Sanford, J. P. (1969). *N. Engl. J. Med.* **281,** 1137–1140.

Kurrle, E. (1981). *Klin. Wochenschr.* **59,** 1085–1089.

Lacey, R. W. (1975). *J. Antimicrob. Chemother.* **1,** 25–37.

LeFrock, J. L., Ellis, C. A., and Weinstein, L. (1979a). *Am. J. Med. Sci.* **277,** 269–274.

LeFrock, J. L., Ellis, C. A., and Weinstein, L. (1979b). *Am. J. Med. Sci.* **281,** 275–280.

Mulligan, M. E., Citron, D. M., McNamara, B. T., and Finegold, S. M. (1982). *Antimicrob. Agents Chemother.* **22,** 226–230.

Myerowitz, R. L., Medeiros, A. A., and O'Brien, T. F. (1971). *J. Infect. Dis.* **124,** 239–246.

Roberts, N. J., and Douglas, R. G. (1978). *Antimicrob. Agents Chemother.* **13,** 214–220.

Rubens, C. E., Farrar, W. E., McGee, Z. A., and Schaffner, W. (1981). *J. Infect. Dis.* **143,** 170–181.

Selden, R., Lee, S., Wang, W. L. L., Bennet, J. V., and Eickhoff, T. C. (1971). *Ann. Intern. Med.* **74,** 657–664.

Sleijfer, D. T., Mulder, N. H., De Vries-Hospers, H. G., Fidler, V., Nieweg, H. O., van der Waaij, D., and Van Saene, H. K. F. (1980). *Eur. J. Cancer* **16,** 859–869.

Sutter, V. L., and Finegold, S. M. (1974). *In* "The Normal Microbial Flora of Man," (F. A. Skinner and J. G. Carr, eds.), pp. 229–240. Academic Press, New York.

Thijm, H. A., and van der Waaij, D. (1979). *J. Hyg.* **82,** 397–405.

van der Waaij, D. (1982a). *In* "Infections in Cancer Patients" (J. Klastersky, ed.), pp. 73–85. Raven Press, New York.

van der Waaij, D. (1982b). *J. Antimicrob. Chemother.* **10,** 263–270.

van der Waaij, D. (1983). *In* "Second International Symposium on Infections in the Immunocompromised Host." (C. S. F. Easmon and H. Gaya, eds.), pp. 55–60. Academic Press, New York.

van der Waaij, D., Berghuis-de Vries, J. M., and Lekkerkerk-van der Wees, J. E. C. (1971). *J. Hyg.* **69,** 405–441.

van der Waaij, D., de Vries, J. M., and Lekkerkerk, J. E. C. (1972a). *J. Hyg.* **70,** 335–342.

van der Waaij, D., Berghuis, J. M., and Lekkerkerk, J. E. C. (1972b). *J. Hyg.* **70,** 605–610.

van der Waaij, D., Vossen, J. M., and Korthals Altes, C. (1973). *In* "Germfree Research; biological effect of gnotobiotic environments" (J. B. Heneghan, ed.), pp. 31–36. Academic Press, New York.

van der Waaij, D., Aberson, J., Thijm, H. A., and Welling, G. W. (1982a). *Infection* **10**, 35–40.
van der Waaij, D., Hofstra, W., and Wiegersma, N. (1982b). *J. Infect. Dis.* **146**, 417–422.
Weinstein, R. A. (1982). *In* "Evaluation and Management of Hospital Infections," (R. Van Furth, ed.), pp. 58–74. Nijhoff, The Hague.
Welling, G. W. (1979). *In* "New Criteria for Antimicrobial Therapy: Maintenance of Colonization Resistance" (D. van der Waaij and J. Verhoef, eds.), pp. 65–71. Excerpta Medica, Amsterdam.
Wiegersma, N., Jansen, G., and van der Waaij, D. (1982). *J. Hyg.* **88**, 221–230.

10 Polyamine inhibitors as antimicrobial agents?

JOHN D. WILLIAMSON and A. STANLEY TYMS

I. INTRODUCTION

Since the aetiology of infectious disease was first understood, it has been an ambition to find chemical agents with selective action against the invasive organism. Antibiotics have now been available for four decades, but their clinical use in the treatment of bacterial infections has become impaired by the emergence of antibiotic-resistant strains. Natural products or synthetic compounds with action suitable for clinical use against other parasites have been hard to find, and this deficiency is most marked in the case of antiviral agents. It is apparent that novel strategies must be considered for the rational design of new chemotherapeutic agents.

The concept of specific chemotherapy was developed originally by Paul Ehrlich more than 80 years ago. Ehrlich was able to show that trypanosomiasis in mice could be cured by treatment with trypan red, but it is pertinent to mention that in this seminal study the phenomenon of drug-resistant organisms was first described. His later development of arsenical compounds for the treatment of syphilis is a model of the rigorous evaluation of many derivatives in order to identify the molecular configuration with the most potent chemotherapeutic effect. Little of value for treatment of bacterial diseases emerged until, in 1935, the dye Prontosil was shown to cure streptococcal infections. Although inactive *in vitro*, patients receiving the drug excreted a breakdown product, sulphanilamide, which had both *in vitro* and *in vivo* effects. The bactericidal action was found to be due to competition between the drug and *para*-aminobenzoic acid, a precursor in the formation of folic acid. This antagonism arises from structural analogy between the two compounds. The antimetabolite acts on a biosynthetic pathway

Medical Microbiology, 4
ISBN 0-12-228004-0

that is peculiar to the prokaryotic cell, since bacteria cannot utilize exogenous folic acid, whereas it is a required vitamin for animals.

Although Fleming's report in 1929 of the bacteriolytic action of penicillin on staphylococci took more than a decade to bear fruit, it is pertinent that his original paper drew attention to the antibiotic's lack of toxicity in humans. It was not until several years after it had been used clinically that the basis for selective, antibacterial action by penicillin was understood. The backbone of bacterial cell walls is composed of polysaccharide chains attached to a tetrapeptide, which is linked in turn by a peptide bridge to another tetrapeptide on an adjacent polysaccharide chain. This essential cross-linking is blocked by penicillin. Since peptidoglycans are not structural components of animal cells, their integrity is unaffected by the antibacterial agent.

The contemporaneous nature of these archetypal discoveries could have led to the subsequent, parallel development of chemotherapeutic agents based on natural products or on synthetic compounds. Certainly the former approach should have been excluded by the large element of serendipity in the discovery of penicillin, but Waksman's discovery of streptomycin, produced by a soil actinomycete, proved to be a watershed in trial-and-error searches for antibiotics. Streptomycin was shown to be active on the ribosomes of bacterial cells but not animal cells. This selective effect added further evidence for the existence of fundamental differences between prokaryotic and eukaryotic cells.

Although random screening of natural products from various microorganisms has been successful in the discovery of other antibacterial agents, such methods have been almost completely ineffectual in the discovery of antiviral agents. The lower protists (bacteria and blue-green algae) have phylogenetic origins different from the higher protists (protozoa, fungi, slime molds and other algae) and metazoan organisms, as reflected in their distinctive physiology. Since animal viruses are parasites resident within and dependent on metazoan metabolism, antibiotics are ineffective. The alternative approach to the development of chemotherapeutic agents based on antimetabolites was profitless for many years, since most proved to be antagonists of metabolites essential for the viability of the host cell. Energy metabolism is an inappropriate target, and the continual turnover of protein and RNA tends to rule out such macromolecules as suitable targets reached through intermediary metabolism. However, active DNA synthesis is associated primarily with mitotic cells, and synthetic nucleoside analogues were found to be effective in the treatment of infections with DNA-containing viruses, particularly members of the herpesvirus group. Although these compounds—for example, 5-iodo-2′-deoxyuridine and 1-β-D-arabinofuranosylcytosine—inhibit steps in the metabolic pathways of both host and viral DNA synthesis, selective inhibition of virus multiplication can be achieved by concentrations of the analogues which are without effect on the host cell. Such discrimination shows that specificity may not be essential, but advantage can be taken of a favourable therapeutic ratio, a principle first appreciated by Paul Ehrlich.

Most recently, a new generation of antiviral compounds—for example, 9-(2-hydroxyethoxymethyl)guanine and *E*-5-(bromovinyl-2′-deoxyuridine)—has been developed that is also based on nucleoside analogues. The action of these compounds is mediated by enzyme activities encoded within the genome of certain DNA-containing viruses, as expressed in the virus-infected cells. Although analogous enzymes are found in normal cells, they show little affinity for the nucleoside analogues. Consequently, virus DNA synthesis is inhibited selectively, since the antiviral effect of the drug is manifest only after it has been acted upon by the virus-specific enzymes.

These examples illustrate the various strategies to be considered in a rational approach to chemotherapy. Infectious agents which are independent entities with metabolic systems widely different from their hosts may be attacked specifically once such distinctions have been recognised. Where such fundamental discrimination is not possible, constituents which are common to the invasive organism and its host may be produced by different metabolic pathways. The formation or utilization of precursors peculiar to the invasive organism may be inhibited selectively by suitable antagonists. Specific action is most difficult to achieve against intracellular organisms whose replication is completely dependent upon the host cell. In such circumstances, metabolic analogues that differentiate quantitatively may be employed provided an acceptable chemotherapeutic ratio is obtained. Finally, the active sites of analogous enzymes may differ sufficiently for specific action to be achieved.

In an elegant dissertation on this subject, Cohen (1979) draws attention to the value of comparative biochemical studies in order to identify the unique metabolic events essential for the viability of aetiological agents of disease. In particular, it is argued that the development of selective chemotherapeutic agents should be directed against proteins or other specific biopolymers with vital structural or metabolic functions in the parasite. It has become apparent in the past two decades that the vital functions of both prokaryotic and eukaryotic cells are dependent on the presence of polyamines. The intracellular concentration of these low-molecular-weight aliphatic bases has been shown to be closely controlled and, although their precise roles are not known at the molecular level, cell growth is inhibited by polyamine depletion. Various inhibitors of polyamine metabolism have been described, but an exciting development has been the recent design of enzyme-activated, irreversible inhibitors. Such compounds have been shown to inhibit the growth of bacteria and animal viruses and, most significantly, a specific chemotherapeutic effect against trypanosomiasis in mice has been obtained (Bacchi *et al.*, 1980).

It is the purpose of this review to describe the metabolic reactions involved in polyamine biosynthesis, since they do not feature significantly in modern textbooks of biochemistry, and to discuss the requirement for these organic cations in the growth of different infectious agents. This will provide a suitable background for further consideration of the chemotherapeutic potential of drugs that either inhibit or perturb the vital functions of polyamines.

II. HISTORICAL BACKGROUND

A brief account of the early history of polyamine chemistry is desirable to introduce these aliphatic bases (Fig. 1) and, incidentally, to explain the origins of their trivial names. Antonie van Leeuwenhock in 1677 had described the separation of clear crystals from human semen, but the name spermine was not applied to such material until more than 200 years later. The chemical structure was determined and the compound synthesised in 1926 by Dudley, Rosenheim, and Starling. A year later the same workers reported the characterization and synthesis of another base isolated from ox pancreas. In view of similarities in occurrence and constitution, the newly discovered polyamine was called spermidine. Its chemical relationship with spermine suggested even at that time that the two compounds were metabolically related. In the late nineteenth century the diamines putrescine and cadaverine had been described in putrefying animal tissue and in cadavers. The formation of these amines by microorganisms was first investigated in 1910 by Ackermann using a synthetic medium consisting of salts, peptone, glucose and a single amino acid inoculated with decomposed pancreas. These studies showed the formation of putrescine from ornithine and cadaverine from lysine. Later work demonstrated their production by pure cultures of identified organisms and, most significantly, the formation of putrescine from arginine. A detailed history of these earlier studies can be found elsewhere (Tabor and Tabor, 1964).

Biochemical studies on the production of amines by bacteria were initiated by Gale (1940), who investigated the decarboxylation of amino acids by strains of *Escherichia coli*. Manometric techniques were used to measure the evolution of carbon dioxide under the action of washed suspensions of bacteria. It appeared that acid conditions were required for decarboxylation to occur: the production of

$$H_2N-CH_2CH_2CH_2CH_2-NH_2 \qquad\qquad H_2N-CH_2CH_2CH_2CH_2-\underset{H}{N}-CH_2CH_2CH_2-NH_2$$

Putrescine   Spermidine

$$H_2N-CH_2CH_2CH_2-\underset{H}{N}-CH_2CH_2CH_2CH_2-\underset{H}{N}-CH_2CH_2CH_2-NH_2$$

Spermine

Fig. 1 Structures of putrescine, spermidine, and spermine.

putrescine from ornithine occurred optimally at pH 5.0 and, at an optimum of pH 4.0, agmatine was formed from arginine, but little activity was obtained at pH 7.2 with either substrate. Gale's paper quotes earlier workers who concluded that the production of amines from amino acids appeared to be a protective mechanism resorted to in high hydrogen-ion concentrations. The induction of such decarboxylase activity has been used subsequently as a taxonomic criterion in the identification of bacteria (Cowan and Steele, 1981).

A more fundamental role for certain amino acid decarboxylases in microorganisms was suggested by the demonstration that putrescine is a growth factor for *Haemophilus influenzae*. Agmatine had some activity, and spermidine and spermine were highly effective, but other amines were totally inactive. These studies by Herbst and Snell (1948) demonstrated the essential nutritive function of "putrefactive amines," and later studies with homologues or analogues confirmed the high degree of specificity in this role of the tetramethylenediamine structure (Guirard and Snell, 1964). A similar requirement for putrescine or spermidine as essential growth factors has been demonstrated with other prokaryotes: *Neisseria perflava* (Martin *et al.*, 1952), *Pasteurella tularensis* (Traub *et al.*, 1955), *Lactobacillus casei* (Kihara and Snell, 1957), *Veillonella alcalescens* (Rogosa and Bishop, 1964) and mycoplasmas (Rodwell, 1967). The requirement for putrescine as a growth factor for a mutant of *Aspergillus nidulans* (Sneath, 1955) and for animal cell culture (Ham, 1965) showed their essential nature in various eukaryotic cells.

The development of sensitive analytical techniques permitted the quantitative determination of polyamines in a wide range of cells and tissues (Bachrach, 1970). It is now recognised that polyamines are ubiquitous in biological materials but, in general, prokaryotes lack spermine and eukaryotes contain relatively small amounts of putrescine (Tabor and Tabor, 1976). Spermine has not been detected in blue-green algae (Ramakrishna *et al.*, 1978), in filamentous fungi (Nickerson *et al.*, 1977), or in certain trypanosomes (Bacchi *et al.*, 1977). Some mycoplasma strains contain significant amounts of putrescine, cadaverine, spermidine and spermine, whereas *Mycoplasma suipneumoniae* has higher amounts of putrescine but no other polyamines (Alhonen-Hongisto *et al.*, 1982).

Polyamines have also been shown to be constituents of virus particles, although their nature was not recognised in the first instance (Hershey, 1957). A year later, however, the previously unidentified materials in T-even bacteriophage were shown to be putrescine and spermine, and it was confirmed that both compounds were derived from arginine (Ames *et al.*, 1958). Later studies showed that the aliphatic bases were carried over with DNA during phenol extraction, and they were present in sufficient amounts to neutralize nearly 50% of the negatively charged phosphate groups of the nucleic acid. Polyamines were not detected in several plant viruses or in poliovirus (Ames and Dubin, 1960). Subsequent studies, however, have shown spermidine and spermine are constituents of some DNA-containing animal viruses: herpes simplex virus (Gibson and Roizman, 1971) and vaccinia virus (Lanzer and Holowczak, 1975). Spermidine and spermine have been reported to be present in adenovirus human type 5 (Shortridge and Stevens, 1973), although this has been disputed (Pett and Ginsberg, 1975). Two RNA-containing animal viruses, influenza and Newcastle disease virus, also contain significant amounts of polyamines (Bachrach *et al.*, 1974).

In view of the cationic nature of polyamines, it is not surprising that they are found in association with anionic macromolecules, but the significance of such interaction has been difficult to interpret. Complexes between prokaryotic or eukaryotic DNA and spermine were shown to result in a stabilized secondary structure as reflected in an increased thermal melting point of the nucleic acid. This effect was dependent on the spermine concentration but independent of the DNA concentration (Mandel, 1962). Conformational studies by X-ray analysis revealed highly stereospecific interactions of spermine or spermidine with eukaryotic DNA (Liquori *et al.*, 1967). Examination of the intracellular distribution of polyamines in *E. coli* showed that the ribosomal fraction contains about 15% of the total polyamine content (Cohen and Lichtenstein, 1960). Putrescine was present in greater amounts than spermidine, but neither was derived from polyamines present in the extracting medium. Ribosomal polyamines were not readily exchangeable, indicating that their presence was not dependent solely on ionic interactions. Addition of spermidine to buffers used in the preparation of bacterial extracts preserved the ribosomal contents, but similar effects could be obtained with inorganic cations. The increased proportion of 100S ribosomes obtained in the presence of polyamines was also found to correlate with the degree of stimulation obtained in a cell-free translation system prepared from *Salmonella typhimurium*. Although certain concentrations of magnesium ions produced a similar effect, optimal conditions were obtained in combination with putrescine and spermidine (Martin and Ames, 1962). Stimulation of the DNA-primed reaction of *Micrococcus lysodeikticus* RNA polymerase (Fox and Weiss, 1964) indicated a further requirement for polyamines in transcription as well as translation, but, again, divalent metal ions were required for maximum activity in this *in vitro* system. It soon became apparent that any indication of the vital functions of polyamines would have to be obtained from experiments using intact cells. In various polyamine auxotrophs of *E. coli* the provision of spermidine was required for RNA synthesis (Raina and Cohen, 1966) and for T4 bacteriophage replication (Dion and Cohen, 1972), but multiple pathways of polyamine synthesis in bacteria (discussed later in this chapter) presented difficulties with this genetic approach.

The association between polyamines and macromolecular synthesis *in vivo* began to emerge more clearly from other, metabolic studies with eukaryotic systems. The accumulation of polyamines during the multiplication of animal cells was first demonstrated in the growth of the chick embryo (Raina, 1963) and the regeneration of rat liver (Dykstra and Herbst, 1965). In the chick embryo, radiolabelling experiments showed that either ornithine or putrescine acted as a precursor in the formation of spermidine and spermine (Caldarera *et al.*, 1965). A subsequent study showed that ornithine decarboxylase activity increased markedly in these rapidly growing tissues (Russell and Snyder, 1968). It is now known that the decarboxylation of ornithine is the only anabolic source of putrescine in animal cells, and this reaction is a key step in the initiation of polyamine biosynthesis. Consequently, study of the mammalian decarboxylase has been the most active area of polyamine biochemistry in recent years (Tabor and Tabor, 1976; Jänne *et al.*, 1978; Pegg and McCann, 1982). All the evidence points towards the general conclusion that an increase in the rate of cell growth is accompanied by an early, dramatic increase in the rate of polyamine biosynthesis.

Conclusive proof of their vital function has been dependent on the development of specific inhibitors of polyamine synthesis. Such compounds have now been available for more than a decade, although the first polyamine inhibitor to be discovered had been used clinically as an antileukaemic agent another decade earlier. Most recently, irreversible inhibitors have been synthesised that are activated specifically by enzymes in the polyamine biosynthetic pathway. Their use has demonstrated unequivocably that polyamine synthesis is essential for the multiplication of both prokaryotic and eukaryotic cells. Similar requirements have been shown for the growth of various aetiological agents of infectious disease. Since these studies are most pertinent to the potential use of polyamine inhibitors as chemotherapeutic agents, they will be discussed in greater detail. First, the metabolic pathways for polyamine biosynthesis will be described.

III. POLYAMINE BIOSYNTHESIS IN PROKARYOTIC ORGANISMS

Although their products had been characterized much earlier, it is only relatively recently that the metabolic pathways of polyamine biosynthesis in prokaryotic organisms have been defined. These studies have shown a diversity of metabolic routes, and it is significant that multiple pathways exist even in the same microorganism. Several pathways originate from the latter part of the arginine biosynthetic pathway, but, as will be seen later, they differ significantly from the metabolic pathways leading to polyamine biosynthesis in eukaryotic cells. The principal pathways of polyamine biosynthesis are shown in Fig. 2.

In *E. coli* there are two major pathways to putrescine, a metabolic precursor of spermidine and spermine. The first route produces putrescine directly by the decarboxylation of ornithine, and a significant event in the characterization of this pathway was the recognition of two ornithine decarboxylases (Morris and

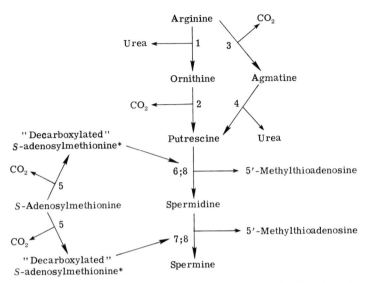

Fig. 2 Principal anabolic pathways of polyamine biosynthesis. Reactions indicated are catalysed by: 1, arginase; 2, ornithine decarboxylase; 3, arginine decarboxylase; 4, agmatine ureohydrolase; 5, S-adenosylmethionine decarboxylase; 6, spermidine synthase; 7, spermine synthase; 8, aminopropyltransferase. *"Decarboxylated" S-adenosylmethionine is the trivial name for S-adenosyl-5'-deoxy-(5')-3-methylthiopropylamine.

Pardee, 1966). In addition to the inducible, degradative enzyme described by Gale (1940), the same activity is expressed by a constitutive, biosynthetic enzyme. Pyridoxal phosphate is an essential cofactor for both enzymes, a requirement also shown by other amino acid decarboxylases. However, the induced and biosynthetic ornithine decarboxylases in *E. coli* are distinguishable by a variety of criteria. Significantly, the degradative activity is optimal at pH 6.9, and the synthetic enzyme is most active at pH 8.1. Both enzymes are activated by nucleotides but with different specificity: guanine triphosphate activates both enzymes, but uridine triphosphate activates the degradative enzyme more effectively. In immunological tests an antiserum prepared against the degradative enzyme did not cross-react with purified biosynthetic ornithine decarboxylase. The latter enzyme activity has been found in a wide variety of *E. coli* strains, but only 1 in 10 produced the degradative enzyme, although most strains had biodegradative decarboxylases against other amino acids (Applebaum *et al.*, 1977).

The second pathway to putrescine in *E. coli* is reached via agmatine, the decarboxylation product of arginine. Again, biodegradative and biosynthetic arginine decarboxylases have been described with optima at pH 5.2 and 8.4, respectively. They are distinguishable also by the absolute requirement for magnesium ions shown by the biosynthetic enzyme. Following the formation of agmatine, specific ureohydrolase activity produces putrescine and urea (Morris and Pardee, 1966).

The existence of two pathways of putrescine biosynthesis in *E. coli* may be explained in relation to control mechanisms of the arginine biosynthetic pathway. Since ornithine is an intermediate for the biosynthesis of arginine, the ornithine pool in repressible strains drops to undetectable levels in growing cultures supplied with exogenous arginine and there is no synthesis of putrescine from ornithine. However, endogenously produced arginine has been shown to be a poor precursor of putrescine in a mutant of *E. coli* lacking ornithine decarboxylase (Morris and Fillingame, 1974). Such evidence has tended to support the idea that there are two arginine pools but only that derived exogenously is available to the biosynthetic arginine decarboxylase. Thus, if the alternative agmatine pathway did not exist, *E. coli* grown in the presence of arginine would become polyamine-starved.

Both forms of ornithine and arginine decarboxylase from *E. coli* have been extensively purified and their physical properties have been determined. An interesting feature has been the demonstration of a multimeric structure and, in each instance, the protomeric unit has a molecular weight of between 75,000 and 85,000. Both the biodegradative and biosynthetic forms of ornithine decarboxylase from *E. coli* consist of two subunits (Applebaum *et al.*, 1977). However, the biosynthetic arginine decarboxylase has 4 subunits, whereas the biodegradative enzyme has 10 subunits (Morris and Fillingame, 1974). The inducible ornithine decarboxylase in *Lactobacillus* sp. *30a* has been purified recently, and monomer, dimer and dodecamer structures were described, although highest enzyme activity was obtained with the dodecameric form. It resembles the inducible arginine decarboxylase from *E. coli* in that each enzyme was dissociated by increase in pH or by decrease in ionic strength (Guirard and Snell, 1980).

The utilization of putrescine as a unit in the biosynthesis of spermidine and spermine had been suggested by earlier studies on their molecular configurations. However, an unexpected observation was the demonstration that methionine is another precursor (Greene, 1957). Detailed studies of spermidine synthesis in cell-free preparations of *E. coli* revealed an allied requirement for magnesium ions and adenosine triphosphate, but the nucleotide could be substituted by *S*-adenosylmethionine (Tabor *et al.*, 1958). It was shown that *S*-adenosylmethionine is enzymatically decarboxylated to produce *S*-adenosyl-5'-deoxy-(5')-3-methylthiopropylamine, and this nucleoside is the source of aminopropyl groups in polyamine biosynthesis. The adenosylmethionine decarboxylase of *E. coli* has been purified to homogeneity and, again, a subunit structure has been described. Each molecule of native enzyme contains 1 or 2 molecules of covalently bound pyruvate, but pyridoxal phosphate is not required as a cofactor for this decarboxylase (Wickner *et al.*, 1970). The prokaryotic enzyme is not activated by putrescine or other low-molecular-weight amines.

The aminopropyltransferase from *E. coli* has been purified, and it is composed of two apparently identical subunits (Bowman *et al.*, 1973). In common with the other enzymes in the polyamine biosynthetic pathway, the enzyme requires intact sulphydryl groups. At neutral pH the synthesis of spermidine from putrescine and decarboxylated *S*-adenosylmethionine is catalysed, but at this pH the further transfer of aminopropyl groups is limited. At pH 8.2 spermidine is still a poor substrate, although at pH 10.0 some formation of spermine does occur. These results show that the aminopropyltransferase from *E. coli* can synthesize both polyamines, but no evidence has been obtained for the separate spermidine and spermine synthases found in eukaryotic cells.

The other product of spermidine biosynthesis, 5'-methylthioadenosine, is produced in stoichiometric amounts, and this nucleoside in moderate concentrations depresses aminopropyltransferase activity. However, a hydrolytic nucleosidase produces adenosine and 5'-methylthioribose, which is utilized in a further reaction to produce methionine (Ferro *et al.*, 1978).

Various mutants of *E. coli* have now been isolated that require exogenous putrescine or spermidine in order to maintain normal growth rates. These requirements have been shown to result from mutations in the genes for enzymes required in polyamine biosynthesis. Genetic studies have shown that the genes for the biosynthetic arginine decarboxylase (*spe A*), agmatine ureohyrolase (*spe B*), biosynthetic ornithine decarboxylase (*spe C*), and *S*-adenosylmethionine synthetase (*met K*) all map in a cluster near 63 minutes on the bacterial chromosome (Cunningham-Rundles and Maas, 1975). The gene for *S*-adenosylmethionine decarboxylase (*spe D*) is located distantly at 2.7 minutes (Tabor *et al.*, 1978). In an agmatine ureohydrolase mutant, putrescine and spermidine biosynthesis by the constitutive pathways is inhibited in the presence of exogenous arginine. It has been shown that the addition of lysine to polyamine-depleted cultures of such auxotrophs results in the synthesis of cadaverine and a spermidine analogue, *N*-3-aminopropyl-1,5-diaminopentane (Dion and Cohen, 1972). The biosynthetic arginine decarboxylase is also subject to feedback inhibition by putrescine and spermidine (Tabor and Tabor, 1976). The precise mechanisms that affect arginine decarboxylase are not known, but ornithine decarboxylase activity is modulated by interaction with macromolecular effectors (Kyriakidis *et al.*, 1978) The modification of ornithine decarboxylase activity in eukaryotic cells has been intensively studied and will be discussed later.

Different metabolic pathways leading to the biosynthesis of polyamines have been described in other microorganisms. The formation of spermidine from putrescine and aspartate has been described in *Micrococcus denitrificans* and *Rhodopseudomonas spheroides* (Tait, 1976). In *Rh. viridis* homospermidine can be synthesized from putrescine and 4-aminobutyraldehyde (Tait, 1979). Putrescine may also be derived in some strains of *E. coli* by the decarboxylation of citrulline to produce carbamoylputrescine (Akamatsu *et al.*, 1978). Agmatine deiminase and putrescine transcarbamoylase in *Streptococcus faecalis* are enzymes in an energy-yielding reaction of some potential (Noon and Barker, 1972). Agmatine ureohydrolase and 4-aminobutyrate aminotransferase are two inducible enzymes in *Klebsiella aerogenes* that degrade agmatine to produce succinate (Friedrich and Magasanik, 1979).

It has been suggested that the further metabolism of polyamines known to occur under certain conditions may constitute a homeostatic mechanism to counter the rise in polycations which would otherwise take place. This proposal arose from the characterization of monoacetylputrescine and two isomeric forms of monoacetylspermidine recovered from growing cultures of *E. coli*. The acetylation of spermidine was enhanced by exogenous spermidine and by high pH (Dubin and Rosenthal, 1960). It has been shown recently that acetylase activity increases shortly after inoculation of cultures and precedes increased ornithine decarboxylase activity (Matsui *et al.*, 1982). Glutathionylspermidine also accumulates in *E. coli* after the logarithmic phase of growth, but its function remains unknown (Cohen *et al.*, 1967). Oxidative deamination in *Serratia marcescens* converts spermidine to 1,3-diaminopropane and pyrroline, but this activity does not occur in *E. coli* (Tabor and Kellog, 1970).

IV. POLYAMINE BIOSYNTHESIS IN EUKARYOTIC CELLS

In contrast to polyamine metabolism in prokaryotic cells, the decarboxylation of ornithine is the only important biosynthetic source of putrescine in animal cells. There is no evidence from studies in such cells or in lower eukaryotes such as fungi, that putrescine can be produced through agmatine following the decarboxylation of arginine (Pegg and McGill, 1979). The formation of spermidine from putrescine in eukaryotes involves the same series of chemical reactions as described previously for prokaryotic polyamine metabolism, but it differs enzymatically in the requirement for a distinct aminopropyltransferase, spermidine synthase. In a further reaction, which is unique to eukaryotic cells, a second aminopropyltransferase, spermine synthase, catalyses the transfer of another aminopropyl group to form spermine. Several studies have shown that spermine is the major polyamine component of nuclei from animal cells, and this has been demonstrated very recently using an *in situ* cell fractionation technique (Mach *et al.*, 1982).

The amino acid substrate of ornithine decarboxylase is an integral part of the Krebs–Henseleit cycle, in which urea and ornithine are produced from arginine by the action of arginase. Since many mammalian cells are unable to synthesize ornithine, its derivation from arginine is an important reaction. In ureotelic animals, arginase activity is not confined to the liver but is found in the kidney, brain, mammary gland, salivary gland and in erythrocytes. Ornithine is not a common constituent of proteins, but the free amino acid may be available in the diet. Under normal conditions, however, only a relatively small amount of ornithine is metabolized through the polyamine pathway, and the majority is utilized in the biosynthesis of proline and other amino acids. Although ornithine decarboxylase activity is low in resting cells, its expression can be markedly enhanced by a wide range of growth stimuli, and high levels of polyamines accumulate, particularly in tumour cells (Jänne *et al.*, 1978).

Ornithine decarboxylase in eukaryotic cells appears to be located in the cytosol. After enucleation of mouse L cells with cytochalasin B, more than 90% of the enzyme activity remained in the cytoplasts with less than 10% in the karyoplasts (McCormick, 1977). The low levels of activity in rat liver nuclei were enhanced after administration of 1-methyl-3-isobutylxanthine, but this was probably due to migration of the cytoplasmic enzyme (Bitonti and Couri, 1981). Fractionation of HeLa cells with the detergent Nonidet P40 resulted in the recovery of ornithine decarboxylase activity exclusively in the cytoplasmic fraction (J. D. Williamson, 1984). These observations confirm other studies that have shown that the enzyme can be recovered from the supernatant after high-speed centrifugation of cells disrupted mechanically. Since a sensitive assay for ornithine decarboxylase activity can be based on the capture of radiolabelled carbon dioxide evolved from [1-^{14}C]ornithine, it is important to ensure that such radioactivity is not released by the action of ornithine-2-oxoacid aminotransferase, an enzyme normally located in the mitochondrial fraction (Murphy and Brosman, 1976). Recently evidence has been obtained in autoradiographic studies with cells from a polychaete that ornithine decarboxylase is not restricted to the cytoplasm but is located in the nucleus, particularly in association with the nucleolus (Emanuelson and Heby, 1982).

Ornithine decarboxylase from rat tissues has been shown to have a molecular weight between 70,000 and 100,000 (Morris and Fillingame, 1974). However, purified enzyme preparations examined under denaturing conditions in polyacrylamide gel electrophoresis have an apparent molecular weight of approximately 50,000, and heat-inactivation studies of the native enzyme showed biphasic kinetics (Obenrader and Prouty, 1977). These results suggest that more than one protein is involved in the catalytic activity of ornithine decarboxylase from rat liver, but it is characteristic of both prokaryotic and eukaryotic ornithine decarboxylase that the catalytic function is both activated and stabilized by certain dithiols. In the absence of such reducing activity the enzymes appear to polymerise, with consequent reduction or loss of enzyme activity. The essential cofactor pyridoxal phosphate can also assist in the stabilization of crude ornithine decarboxylase preparations.

Recent studies have provided information on the control and regulation of ornithine decarboxylase in mammalian cells. This enzyme activity has been shown to increase markedly in many different systems in response to various inducers of cell growth and to decline rapidly to very low levels in resting cells. The enzyme has an extremely short half-life of about 20 minutes: similar values were determined from the rate of decline in activity following inhibition of protein synthesis with cycloheximide and by direct measurement of the enzyme protein in an immunological assay (Jänne *et al.*, 1978). It had been assumed that such properties provide a simple basis for regulation of ornithine decarboxylase through low-molecular-weight effector molecules producing changes in the kinetics of the enzyme's reactions. Although its activity is inhibited competitively by putrescine, and to a lesser extent by spermidine or spermine, the characteristics of such effects are not consistent with feedback inhibition by product formation. It is now known that a novel mechanism for regulation of ornithine decarboxylase activity is affected in animal cells by a protein which reacts specifically with the enzyme (Heller *et al.*, 1976). This macromolecular effector, or "antizyme," has an approximate molecular weight of 25,000 and is induced by putrescine, spermidine and spermine or their analogues, such as 1,3-diaminopropane. Most recently an "antizyme inhibitor" has been described which specifically inhibits antizyme and reactivates ornithine decarboxylase inactivated by antizyme (Fujita *et al.*, 1983). Evidence for positive and negative effectors has also been obtained in prokaryotic systems (Kyriakidis *et al.*, 1978).

Although antizyme has been detected in a number of mammalian cell systems, it may not be the only regulatory mechanism for ornithine decarboxylase in eukaryotes. Using a clone of rat HTC cells with a more stable enzyme activity than in parental cells, regulation can be achieved by dose-dependent treatment of such cells with putrescine (McCann *et al.*, 1979). When the culture medium was supplemented with 10^{-5} M putrescine, a concentration lower than the estimated intracellular levels, enzyme activity was reduced but not by antizyme action. In contrast, the addition of 10^{-2} M putrescine effected the release of bound antizyme and initiated antizyme synthesis. The response to the lower concentration of putrescine suggests a control mechanism involving cell surface receptors and the production of adenosine-3',5'-cyclic monophosphate, cyclic AMP. Protein kinase activity, which is dependent on cyclic AMP, is implicated in this exogenously activated mechanism, since mutants of the S49 lymphoma cell line deficient in protein kinase, unlike parental cells, do not respond to stimulation with cyclic nucleotides by the induction of ornithine decarboxylase (Hochman *et al.*, 1978).

A further mechanism for the modulation of ornithine decarboxylase has been recognised by the chromatographic separation of ionically distinct forms of the enzyme. This phenomenon was first described with the lower eukaryote *Physarum polycephalum* (Mitchell *et al.*, 1978). A protein factor, activated by cellular spermidine, modified the charge and activity of the enzyme. Multiple ionic forms of ornithine decarboxylase from rat HTC cells have also been reported (Mitchell and Mitchell, 1982). In the mammalian system three peaks of enzyme activity were recovered from modified cellulose ion-exchange resins, but the separated enzyme forms were indistinguishable with respect to activation by ornithine or pyridoxal phosphate. Other properties supported the proposition that the three species of enzyme protein represent one gene product. Their sequential appearance during enzyme induction suggests an association with the rapid turnover of ornithine decarboxylase, but differential intracellular location has not been excluded.

It is apparent from the studies just described that the activity of ornithine decarboxylase in animal cells is closely controlled. In addition to the rapid turnover of enzyme protein, its expression can be modulated by antizyme or by posttranslational modification. The physiological significance of these various effects on the key enzyme in eukaryotic polyamine metabolism is unclear, but their presence in a variety of systems, including prokaryotic cells, argues strongly against their artificiality. The fact that ornithine decarboxylase is subject to fine regulation by such a diversity of mechanisms (McCann, 1980) is, perhaps, a significant reflection of the parallelism between polyamine metabolism and cell growth (Jänne *et al.*, 1978; Pegg and McCann, 1982).

The utilization of putrescine for the formation of spermidine in eukaryotic cells involves a series of enzyme reactions which are similar to those described earlier for prokaryotes. Again, the aminopropyl group is derived from *S*-adenosylmethionine after its decarboxylation by an enzyme activity recoverable in the high-speed supernatants from extracts of animal tissues. Unlike *S*-adenosylmethionine decarboxylase from *E. coli,* the rat liver enzyme is not activated by magnesium ions, and a further distinction from the prokaryotic enzyme is the activation by putrescine exhibited by the purified mammalian enzyme. A similar effect, but to a lesser extent, can be obtained with spermidine and the putrescine analogue 1,3-diaminopropane. Two lower eukaryotes, the slime molds *Physarum polycephalum* (Mitchell and Rusch, 1973) and *Dictyostelium discoideum* (Stevens *et al.*, 1978), contain *S*-adenosylmethionine decarboxylase activity which is unaffected by putrescine and inhibited by magnesium ions. Pyridoxal phosphate is not required as a cofactor by analogous enzyme activities in either prokaryotic or eukaryotic cells, but pyruvate is the prosthetic group of *S*-adenosylmethionine decarboxylases from both *E. coli* and rat liver.

S-Adenosylmethionine decarboxylase has been purified from a variety of animal tissues, most recently from calf liver (Seyfried *et al.*, 1982). The purified enzyme migrated in polyacrylamide gel electrophoresis under denaturing conditions as a major band with a molecular weight of 32,000. Its sedimentation in sucrose gradients is consistent with a dimeric structure for the native enzyme, and a molecular weight of 70,000 has been reported for the rat liver enzyme (Pegg, 1977).

An antiserum prepared against the calf liver enzyme cross-reacted with *S*-adenosylmethionine decarboxylase from bovine lymphocytes, and these specific immunoglobulins have been used in affinity chromatography to study regulation of the enzyme activity during lymphocyte mitogenesis (Seyfried *et al.*, 1982). The system is characterized by a biphasic induction of enzyme activity following mitogen stimulation of resting lymphocytes. There is an initial plateau reached 10 hours after transformation and a second increase at 20 hours, which is concomitant with the initiation of DNA synthesis in these cells. The rate of enzyme synthesis in activated lymphocytes was studied by labelling the cells with [^{14}C]leucine and recovery of the radioactive enzyme by affinity chromatography. The rate of incorporation of radiolabel into the purified enzyme was found to increase approximately 10-fold during the first 10 hours, but it remained relatively constant at later times. This increase in protein synthesis was accompanied by a 10-fold increase in enzyme activity, which at 6 hours had a half-life of approximately 80 minutes. The analogous enzyme in rat tissue has a half-life of 50 minutes calculated from the rate of decline after inhibition of protein synthesis by cycloheximide and a slightly longer half-life of 65 minutes under such conditions when the enzyme protein was measured immunologically (Pegg, 1979). However, the *S*-adenosylmethionine decarboxylase protein in bovine lymphocytes had a longer half-life of 170 minutes during the second phase after mitogen activation, and this latter period is characterized by a further twofold increase in enzyme activity. These results show that the biphasic pattern correlates with increased protein synthesis in the first phase and with increased enzyme stability in the second phase.

There are indications of other mechanisms for control of *S*-adenosylmethionine decarboxylase in mammalian cells. An increase in the levels of putrescine through the stimulation of ornithine decarboxylase produces a marked increase in *S*-adenosylmethionine decarboxylase activity (Tabor and Tabor, 1976). However, inhibitors of ornithine decarboxylase (discussed later in this chapter) appear to stimulate *S*-adenosylmethionine decarboxylase activity in Ehrlich ascites tumour cells even though the intracellular putrescine and spermidine concentrations are decreased (Alhonen-Hongisto, 1980). Such stimulation involved increased enzyme stability and enhanced enzyme synthesis. Low concentrations of exogenous spermidine or spermine repressed this activity, and a similar effect, albeit delayed, was obtained with putrescine. The intracellular concentrations of decarboxylated *S*-adenosylmethionine may also influence *S*-adenosylmethionine decarboxylase activity (Mamont *et al.*, 1982).

There are two aminopropyl transferases involved in spermidine and spermine production in eukaryotic cells, designated spermidine synthase and spermine synthase, respectively. The quantity of each synthase activity in various tissues is inversely related, but both activities are usually greater than either ornithine decarboxylase or *S*-adenosylmethionine decarboxylase. Both synthases are also more stable enzymes, with half-lives of several hours, and neither enzyme requires a cofactor nor possesses a prosthetic group for its activity. Each native enzyme from bovine brain has a dimeric form with total molecular weights of 70,000 and 80,000 for spermidine synthase and spermine synthase, respectively, values which are comparable with analogous enzymes from rat prostate (Raina *et al.*, 1983). Unlike spermidine synthase, the activity of purified spermine synthase is inhibited by 1 mM 5'-deoxy-5'-methylthioadenosine, the other product of the aminopropyltransferase reaction (Hibashami and Pegg, 1978). A specific phosphorylase present in normal cells, but absent from certain malignant tumour cell lines, recovers the purine base together with 5-methylthioribose-1-phosphate (Williams-Ashman *et al.*, 1982). A high rate of degradation makes it unlikely that the nucleoside product plays an important regulatory role in polyamine biosynthesis. Further control may be exerted by putrescine, since this substrate for spermidine synthase is a competitive inhibitor of spermidine in its reaction with spermine synthase (Hannonen *et al.*, 1972). Finally, it is interesting that although separate spermine synthase activity is not present in *E. coli*, the prokaryotic aminopropyl transferase is able to form both spermidine and spermine from putrescine. There is no evidence at present, however, for physical complexes formed by the eukaryotic enzymes during polyamine biosynthesis (Raina *et al.*, 1983).

V. POLYAMINE INHIBITORS

During the past 10 years a large number of compounds have been described that are effective inhibitors of polyamine biosynthesis in both prokaryotic and eukaryotic cells (Jänne *et al.*, 1978; Pegg and McCann, 1982). Their inhibitory effects are directed against various events in the polyamine metabolic pathways, but they may be categorized as follows: compounds with action against appropriate enzymes, the amino acid decarboxylases, S-adenosylmethionine decarboxylase or spermine and spermidine synthases; antagonists of pyridoxal phosphate, the essential cofactor in certain decarboxylation reactions; or, effectors of the macromolecular inhibitors ("antizymes") of ornithine decarboxylase. Apart from a few important exceptions, most polyamine inhibitors have been based on analogues or homologues of the substrates acted on by enzymes in the polyamine biosynthetic pathways. An exciting new development has been to design inhibitors with latent reactive groupings which are activated specifically by the normal catalytic action of the enzyme. Such catalytic, irreversible inhibition may be based on either the normal substrate or its product. Several halogenated congeners of arginine, ornithine and putrescine have been synthesized which act as such "suicide" enzyme inhibitors (Sjoerdsma, 1981). These compounds are the most potent inhibitors, to date, of putrescine and spermidine formation in living cells.

The availability of specific inhibitors has made it possible for the first time to achieve polyamine deprivation *in vivo* and, consequently, to investigate the physiological roles of putrescine, spermidine and spermine. A large number of investigations have now been made on the effects of polyamine inhibitors on cell growth and division, on cell differentiation and on embryonic development. Such information is invaluable in any assessment of the chemotherapeutic potential of those polyamine inhibitors that have been shown to be active against pathogenic organisms. First, the molecular basis of their action as polyamine antimetabolites will be described.

A.   Inhibitors of ornithine and arginine decarboxylase

α-Methylornithine was one of the first inhibitors of ornithine decarboxylase to be synthesized. The analogue was found to be a potent, competitive inhibitor of mammalian ornithine decarboxylase with respect to ornithine, and its inhibitory effect was not reversed by increasing the concentration of pyridoxal phosphate (Abdel-Monem *et al.*, 1974). Other evidence, however, suggests that the extent of inhibition of ornithine decarboxylase from *Lactobacillus* is influenced by the concentration of the cofactor (O'Leary and Herreid, 1978). These results foreshadowed later studies which have demonstrated different responses by prokaryotic and eukaryotic ornithine decarboxylases to the inhibitory effect of ornithine analogues.

α-Difluoromethylornithine was the first compound to be described with the property of catalytic irreversible inhibition of mammalian ornithine decarboxylase. The proposed mechanism of action requires that the halogenated derivative of α-methylornithine and pyridoxal phosphate form an aldimine derivative which is decarboxylated by the enzyme. This results in the production of reactive imines that alkylate a nucleophilic residue at or near the active site to covalently bind the inhibitor to the enzyme (Metcalf *et al.*, 1978). Evidence for this mechanism is obtained from the failure to recover enzyme activity after prolonged dialysis and by the protective effects of ornithine or putrescine against inhibition of the native enzyme by α-difluoromethylornithine.

Although an effective inhibitor of the eukaryotic enzyme, α-difluoromethylornithine is ineffective against the ornithine decarboxylase from *E. coli*. However, the prokaryotic enzyme from *Pseudomonas aeruginosa* is sensitive to inhibition by the compound (Kallio and McCann, 1981). Both ornithine decarboxylase from *E. coli* and from *P. aeruginosa* are inhibited by α-monofluoromethylornithine, another catalytically activated, irreversible inhibitor (Bitonti *et al.*, 1982). The latter compound also inactivates ornithine decarboxylase from rat liver (Kollonitsch *et al.*, 1978).

α-Monofluoromethylputrescine is an analogue of putrescine, the product of ornithine decarboxylase, and it inhibits irreversibly eukaryotic ornithine decarboxylase (Seiler *et al.*, 1978). Unlike α-difluoromethylornithine, α-monofluoromethylputrescine is an effective inhibitor of ornithine decarboxylase from *E. coli* but a poor inhibitor of the analogous enzyme from *P. aeruginosa* (Kallio *et al.*, 1982). These selective effects point towards important differences in the action of analogous enzymes, but the molecular basis for such discrimination is not known.

Putrescine biosynthesis in prokaryotic organisms can occur by an alternative pathway through agmatine, the decarboxylation product of arginine. α-Difluoromethylarginine has been shown to be a specific, irreversible inhibitor of arginine decarboxylase from *E. coli* and *P. aeruginosa* (Kallio *et al.*, 1981). This inhibitor may be predicted to have a selective action against prokaryotic organisms, since putrescine is derived from arginine through ornithine by the action of arginase in eukaryotic cells.

An unexpected result of the inhibition of ornithine decarboxylase in mammalian cells by α-methylornithine or α-difluoromethylornithine was an increase in the activity of S-adenosylmethionine decarboxylase after prolonged exposure to the inhibitor (Mamont *et al.*, 1978). With prokaryotic cells, a combination of α-monofluoromethylornithine and α-difluoromethylarginine reduced the putrescine concentration by 86% in *E. coli* and 34% in *P. aeruginosa*, but there were 42% and 20% increases, respectively, in intracellular spermidine concentrations (Bitonti *et al.*, 1982). These phenomena are contrary to the presumed consequences of putrescine deprivation, since the diamine stimulates eukaryotic S-adenosylmethionine decarboxylase activity *in vitro* and is also a precursor of spermidine biosynthesis in both prokaryotic and eukaryotic cells. As discussed earlier, however, compensatory mechanisms affected by putrescine availability have been shown to modulate S-adenosylmethionine decarboxylase activity in mammalian cells (Alhonen-Honigsto, 1980; Mamont *et al.*, 1982). Such considerations point toward the need to use combinations of inhibitors in order to achieve more effective depletion of polyamines in living cells.

B.   Antagonists of pyridoxal phosphate

Canaline, the oxyamino analogue of ornithine, has been shown to be an effective inhibitor of mammalian ornithine decarboxylase (Rahiala *et al.*, 1971). The compound forms a Schiff base product with pyridoxal phosphate, and it is this reaction with the essential cofactor which is responsible for the inhibitory effect. Other reactions dependent on pyridoxal phosphate are inhibited by a similar mechanism, and consequently, canaline is not a specific inhibitor of ornithine decarboxylase. Synthesis of the compound has proved difficult, but canaline can be obtained by the action of arginase on canavanine, the oxyguanidium analogue of arginine (Williamson and Archard, 1974). The antiviral effect of canaline is reversible by pyridoxal phosphate (Archard and Williamson, 1974; Williamson and Archard, 1976).

C. Effectors of ornithine decarboxylase activity

Putrescine has been known for some time to be a strong inhibitor of ornithine decarboxylase activity *in vivo,* but the conditions of such inhibition were not paralleled with the free enzyme (Pett and Ginsberg, 1968). Other diamines were shown subsequently to behave similarly, and 1,3-diaminopropane or its close derivatives were shown to be the most potent (Pösö and Jänne, 1976). The diamine inhibitors did not appear to act by product inhibition, but enzyme inactivation occurred very rapidly in cell cultures or in animal models, although protein synthesis was required for expression of the inhibitory effect. Such properties are now known (see Section IV) to be consistent with the induction of macromolecular inhibitors of ornithine decarboxylase ("antizymes") by diamine treatment of animal cells (Heller *et al.,* 1976). Although 1,3-diaminopropane and cadaverine elicited antizyme formation as efficiently as putrescine in rat HTC cells, the homologous diamines blocked ornithine decarboxylase activity by another mechanism, but less effectively than putrescine (McCann *et al.,* 1980). In common with other diamine inhibitors, 1,3-diaminopropane can also activate *S*-adenosylmethionine decarboxylase (Alhonen-Hongisto, 1980), and it is conceivable that in certain circumstances the diamine may substitute the requirement for natural polyamines.

D. Inhibitors of *S*-adenosylmethionine decarboxylase

Methylglyoxal bis(guanylhydrazone) (MGBG; mitoguazone) had been used clinically in the treatment of acute myeloblastic leukaemia before it was recognised as a polyamine antimetabolite. In an attempt to alleviate its toxicity, antagonism between MGBG and spermidine was demonstrated using an experimental *in vivo* model, but it was nearly a decade later that MGBG was shown to be an extremely effective inhibitor of mammalian *S*-adenosylmethionine decarboxylase. The action appears to be directed primarily at the putrescine-activated enzyme typical of eukaryotic cells, since much higher concentrations of MGBG are required to inhibit the magnesium-activated *S*-adenosylmethionine decarboxylase in prokaryotic cells (Williams-Ashman and Schenone, 1972).

Since the discovery of its antiproliferative activity, MGBG has been studied intensively, with the result that there is a vast amount of information from both *in vivo* and *in vitro* systems. MGBG has been shown to block the formation of spermidine and spermine in a variety of mammalian cell cultures, but the intracellular concentration of putrescine increased concomitantly. However, it has proved difficult to prevent polyamine accumulation in whole animals; in addition, MGBG stabilizes *S*-adenosylmethionine decarboxylase against intracellular degradation. Since the inhibitory effect of MGBG is competitive and reversible, removal of the compound by dialysis of tissue extracts prepared from treated animals results in a marked increase in the enzyme activity assayed. Structural analogy is the probable basis both for the common uptake system shared with spermidine and for some other effects of MGBG that may result in the direct displacement of natural polyamines from their intracellular binding sites (Jänne *et al.*, 1978; Pegg and McCann, 1982).

E.   Inhibitors of spermidine and spermine synthases

1,3-Diaminopropane inhibits the formation of spermine catalysed by spermine synthase from rat prostate (Hibasami and Pegg, 1978), and dicyclohexylammonium sulphate has been shown to be an inhibitor of spermidine synthase from eukaryotic cells (Hibasami *et al.*, 1980) and prokaryotic cells (Bitonti *et al.*, 1982). The precise modes of action of these inhibitors are not known. A transition-state analogue, *S*-adenosyl-1,8-diamino-3-thiooctane, is a potent inhibitor of spermidine synthase (Tang *et al.*, 1980) which blocks spermidine synthesis in mammalian cells (Pegg *et al.*, 1982). Bacterial aminopropyltransferases are also inhibited by the drug, but it was less effective than dicyclohexylamine in reducing spermidine levels in bacterial cells (Pegg *et al.*, 1983).

F.   Polyamine inhibitors, cell growth and differentiation

The information provided above is not intended to be a comprehensive list, since it has been abbreviated by one important consideration: that these reversible and irreversible inhibitors should also prevent polyamine biosynthesis in whole cells. One of the first studies with cell cultures investigated the effect of methylglyoxal bis(guanylhydrazone) (MGBG) on lymphocyte transformation (Fillingame *et al.*, 1975). This drug inhibited the accumulation of polyamines, which was observed in control cultures of bovine lymphocytes, but was without effect on protein synthesis or the synthesis and processing of RNA. In the absence of spermidine and spermine biosynthesis, however, there was a 60% reduction in the incorporation of [methyl-^{3}H]thymidine into DNA, although the proportion of labelled cells detected by autoradiography did not alter significantly. The inhibitory effect of MGBG on DNA synthesis could be reversed by the exogenous provision of spermidine. Treatment with MGBG resulted also in a 60% decrease in the population of cells undergoing division, as measured by the appearance of mitotic figures in the presence of colcemid. These results suggest that polyamine deprivation does not affect the progression through the cell cycle to the *S* phase, but inhibits the rate of DNA replication. Inhibition of *S*-adenosylmethionine decarboxylase by MGBG results in an accumulation of putrescine, and it is conceivable that residual DNA synthesis observed in the absence of spermidine and spermine biosynthesis could be due to enhanced levels of the diamine. Alternatively, the excess putrescine in the presence of MGBG could inhibit DNA synthesis. Such limitations were overcome by the subsequent availability of inhibitors of ornithine decarboxylase which block the initial event in polyamine biosynthesis in eukaryotic cells.

In growing rat HTC cells, putrescine concentrations show a biphasic increase paralleled by similar changes in ornithine decarboxylase activity (McCann *et al.*, 1975). In the presence of α-methylornithine these increases were blocked and putrescine levels rapidly declined, but there was a lag before spermidine concentrations decreased. In these cells DNA synthesis was unaffected for one generation period in the presence of the polyamine inhibitor but declined subsequently with a concomitant decrease in the proportion of cells in mitosis (Mamont *et al.*, 1976). When the α-methylornithine block was reversed by the addition of putrescine, spermidine, or spermine, cell proliferation resumed immediately. The growth of rat HTC cells was inhibited similarly by α-difluoromethylornithine, but this irreversible inhibitor has a more effective action against cell proliferation than the competitive inhibitor in other cell lines (Mamont *et al.*, 1978). The use of these inhibitors in subsequent studies has confirmed the importance of polyamines in the cell cycle, especially their ability to affect new DNA synthesis (Pegg and McCann, 1982).

The effect of polyamine inhibitors on cell differentiation has been studied in a variety of systems but most extensively with explant cultures of mammary epithelium obtained from pregnant mice (Oka *et al.*, 1981). When maintained in the presence of insulin, cortisol, and prolactin, these organ cultures synthesize the milk proteins casein and α-lactalbumin. It was established that arginase, ornithine decarboxylase, *S*-adenosylmethionine decarboxylase, and spermidine synthase activities were all increased in response to the hormone treatment. Furthermore, radiotracer studies demonstrated a temporal correlation between enhanced arginase activity and the utilization of arginine for the production of spermidine. In the presence of MGBG, the synthesis of milk proteins was inhibited, and this effect was reversed by the addition of spermidine but not by putrescine or spermine. This requirement for spermidine can be distinguished from the need for polyamines in cell growth (Oka, 1974). By comparison, α-difluoromethylornithine prevented the proliferation but not differentiation of human promyelocytic leukaemic cells (Luk *et al.*, 1982).

Amongst the various inhibitors of ornithine decarboxylase, the "suicide enzyme inhibitors" may be expected to show low toxicity by virtue of the precision of their action. The growth of different murine tumours is inhibited by α-difluoromethylornithine, and marked antitumour activity can be obtained during simple administration of the compound as a solution in drinking water (Sjoerdsma, 1981). In such experiments treatment was accompanied by reduced ornithine decarboxylase activity and decreased polyamine concentrations, but no toxic effects were detected with this drug regimen. However, an interesting effect of α-difluoromethylornithine on embryogenesis has been described. If the polyamine inhibitor is administered during the pro-oestrus period, ovulation is unaffected and the course of any pregnancies resulting from mating proceed normally. However, treatment on days 6–8 after fecundation was without effect on implantation, but subsequent embryonic development was totally inhibited. This critical period of treatment to obtain an effect on embryogenesis coincided with the period when ornithine decarboxylase activity and polyamine levels increased markedly in the uteri of control pregnant mice (Fozard and Koch-Weser, 1982).

VI. ANTIMICROBIAL ACTION OF POLYAMINE INHIBITORS

A. Antiviral action

Methylglyoxal bis(guanylhydrazone) (MGBG) was the first polyamine inhibitor to be shown to have antiviral properties (Ferrari *et al.*, 1964). Although the antitumour action of MGBG was known at the time, it was several years before its mode of action as a polyamine inhibitor was recognised. The drug inhibited the replication of poliovirus type 1, Coxsackie B3 virus and echo virus 6 in human amnion cells, but a less marked effect was obtained against vaccinia virus. It was shown that the antiviral action was not directed against the virus particle but against the virus-infected cell, and concentrations of MGBG that completely inhibited the growth of poliovirus did not prevent the multiplication of human amnion cells. This selective action of MGBG was confirmed in a later study using vaccinia virus-infected chick embryo fibroblasts maintained under an agar overlay so that virus growth resulted in the formation of focal lesions or plaques. If MGBG at a concentration of 50 μg/ml was allowed to diffuse into the infected cultures from wells cut into the agar, a small toxic zone surrounded by a large, plaque-free zone was observed (Küchler *et al.*, 1968). This technique subsequently became widely used for the quantitative measurement of antiviral activity after it was modified by the direct incorporation of the inhibitor at various concentrations into the overlay medium supplied to virus-infected cultures. The ED_{50} values for antiviral compounds can then be determined from plots of the percentage plaque reduction against the log_{10} molar concentration of the inhibitor (Collins and Bauer, 1977).

   Vaccinia virus has been used as a model in various studies of antiviral compounds primarily because of its ready growth in different cell systems, but another advantage lies in the available detailed knowledge of the molecular biology of this virus. It is possible in certain circumstances, therefore, to explain the mode of action of antivaccinial drugs in terms of their effect on specific molecular events in the vaccinia growth cycle. In common with other DNA viruses, the replication of vaccinia virus in HeLa cells is inhibited by the withdrawal of arginine from medium supplied to infected cultures (Archard and Williamson, 1971). It has been pointed out earlier that the formation of ornithine from arginine by the action of arginase may be regarded as the initial step for polyamine biosynthesis in mammalian cells (Pegg and McCann, 1982). The importance of arginine in vaccinia virus replication is indicated by its bio-synthesis using virus-specific enzymes in infected cultures supplied with cit-rulline in place of arginine (Cooke and Williamson, 1973; Williamson and Cooke, 1973). Although the amino acid is also required for the synthesis of viral proteins containing arginyl residues, it is now known that arginine is the essential source of ornithine for polyamine biosynthesis in vaccinia-infected cells (Obert *et al.*, 1980).

The utilization of ornithine for the biosynthesis of spermidine and spermine during the replication of vaccinia virus was first demonstrated by radiotracer studies (Lanzer and Holowczak, 1975). Purified virions from HeLa cells pre-labelled with [³H]ornithine were found to contain labelled polyamines with spermine apparently concentrated in the nucleoid, which contains the virion DNA, since a higher ratio of radioactively labelled spermine to spermidine was obtained with viral core preparations compared with complete virions. In order to measure the effect of virus replication on the synthesis of polyamines, Lanzer and Holowczak (1975) also monitored the metabolic fate of [³H]ornithine added to HeLa cultures at various times after infection. In view of the rapid inhibition of host protein synthesis in HeLa cells infected with vaccinia virus and the remarkably short half-life of ornithine decarboxylase in animal cells, it was an unexpected finding that radiolabelled polyamines were recovered from infected cells when the [³H]ornithine was added as late as 6 hours postinfection. This apparent paradox was resolved by the demonstration that ornithine decarboxylase activity increases markedly in HeLa cells after infection with vaccinia virus (Hodgson and Williamson, 1975). The physicochemical properties of such ac-tivity together with certain features of its control provided strong evidence for a new enzyme encoded by the viral genome. The expression of *S*-adenosylmethio-nine decarboxylase activity also increases in vaccinia-infected HeLa cells (Hodgson, 1976), and these studies together show *de novo* synthesis of spermi-dine and spermine during the replication of vaccinia virus.

Apart from a possible structural role, polyamines appear to be necessary for other events in vaccinia virus replication. The production of infectious progeny virus is also prevented by the withdrawal of arginine from vaccinia-infected KB cells, but the early sequential stages of adsorption, penetration, uncoating, early virus-specific mRNA synthesis and viral DNA synthesis are unaffected. The synthesis of late virus-specific mRNA normally follows these events, but such transcription did not occur in the absence of arginine. However, this requirement for arginine could be replaced by ornithine or the polyamines derived from its metabolism by the eukaryotic pathway (Obert *et al.*, 1980). In addition to a function in the formation of certain viral mRNA species, these studies also demonstrated a further requirement for polyamines in the maturation of vaccinia virions. Immature particles without electron-dense cores were seen by electron microscopy in sections from vaccinia-infected KB cells deprived of arginine, but the addition of ornithine, putrescine, spermidine or spermine to such cultures permitted the condensation of electron-dense nucleoprotein material in the immature particles. This requirement for polyamines in the replication of vaccinia virus is redolent of the stabilization by spermidine of condensed DNA conformations in the packaging process of bacteriophage replication (Cohen and McCormick, 1979).

The essential nature of polyamine biosynthesis in vaccinia-infected cells has been confirmed by the antiviral effect of polyamine inhibitors. In accord with earlier studies, a progressive reduction in virus yield was obtained with vaccinia-infected HeLa cells treated with increasing concentrations of MGBG (Williamson, 1976). The maximal inhibitory action obtained with 0.5 mM MGBG resulted in a 70% reduction in virus yield but complete reversal of this effect could be obtained by a further addition of 1.0 mM spermidine to the culture medium at the time of infection. Although viral DNA synthesis appeared to be unaffected in the presence of the inhibitor of S-adenosylmethionine decarboxylase, there was a reduction in the formation of virus-specific, DNA-containing inclusions in the cytoplasm of infected cells. This effect is consistent with the requirement for polyamines in the maturation of vaccinia virus in infected KB cells observed by Obert and his colleagues (1980). In addition, the replication of vaccinia virus is blocked by the inhibitors of ornithine decarboxylase, α-methylornithine, and α-difluoromethylornithine and by 1,3-diaminopropane, an inducer of ornithine decarboxylase antizyme or other inhibitory mechanisms (Tyms *et al.*, 1983). These most recent results also serve to illustrate two important considerations in all studies of antiviral compounds. Firstly, a drug-resistant population of vaccinia emerged after passage of the virus in MGBG-treated HeLa cells. Secondly, the nature of the host-cell system influenced the quantitative aspect of the antiviral effect. In HeLa cells, the MGBG-sensitive vaccinia virus gave an ED_{50} of 330 μM by the virus yield method, but the sensitivity to the drug of the virus stock was 100-fold greater in MRC-5 cells, a human diploid fibroblast line. The MGBG-resistant virus, by comparison, was much less sensitive to the drug in either cell culture system. Both virus populations, however, were sensitive to the antiviral effect of α-difluoromethylornithine with similar ED_{50} values of 5.9 mM and 4.4 mM in HeLa or MRC-5 cells, respectively (Tyms *et al.*, 1983).

Similar studies of polyamine metabolism and the effect of polyamine inhibitors in virus replication have been made with other important human pathogens. In fact, the first indication that animal viruses utilize polyamines for structural purposes was obtained with purified herpes simplex virions (Gibson and Roizman, 1971). Due to the physical nature of all herpesviruses, the virion envelope can be removed by treatment with detergent and urea to obtain naked nucleocapsids. Using this technique of controlled degradation with purified herpes simplex virus type 1 (HSV-1) virions, Gibson and Roizman (1971) showed that spermidine is removed selectively with the virus envelope, and spermine is preferentially associated with the nucleocapsid. This distribution of polyamines is reminiscent of that described earlier for vaccinia virus. The precise function of polyamines in the herpes virion is unknown, but it is estimated that the spermine content of HSV-1 is sufficient to neutralize nearly 50% of the viral DNA phosphate (Cohen and McCormick, 1979).

In view of the structural association of polyamines with HSV, it is perhaps surprising that several studies have shown that the synthesis of polyamines from ornithine is inhibited in cells infected with this virus. Gibson and Roizman (1971) demonstrated the recovery of radiolabelled polyamines in purified virions from continuous human cells (HEp-2) supplied with radioactive ornithine before infection but not when the labelled precursor was added after infection. The synthesis of spermidine and spermine from putrescine in mouse L cells was also shown to be inhibited by HSV-1 infection (McCormick and Newton, 1975). Polyamine turnover during HSV-1 replication was studied further by labelling HeLa and L cells with radioactive spermidine or spermine before infection and measuring subsequent changes in the specific activity of the polyamine pools after infection. Since the specific activities of spermidine and spermine did not change in infected cells, their synthesis may cease after HSV-1 infection (McCormick, 1978). In fact, it appears that cells of murine origin lose nearly all their cell polyamines during HSV replication (McCormick, 1978; Tyms *et al.*, 1983), but there is little or no leakage from HeLa cells (McCormick, 1978) or BHK_{21} C13 cells (Wallace and Keir, 1981). It is interesting that HSV-1 multiplies 20 times more efficiently in HeLa cells than in L cells, but the exogenous provision of spermidine or spermine did not increase the virus yield in either cell system. Similarly, infection of MRC-5 cells with the genital strain of herpes simplex virus (HSV-2) prevented the synthesis of spermidine and spermine from ornithine (Tyms *et al.*, 1979). These varied observations appear to be consistent with the failure to produce putrescine as a result of the loss of ornithine decarboxylase activity which occurs after HSV-1 or HSV-2 infection of mammalian cells (Gibson and Roizman, 1973; Isom, 1979).

In spite of the inhibition of their biosynthesis by the anabolic pathway after HSV infection, spermidine and spermine have been shown to be effectors of different enzymes encoded by the HSV genome. Both HSV-1 and HSV-2 DNA polymerases were found to be stimulated by either polyamine in *in vitro* assays (Ostrander and Cheng, 1980; Wallace *et al.*, 1980). Conversely, the DNase activity induced after infection with either virus was inhibited by spermidine or spermine. This viral enzyme has both exonuclease and endonuclease activity, but the endonuclease is more sensitive to the inhibitory effects of spermine (Hoffman and Cheng, 1979). These different effects on DNA polymerase and DNase activities are reflected in the regulatory role played by polyamines in the cell-free synthesis of HSV DNA (Francke, 1978). In an unfractionated cell lysate prepared from HSV-1-infected BHK cells, DNA synthesis results in the formation of viral genome-size products. However, in purified nuclear preparations of infected cells, repair-type DNA synthesis only was carried out, but this was complicated by extensive endonucleolytic and exonucleolytic activity. The nuclear system was found to lack polyamines, whereas putrescine, spermidine and spermine were present in the whole cell lysate. Addition of spermidine or spermine to the nuclear preparation inhibited the nuclease activity and resulted in a larger product with sedimentation characteristics of viral DNA, but too-high concentrations of the polyamines inhibited DNA synthesis. The pertinence of these studies is shown by the fact that the optimal concentrations of polyamines required for HSV DNA replication *in vitro* were close to the intracellular polyamine concentrations in infected cells (Francke, 1978).

The requirements for polyamines in HSV replication demonstrated *in vitro* seem to be inconsistent with the inhibition of ornithine and putrescine utilization in infected cells. Indeed, the drastic reduction of host protein synthesis after HSV infection (Roizman, 1978) will result in a rapid loss of both ornithine decarboxylase and *S*-adenosylmethionine decarboxylase activities due to the short half-lives of both enzymes. Such considerations can explain the lack of antiviral action by α-methylornithine against HSV-1 or HSV-2 (Tyms *et al.*, 1979). An effect by α-difluoromethylornithine against the growth of HSV-2 in BHK-21 cells has been reported but only after treatment of the cell cultures with the compound for 3 days prior to infection. Although the antiviral effect was very limited, its reversal by concomitant treatment with spermidine suggests some specificity (Tuomi *et al.*, 1980). Treatment of MRC-5 cells or primary mouse embryo fibroblasts with α-difluoromethylornithine, however, failed to produce any antiviral effect detectable by the plaque reduction method in spite of the fact that the experimental procedure exposes the majority of cells to the compound before infection (Tyms *et al.*, 1983). There may, of course, be sufficient quantities of spermidine and spermine extant in the cells at the time of infection to satisfy the polyamine requirements for virus replication. However, the growth of HSV-2 in both human and murine cells is inhibited by MGBG but only when the cell cultures are treated with the drug both prior to and during infection (Tyms *et al.*, 1983). Since *S*-adenosylmethionine decarboxylase activity may be expected to be lost rapidly due to the effect of HSV infection on host-cell protein synthesis, this antiviral effect of MGBG is surprising and suggests that the drug may have another mode of action against polyamine metabolism. Such a possibility can be discerned in other quantitative studies of polyamine levels in uninfected and HSV-infected cells.

A persistent phenomenon that is not compatible with virus-mediated inhibition of polyamine synthesis is the increased intracellular concentration of spermidine relative to spermine, which is consequent upon HSV infection. In HEp-2 cells the ratio spermidine:spermine changed from 0.85 to 1.56 after infection. There was also an unexplained decrease in the specific activities of polyamines recovered from infected cells that had been provided with [³H]ornithine for 18 hours prior to infection (Gibson and Roizman, 1973). In BHK-21 cells infected with HSV-1, there was no change in the spermine concentrations, but there was a small increase in spermidine (Francke, 1978). A large increase in putrescine was also measured, considered to be due to the virus-mediated inhibition of host protein synthesis resulting in a lack of cellular enzymes to process putrescine to higher polyamines, but such an effect should also inhibit anabolic putrescine production. Another study in HSV-1-infected BHK-21 cells showed an increase in the spermidine:spermine ratio from 0.66 at 3 hours postinfection to 1.09 at 24 hours postinfection (Wallace and Keir, 1981). Although infection completely prevented the excretion of polyamines, the intracellular concentration of spermidine remained unchanged while the concentration of spermine decreased. The possibility that such a reduction may be due to the oxidation of spermine to spermidine and/or putrescine was suggested. Such a catabolic route has, in fact, been described recently in rat tissues (Pegg and McCann, 1982). The polyamine interconversion is dependent, firstly, on the activity of spermidine N^1-acetyltransferase and, in view of the intranuclear site of HSV-1, it is significant that the chromatin-bound enzyme can acetylate both spermidine and spermine. Secondly, polyamine oxidase can cleave the acetyl derivatives to produce putrescine or spermidine in accord with the appropriate substrate.

The proposition that catabolic reactions may produce spermidine and putrescine from spermine in infected cells is supported by the effect of MGBG on HSV replication. Aminoguanidine is a known inhibitor of both diamine oxidase and polyamine oxidase (Seiler *et al.*, 1983) and the reactive group is doubly present in the MGBG molecule. Concentrations of MGBG that significantly reduced the synthesis of spermidine and spermine from putrescine in uninfected cells had no effect on the replication of HSV-1 or HSV-2 when added shortly before or at the time of infection (McCormick and Newton, 1975; Tyms *et al.*, 1979). As discussed previously, MGBG does prevent the growth of HSV-2 provided it is present both before and after infection (Tyms *et al.*, 1983). This antiviral effect is consistent with a preliminary reduction in spermidine and spermine levels by its effect on *S*-adenosylmethionine decarboxylase in the uninfected cells so that there is insufficient intracellular free polyamine to support virus replication at the time of infection. If spermine is utilized for the production of spermidine and putrescine after infection, the continued presence of MGBG will inhibit HSV-2 replication. In such circumstances it is possible that the antiviral effect of MGBG is due to its action on the polyamine oxidase activities that are essential in the catabolic polyamine pathway. It is important that the actual mechanism of antiviral action by MGBG against HSV-2 should be determined.

Human cytomegalovirus (CMV) is also a member of the herpesvirus group, but this virus has marked species specificity so that productive infection is limited to human cells. In MRC-5 cells infected with human CMV, the eclipse phase leading to the initial appearance of infectious progeny virus lasts for about 36 hours, but the infected cells continue to produce virus for at least 9 days, under one-step growth conditions (Tyms and Williamson, 1980). Such longevity and the marked stimulation of host cell macromolecular synthesis after human CMV infection are in marked contrast to the cytocidal nature of HSV replication, which is complete by 24 hours in many host cell systems.

Polyamine synthesis is markedly stimulated in MRC-5 cells infected with human CMV. Incorporation of [^{14}C]putrescine was shown to increase immediately after infection and maximal levels were attained following the production of infectious progeny virus. There were parallel, kinetic changes in the utilization of putrescine in the production of spermidine and spermine (Tyms and Williamson, 1980). The intracellular concentrations of spermidine and spermine in infected cells at 3 days postinfection were 1.5- and 12.4-fold higher, respectively, than in uninfected, control cells (Tyms and Williamson, 1982). This accumulation of spermine in MRC-5 cells after infection with human CMV strain AD 169 resulted in a progressive decrease in the spermidine:spermine ratio compared with an increased ratio in uninfected cells. Such qualitative differences were apparent throughout the virus growth cycle until at least 5 days postinfection (Tyms *et al.*, 1983). In a separate study using whole human embryo (Flow 5,000) cells, ornithine decarboxylase activity was shown to increase from 12 hours after infection with the same strain of human CMV (Isom, 1979). Maximal stimulation of enzyme activity was obtained with a multiplicity of infection calculated to infect all cells in the monolayer cultures. The specific nature of this effect was demonstrated by the failure to obtain increased ornithine decarboxylase activity in cells exposed to virus either inactivated with ultraviolet light or neutralized with antiviral antibody. Regulation of ornithine decarboxylase in the human embryo cells changed after infection so that its activity became less susceptible to inhibition by higher concentrations of spermidine or spermine (Isom, 1979; Isom and Backström, 1979). Such enzyme activity is compatible with the accumulation of polyamines after human CMV infection, but it is not known if these qualitative and quantitative changes are due to virus-coded enzymes. However, the stimulation of ornithine decarboxylase activity by human CMV was markedly inhibited by phosphonoacetic acid, a specific inhibitor of the viral DNA polymerase. It has been suggested that the polymerase, in addition to its catalytic activity, may have a regulatory function in the control of the virus-induced ornithine decarboxylase activity (Isom, 1979).

The growth of human CMV in MRC-5 cells can be prevented by different inhibitors of polyamine biosynthesis. Utilization of ornithine or putrescine for the synthesis of spermidine and spermine after infection was blocked by α-methylornithine or MGBG at concentrations that completely inhibited the production of infectious progeny virus (Tyms *et al.*, 1979). The same concentrations of the polyamine inhibitors also prevented the formation of intranuclear, DNA-containing inclusions which are the sites of viral DNA synthesis in infected cells. It was concluded that virus-specific DNA synthesis also requires concomitant polyamine biosynthesis. Such conclusions were disputed in a later study which failed to show any antiviral effect by α-methylornithine or α-difluoromethylornithine on the replication of human CMV strain AD 169 in Flow 5,000 cells (Isom and Pegg, 1979). The authors claimed that concentrations of the compounds which inhibited the virus-induced increase in ornithine decarboxylase activity failed to block the synthesis of viral DNA or the production of infectious progeny virus. It is pertinent that the virus stocks used in the studies by Isom and Pegg (1979) were derived from cell-associated virus without purification to reduce the high concentrations of polyamines associated with human CMV-infected cells (Tyms and Williamson, 1982). In addition, the cells used to study the antiviral effect had been grown in the presence of the inhibitors of ornithine decarboxylase for several days prior to infection, conditions known to stimulate *S*-adenosylmethionine decarboxylase activity (Mamont *et al.*, 1978). Consequently, polyamine concentrations sufficient to support virus replication may have been attained in the Flow 5,000 cells in spite of the inhibition of ornithine decarboxylase activity.

The effect of α-difluoromethylornithine on the replication of human CMV strain AD 169 has been examined in MRC-5 cells using washed extracellular virus, and the polyamine inhibitor was added at the time of infection. Both the formation of intranuclear, DNA-containing inclusions and the production of infectious progeny virus were inhibited (Tyms and Williamson, 1982). The absence of any toxic effect was shown by the restoration of virus growth after removal of the inhibitor at 5 days after infection. In the same study the antiviral action of MGBG was demonstrated against eight strains of human CMV using the plaque reduction technique, and the compound was far more potent than antiviral compounds used clinically against CMV infections. These observations show that polyamine metabolism is essential for the replication of human CMV and polyamine inhibitors may be suitable drugs for the treatment of CMV infections.

A major limitation in the study of potential antiviral agents against human CMV infections is the highly specific nature of the host. Consequently, there is no animal model of the human disease although there are a number of related animal viruses that behave like human CMV. The murine CMV *in vivo* is considered to be a valid and practical model for studies related to human CMV infection and disease (Hudson, 1979). The replication of murine virus in cultures of primary mouse embryo fibroblasts appeared insensitive to the antiviral effect of α-difluoromethylornithine. Likewise, the replication of vaccinia virus is insensitive to the same drug in the mouse cells even though the virus is sensitive in human cell cultures. Contrariwise, MGBG is a potent inhibitor of murine CMV. The specificity of this antiviral effect was substantiated by the observation that intracellular concentration of polyamines, and in particular the spermine:spermidine ratio, was increased after infection with the murine virus (Tyms *et al.,* 1983). The suitability of murine CMV as an *in vivo* model to study the chemotherapy of cytomegalovirus infections by polyamine inhibitors is currently under investigation in this laboratory.

It is, perhaps, significant that the animal deoxyriboviruses whose replication is known to be affected by polyamine depletion—vaccinia, HSV-1, HSV-2 and human CMV—also show an essential requirement for arginine (see Tyms and Williamson, 1980). The replication of adenovirus type 5 is also arginine-dependent, but this virus does not induce ornithine decarboxylase activity even though infection of quiescent rodent cells results in a $G1$- to S-phase progression. This induction of host-cell DNA synthesis was accompanied by an increase in thymidine kinase activity. The increase in this enzyme activity after infection was inhibited by MGBG but not by α-methylornithine (Cheetham and Bellett, 1982). The uncoupling of ornithine decarboxylase from the other periodic enzymes involved in DNA synthesis is interesting. Further evidence for the independence of adenovirus type 5 replication from polyamine biosynthesis is provided in a recent report by Cheetham *et al.* (1982). The authors showed that chromosome damage caused by adenovirus infection of rodent cells can be prevented by the provision of exogenous spermine or by the inhibition of the oxidative degradation of endogenous spermine by treatment with aminoguanidine. It is suggested that infection with this virus results in a spermine deficiency, which encourages an increase in endonuclease activity, resulting in chromosome damage. However, infection of primary mouse embryo cells with polyoma virus, a papovavirus, also causes a progression into the S-phase of the cell cycle, but this is accompanied by a biphasic stimulation of both ornithine decarboxylase activity and S-adenosylmethionine decarboxylase activity. These changes occurred in polyoma-infected cells in the absence of viral or cellular DNA synthesis (Goldstein *et al.,* 1976).

Apart from the early studies with MGBG (Ferrari *et al.,* 1964), little is known of the requirements for polyamines in the replication of animal riboviruses. Treatment of BHK-21 cells with α-difluoromethylornithine for 3 days prior to infection with Semliki Forest virus results in a hundred-fold reduction in infectivity titres at 8 hours postinfection, compared with untreated control cultures and a marked decrease in the activity of viral RNA polymerase. Both effects were reversible by the addition of spermidine 24 hr before infection (Tuomi *et al.,* 1980). An unexplained phenomenon is the increased yield of poliovirus obtained by superinfection of human CMV-infected cells, which may be related to enhanced polyamine levels (Furukawa *et al.,* 1978).

B. Antibacterial action

The characterization of putrescine as a growth factor for *Haemophilus influenzae* and the substitution of this requirement by spermidine or spermine were the first indications of an essential nutritive function of polyamines in prokaryotic cells (Herbst and Snell, 1948). Other bacteria have been shown subsequently to exhibit a similar dependence on the availability of polyamines whilst some studies have also demonstrated the physiological importance of polyamines in bacterial growth. For example, both mRNA and protein synthesis in an *E. coli* auxotroph were found to be dependent on the provision of exogenous spermidine. The structural specificity of this requirement was established using spermidine homologues (Jorstad *et al.*, 1980). Polyamine auxotrophs of *E. coli* have been constructed which are also unable to synthesize putrescine, and the passage of these mutants in the absence of polyamines results in a reduction of their growth rate to about one third of that obtained in medium supplemented with polyamines. This lower growth rate of polyamine-deficient strains can be maintained indefinitely, and their ability to support the replication of T-bacteriophage is unimpaired (Hafner *et al.*, 1979). These phenotypic characters were retained by mutants unable to synthesize cadaverine in addition to their deficiencies in putrescine and spermidine biosynthesis (Tabor *et al.*, 1980). An absolute requirement for polyamines has been described recently, however, in certain *E. coli* strains constructed by transduction of streptomycin resistance (Tabor *et al.*, 1981). Although the parental strain lacked ornithine decarboxylase, arginine decarboxylase, and agmatine ureohydrolase activities, it grew slowly in the absence of exogenous polyamines, but the rps L9 transductant ceased to grow shortly after resuspension in polyamine-free medium. The rps L mutation affects the S12 ribosomal protein, and the stabilization of bacterial ribosomes by polyamines is well known (Cohen and Lichtenstein, 1960). However, the rps L gene has an effect on decreasing ambiguity in translation, so the vital function(s) of polyamines in these bacterial mutants cannot be defined precisely.

In spite of prokaryotic cell dependence upon polyamines and in contrast to eukaryotic cells, it has not been possible to inhibit bacterial growth with any specific inhibitor of ornithine decarboxylase. Such failure is due to the presence of multiple pathways of polyamine biosynthesis in prokaryotic cells so that putrescine can be derived from precursors other than ornithine. Consequently, bacterial growth is unaffected by treatment with inhibitors of ornithine decarboxylase alone, since there is a concomitant increase in arginine decarboxylase activity (Kallio and McCann, 1981). A combination of α-monofluoromethylornithine, an irreversible inhibitor of ornithine decarboxylase, and α-difluoromethylarginine, an inhibitor of arginine decarboxylase, still failed to prevent the growth of either *E. coli* or *P. aeruginosa,* despite marked reductions of appropriate enzyme activities in bacteria grown in the presence of the inhibitors (Bitonti *et al.*, 1982). Such treatment reduced the putrescine content by 86% in *E. coli* and by 34% in *P. aeruginosa* but, rather unexpectedly, the spermidine content actually increased in these organisms by 42% and 20%, respectively. Marked reductions in the intracellular content of both putrescine and spermidine were obtained only by simultaneous treatment with a third drug, dicyclohexylammonium sulphate, which is a competitive inhibitor of spermidine synthase. With multiple drug treatment the spermidine content decreased by 50% in *E. coli* and by 95% in *P. aeruginosa* with parallel reductions in putrescine content of 66% and 80%, respectively. Dicyclohexylammonium sulphate alone at a 10 mM concentration reduced the spermidine content by 15% in *E. coli*, whereas a dramatic decrease of 92% was obtained in *P. aeruginosa* incubated with 5 mM dicyclohexylammonium sulphate.

Further experiments showed that the various effects of these three polyamine inhibitors on the intracellular polyamine concentrations correlated with changes in bacterial growth (Bitonti *et al.*, 1982). Growth rates were unaffected by any drug alone, apart from a small reduction in the growth of *P. aeruginosa* in the presence of dicyclohexylammonium sulphate, reversed by a combination of putrescine and spermidine. The growth of bacteria treated with the dual combination of α-monofluoromethylornithine and α-difluoromethylarginine was the same as in control cultures. The three drugs together, however, gave a 3-fold decrease with *E. coli* and a 6-fold decrease with *P. aeruginosa* as measured by the number of bacteria during the exponential growth phase. This inhibitory action against *P. aeruginosa* could be reversed by 5 mM putrescine added to the growth medium containing the three drugs, but 0.1 mM putrescine was sufficient to reverse their action against *E. coli*. Complete reversal of growth inhibition of both bacteria could be obtained with 0.1 mM spermidine, but a substantial increase in the intracellular putrescine content under such conditions strongly suggests that the exogenous spermidine was used for putrescine production. Such experiments provide confirmation that the inhibitory effect on bacterial growth of the three drugs in combination is, indeed, due to their action on polyamine biosynthesis.

The genetic studies with polyamine auxotrophs and the metabolic studies with polyamine inhibitors together show that bacterial growth is not inhibited completely by exhaustive deprivation of putrescine and spermidine. The reduced growth rate in the absence of polyamines may still be sufficient to maintain the pathogenic potential of the bacterium and, in such circumstances, polyamine inhibitors will not have a direct chemotherapeutic effect. However, it is clear that polyamines are essential for optimal bacterial growth and they have important roles, albeit ill defined, in the mechanisms of transcription and translation in prokaryotic cells. Any compound, ideally based on polyamine analogues, which perturbs these physiological functions would be expected to have a synergistic action with other inhibitors of polyamine biosynthesis against the growth and viability of bacterial cells. Although this strategy is still a theoretical proposition for other microorganisms, it is already available for the chemotherapeutic treatment of certain protozoal infections, particularly trypanosomiasis.

C. Antiprotozoal action

Although polyamines have been known for some time to be constituents of viruses and bacteria, their presence in parasitic protozoa is a relatively recent discovery (Bacchi *et al.*, 1977). Both putrescine and spermidine were found in *Trypanosoma brucei*, *Trypanosoma mega*, *Crithidia fasciculata*, and *Leptomonas* sp., but spermine was not detected. Growing cultures of *Leptomonas* sp. accumulate both putrescine and spermine, and the utilization of putrescine for polyamine biosynthesis has been demonstrated with promastigotes, the extracellular form of *Leishmania tropicana major* (Bachrach *et al.*, 1979b). Ornithine decarboxylase activity increases during both the growth of promastigotes in culture and in mouse macrophages infected with amastigotes, the intracellular form of the leishmanial parasite. Enhanced putrescine and spermidine levels were also found in the skin and the spleen of mice infected with *Leishmania tropicana major* (Bachrach *et al.*, 1981).

Apart from their association with the growth of protozoal parasites, polyamines have been shown to activate certain trypanosomal enzymes. An NAD--linked enzyme, L-α-glycerophosphate dehydrogenase, in *Trypanosoma brucei* requires spermidine for full activity (Lambros and Bacchi, 1976). This enzyme catalyses the reversible conversion of dihydroxyacetone to L-glycerophosphate, which, together with a second enzyme, L-α-glycerophosphate oxidase, is active in the energy metabolism of trypanosomes. The importance of these enzymes to the viability of the parasite is reflected in the trypanocidal action of ethidium, which, at high concentrations, inhibits the α-glycerophosphate of *Trypanosoma brucei* (Lambros *et al.*, 1977). Ethidium and spermidine have similar molecular configurations, and it is conceivable that they compete for common binding sites on the enzyme. Apart from these enzymes involved in anaerobic glycolysis, a DNA polymerase from *Trypanosoma brucei* is also activated by polyamines (Marcus *et al.*, 1980).

It was established from these biochemical studies that the metabolic pathway of polyamine biosynthesis in a variety of protozoal parasites is similar to other eukaryotic cells. The induction of ornithine decarboxylase activity with maximal activity during the log phase and the subsequent accumulation of putrescine and spermidine in growing cultures are strong indications of the vital nature of polyamine synthesis in these organisms. Such conclusions are supported by the activation by spermidine of enzymes which are essential for energy metabolism and for cell multiplication. These requirements provided the basis for a proposition by Cohen (1979) that polyamine metabolism is a suitable target for the chemotherapy of protozoal parasites. Indeed, MGBG had been shown to cure infections with *Trypanosoma equiperdum* (Jaffe, 1965) or with leishmanial parasites (Bachrach *et al.*, 1979a), and it may be presumed that such chemotherapeutic action is based on the inhibition of spermidine synthesis. The development of other highly specific inhibitors has provided compelling evidence that polyamine depletion is, indeed, the basis for antiprotozoal action of such compounds. In recent studies α-difluoromethylornithine either alone or in combination with bleomycin has been shown to cure mice infected with virulent, rodent-adapted trypanosomes (Bacchi *et al.*, 1980; McCann *et al.*, 1981a). The mechanisms of this trypanocidal action will be discussed in some detail, since they can serve as models for the use of polyamine inhibitors in the treatment of other parasitic infections.

VII. CLINICAL POTENTIAL OF POLYAMINE INHIBITORS AS CHEMOTHERAPEUTIC AGENTS

It is ironic that some 80 years have passed since Paul Ehrlich demonstrated that trypanosomal infections in mice could be cured by treatment with trypan red, yet the trypanosomiases are still significant diseases of man and other animals. There are many reasons for this situation, but it highlights the need for new approaches to the development of trypanocidal drugs. In 1980 Bacchi and his colleagues showed that α-difluoromethylornithine given as a 1% solution in drinking water can cure mice infected with a virulent rodent passaged strain of *Trypanosoma brucei brucei*. Infection resulted in death about 5 days after inoculation with 5×10^5 parasites, but the organisms disappeared rapidly from the blood of mice treated with the drug for 3 days. Treatment was started 24 hours after infection. Animals cured of established infections remained free from parasites for at least 30 days after the deaths of untreated animals. There was no evidence of cryptic infections in the brains of cured animals, and no toxic effects were observed even in animals treated for 6 days with 2% solutions of the drug. It is interesting that α-methylornithine, the competitive inhibitor of ornithine decarboxylase, did not protect infected mice.

   The action of α-difluoromethylornithine against ornithine decarboxylase activity in the protozoan parasite was investigated through its effect on the utilization of [^{3}H]ornithine in culture forms of *T. brucei brucei* (Bacchi *et al.*, 1980). The formation of radiolabelled putrescine was inhibited markedly in the presence of the drug and, in further experiments using cell-free extracts of the organism, 10–25-μM concentrations also effected a marked reduction in the utilization of the radiolabelled precursor. Studies in infected rats showed marked reductions in the intracellular putrescine and spermidine content of the parasites after drug treatment, although spermine levels increased. Such effects on polyamine metabolism were accompanied by further changes in trypanosomal macromolecular synthesis and morphology. The sensitivity of the parasite to α-difluoromethylornithine is due to the rapid uptake of the drug, resulting in higher intracellular concentrations compared with those in mammalian cells (Bacchi *et al.*, 1983). These results show that ornithine is the sole source of putrescine for polyamine biosynthesis in *T. brucei brucei* and the chemotherapeutic effect of α-difluoromethylornithine is directed against the organism's ornithine decarboxylase. The specificity of such action is shown by the reversal of the drug's curative effect in infected animals by the simultaneous administration of putrescine, spermidine or spermine (Nathan *et al.*, 1981). The antiprotozoal action of α-difluoromethylornithine has also been demonstrated with *T. brucei rhodesiense* (McCann *et al.*, 1981b) and *Eimeria tenella* (Hanson *et al.*, 1982). The coccidial infection in 2-week-old chickens was prevented by treatment both before and after infection with the drug provided in drinking water at concentrations as low as 0.0625%. Such prophylactic treatment allowed normal gains in body weight, showing, again, the lack of toxic side effects. Injection of putrescine into the abdominal cavity of chickens given 0.5% α-difluoromethylornithine in the drinking water completely reversed the anticoccidial action of the drug. Effective prophylactic treatment against coccidiosis did not affect the acquisition of immunity, as indicated by subsequent resistance to further infection (Hanson *et al.*, 1982).

The susceptibility of other protozoal parasites to the polyamine inhibitor, however, appears to depend on the stage of the life cycle. The effect of α-difluoromethylornithine against *Plasmodium berghei* in mice was restricted to the exoerythrocytic schizogeny (Gillet *et al.*, 1982). Such discriminatory action was also observed *in vitro* with cultures of *P. falciparum* (McCann *et al.*, 1981b). The drug had a significant effect on the ability of the parasites to undergo schizogony, but the attachment of merozoites and their penetration of erythrocytes was unaffected. These different effects may be related to the site of infection and also, possibly, to high ornithine levels in erythrocytes due to the presence of arginase. Alternatively, the susceptibility of ornithine decarboxylase to α-difluoromethylornithine may change during the life cycle of the parasite or the organism may possess other pathways for the synthesis of polyamines. However, it is clear that some protozoal parasites can utilize only one route, from ornithine, for the synthesis of putrescine, and this essential requirement is the metabolic basis for the antiprotozoal action of polyamine inhibitors. This conclusion is supported by the suppression of parasitaemia obtained by treatment with MGBG of other trypanosomal infections in mice (Nathan *et al.*, 1979).

In addition to its direct action against ornithine decarboxylase, α-difluoromethylornithine acts synergistically with the antitumour antibiotic bleomycin to cure acute *T. brucei brucei* infections in mice (McCann *et al.*, 1981a). At least 1% α-difluoromethylornithine in drinking water or 3.0 mg bleomycin/kg by intraperitoneal injection was required for effective treatment, but similar results could also be obtained with 4-fold and 12-fold lower concentrations, respectively, administered simultaneously. The lower concentration of either drug alone prolonged survival, but the treated mice eventually succumbed to the infection. In combination therapy, the α-difluoromethylornithine concentration appears to be the more important, since small increments in its dosage together with 0.25 mg bleomycin/kg resulted in marked increases in survival time by comparison with increases in bleomycin dosage at a constant concentration of the polyamine inhibitor. Predictably, the curative action of the drug combination was prevented by the simultaneous administration of putrescine, spermidine or spermine, but two putrescine homologues, 1,3-diaminopropane and cadaverine, were without effect. Since the synergistic action could also be obtained if α-difluoromethylornithine were given before bleomycin, but not if the drugs were given in reverse order, it is apparent that polyamine depletion is a prerequisite for the enhanced effect of bleomycin. An important biological consequence of the combined therapy is the ability to cure semichronic infections with *T. brucei brucei* in the central nervous system of outbred mice, although neither α-difluoromethylornithine nor bleomycin alone is effective against such infections (Clarkson *et al.*, 1983).

It is tempting to speculate that synergism between α-difluoromethylornithine and bleomycin is due to the perturbation of the normal physiological function(s) of polyamines. The chemical structures of several bleomycin antibiotics have been determined and the terminal amines of bleomycin A5 and bleomycin A6 are spermidine and spermine, respectively. These antibiotics bind to DNA, causing the double-strand scission that accounts for their cytotoxic action (Umezawa, 1983). Bleomycin alone inhibits nuclear division and causes malformation of the nucleus and disruption of microtubule infrastructure in *T. brucei gambiensi:* these effects are reversible by spermidine or spermine but not by putrescine (Bacchi *et al.*, 1982). Since polyamines are known to stabilize native nucleic acid and protein–nucleic acid complexes, it is possible that polyamine deprivation facilitates the cytotoxicity of those drugs whose action is directed to the target molecule by a polyamine prosthetic group. In addition to bleomycin, the curative effect of other drugs—for example, amicarbalide and imidocarb—in trypanosomal infections has been shown to be reversed by spermidine or spermine, but not putrescine (Bacchi *et al.*, 1981). These trypanocidal drugs did not impair the uptake of exogenous polyamines or affect the utilization of labelled precursors for putrescine and spermidine biosynthesis in intact trypanosomes from rat blood. Again, the molecular configuration of these drugs has structural analogies with spermidine or spermine, and their action appears to be directed against polyamine function(s).

The cytotoxic action of other drugs in combination with polyamine inhibitors has also been demonstrated in mammalian cells. Cytosine arabinoside, a nucleoside analogue, is an effective inhibitor of DNA synthesis which exerts its effect on cell growth during the *S*-phase of the cell cycle. Treatment of HeLa cells, a human cell line derived from a cervical carcinoma, with α-difluoromethylornithine and cytosine arabinoside had a marked cytocidal effect, whereas the same drug combination was ineffective against WI-38 cells, a diploid cell line derived from human embryonic lung. This discriminatory action appears to be due to the arrest of the diploid human cells in *G*1 as a result of polyamine depletion. Unlike the tumour cells, this prevents their entry into the *S*-phase and, therefore, protects against the cytotoxic effect of cytosine arabinoside (Sunkara and Rao, 1981). It is not clear whether such discrimination is based on quantitative or qualitative differences between the polyamine requirements of normal and tumour cells. Similarly, the cytotoxic effect of 1,3-bis(2-chloroethyl)-1-nitrosourea against the murine glioma 26 and the rat 9L intracerebral tumours was significantly enhanced in experimental animals pretreated with α-difluoromethylornithine. Although the polyamine inhibitor alone was ineffective, the consequential polyamine depletion resulted in a significant increase in the survival of animals given a single dose of the cytotoxic drug (Marton *et al.*, 1981). In contrast to these studies, pretreatment with α-difluoromethylornithine significantly decreases the cytotoxic effect of *cis*-diamminedichloroplatinum against rat 9L brain tumour cells in culture. This difference has been explained in terms of the effect of polyamine deprivation on DNA structure (Oredsson *et al.*, 1982). The removal of polyamines from DNA can make this macromolecule more accessible to chemical action so that its alkylation by the nitrosourea derivative is enhanced. Conversely, an alteration in the physical structure of DNA due to polyamine deprivation would impair the cross-linking reaction with *cis*-platinum, since precise spatial apposition is required for the formation of platinum–DNA complexes.

It is very pertinent to their potential use in other human disease states that two polyamine inhibitors have been shown to act synergistically in the treatment of childhood leukaemia. Both advanced lymphoblastic and myeloblastic leukaemias responded rapidly to the sequential administration of α-difluoromethylornithine and MGBG (Siimes *et al.*, 1981). Polyamine deprivation due to inhibition of ornithine decarboxylase activity primes the leukaemic cells to greatly enhanced uptake of MGBG so that intracellular concentrations of 1.5 m*M* or higher are reached. Apart from its action against polyamine biosynthesis, MGBG at such high concentrations has other effects which are cytotoxic. The regimen based on combined drug therapy was more effective than either drug alone, and side-effects were either absent or mild. These exciting clinical studies are also important in terms of the mechanism of therapeutic action at the molecular level, since structural similarities with spermidine suggest that MGBG may act as a metabolic analogue.

VIII. FUTURE DEVELOPMENTS

The efficacy of polyamine inhibitors in the treatment of protozoal infections together with their clinical use for the treatment of childhood leukaemia are two important factors that augur well for other chemotherapeutic applications. Various strategies can be envisaged, but it is important that they are matched to particular properties of the pathogen. The chemotherapy of bacterial infections using polyamine inhibitors is complicated by multiple pathways of putrescine biosynthesis found in prokaryotic cells in culture. However, various factors in the infected host—for example, the suppression of ornithine production by exogenous arginine—may affect the expression of particular pathways in the bacterium. Consequently, the combination of polyamine inhibitors required to prevent bacterial growth on artificial culture media may not be necessary for the control of natural infections. Since enzymes such as arginine decarboxylase and agmatine ureohydrolase are unique to prokaryotic cells, any inhibitors of their activity will show selective action against bacterial pathogens in an animal host.

It is an important stricture that the pertinence of any *in vitro* studies on pathogenic organisms should be extrapolated with care into the quite different context of the diseased host. This limitation applies most particularly to extracellular microorganisms but less so to intracellular parasites such as viruses, since the replication of any virus is intimately dependent on the metabolism of the host cell. Apart from some unique enzymes associated primarily with nucleic acid synthesis, other functions encoded within the genome of many viruses are restricted to the structural components of progeny virions. Such economy of genetic information is not shown by the poxviruses, and enzymes associated with polyamine metabolism are expressed in vaccinia-infected cells which are qualitatively distinct from analogous activity in uninfected cells. The growth of vaccinia virus in cell cultures could be blocked by various polyamine inhibitors but, with the eradication of smallpox, there are no longer any related viruses of significance which cause human disease. However, the growth of other clinically important viruses has been shown to be inhibited by polyamine deprivation, and two examples can illustrate in different ways the potential of antiviral chemotherapy based on polyamine inhibitors.

Human cytomegalovirus (CMV) is the most common aetiological agent in congenital infections and a significant cause of handicap in the newborn. This may be due to a primary virus infection in the mother, but the virus can also exist in a latent state and its reactivation during pregnancy may result in congenital perinatal or postnatal infections. Although such infections are usually asymptomatic, human CMV can produce severe, sometimes fatal, disease in the neonate. This is particularly the case in a newborn without maternal antibody who may acquire infection from blood transfusion products. Human CMV infection is also a major problem as a cause of disease in the immunocompromised host. Recent reviews have discussed human CMV infections in the foetus and neonate (Tyms, 1982) and in transplant patients (Betts, 1982).

Nucleoside analogues such as adenosine arabinoside, cytosine arabinoside, or 5-iodo-2'-deoxyuridine (idoxuridine) have been used clinically to treat disease caused by human CMV, particularly in the neonate, but there is still no established therapy (Bauer, 1977). Most recently acyclovir has become available, but human CMV does not encode a virus-specific thymidine kinase, the key enzyme activity for selective phosphorylation of the acyclic nucleoside in herpes simplex virus-infected cells. Consequently, the replication of human CMV is relatively insensitive to acyclovir in cell culture, although the degree of sensitivity appears to be strain-dependent (Tyms *et al.*, 1981). Marked species specificity has precluded any assessment of drug therapy in experimental animal models of the human disease, but recently data have become available from clinical trials. Human CMV is the most common cause of infection in renal transplant patients, resulting in serious complications and up to 20% of deaths. Treatment with acyclovir resulted in a significantly faster rate of improvement in renal transplant patients with various forms of CMV disease compared with placebo-treated controls but the mortality rate in the two groups was statistically indistinguishable. Acyclovir did not prevent virus excretion in the throat or urine and, although viraemia ceased during treatment, virus was also recovered from the blood after the drug therapy was completed (Balfour *et al.*, 1982). A second clinical trial of acyclovir has been carried out with bone-marrow transplant patients suffering from CMV pneumonia (Wade *et al.*, 1982). This condition occurred in at least 20% of such allograft recipients with a 90% or higher mortality rate, but treatment with acyclovir was without effect even in patients with plasma levels of the drug above concentrations shown previously to be effective in other *in vitro* studies.

It is apparent that, at the present time, there is no satisfactory treatment for human CMV infections, but polyamine inhibitors may provide an alternative basis for chemotherapy. A recent study has shown that MGBG inhibits plaque production in MRC-5 cells by either laboratory strains or clinical isolates of human CMV (Tyms and Williamson, 1982). The median ED_{50} value of the polyamine inhibitor was 50-fold and 10-fold lower, respectively, than either acyclovir or idoxuridine. Human CMV replication was also inhibited by treatment of infected cells with α-difluoromethylornithine at concentrations without overt cytotoxic effect in uninfected cultures. Further studies in an *in vivo* system have been encouraged by the increased intracellular levels of spermidine and spermine found in cell cultures infected with murine CMV and by the sensitivity of this virus to MGBG (Tyms *et al.*, 1983). It is questionable, however, whether murine CMV infection is a pertinent model of the human disease. Consequently, an evaluation of the chemotherapeutic potential of polyamine inhibitors may have to be made by clinical trial. The use of MGBG and α-difluoromethylornithine in the treatment of childhood leukaemias (Siimes *et al.*, 1981) and other proliferative diseases in humans (Sjoerdsma, 1981) has provided pharmacokinetic data that could be used to develop a suitable drug regimen. In the clinical trials with acyclovir an important difference between the two transplant conditions is the relative impairment of immunological competence in renal allograft recipients compared with total immunosuppression in bone-marrow transplant patients. Since the antiviral effect of either polyamine inhibitor is not virucidal, further recovery from CMV disease after any successful chemotherapeutic treatment is likely to be dependent on acquired immunity. The apparent lack of any immunosuppressive effect by α-difluoromethylornithine during successful prophylactic treatment against coccidiosis in chickens (Hanson *et al.*, 1982) must be interpreted very cautiously in view of the differences between avian and primate immune systems. However, recent studies in murine model systems have shown that administration of α-difluoromethylornithine actually enhances haematopoiesis (Niskanen *et al.*, 1983). This effect can be explained by the requirements for polyamine metabolism in subpopulations of regulatory cells (Sharkis *et al.*, 1983). The catalytically activated, irreversible inhibitor has very low toxicity (Sjoerdsma, 1981), whereas MGBG can be toxic at high concentrations, although careful monitoring of blood levels can guard against undesirable side-effects (Siimes *et al.*, 1981). It is apparent that polyamine inhibitors have many properties that are suitable for their chemotherapeutic use in treatment of human CMV infections.

Unlike human CMV, HSV-1 and HSV-2 are extremely susceptible to the antiviral action of acyclovir. Their sensitivity is dependent on two enzymes encoded by the virus genomes expressed in infected cells, thymidine kinase and DNA polymerase. Newly cloned populations of HSV yield acyclovir-resistant mutants under nonselective conditions at a frequency ranging from 0.01 to 0.2% of the total virus population. This high frequency of mutation occurs primarily in the thymidine kinase gene, although mutations in the viral DNA polymerase gene have also been described (Coen *et al.*, 1982). Viruses that fail to induce TK activity can be cross-resistant to other drugs, such as bromovinyldeoxyuridine or idoxuridine, which must be phosphorylated before their antiviral action is expressed. Resistance to acyclovir can be developed *in vivo* by repeated passage of virus isolated from mice undergoing low continuous oral acyclovir therapy (Field *et al.*, 1982). Acyclovir-resistant HSV has also been isolated from immunodeficient children during treatment for severe orofacial infections. In one study the drug-resistant virus also became resistant to bromovinyldeoxyuridine, but sensitivity to adenine arabinoside was retained (Schnipper *et al.*, 1982).

Nucleoside analogues were developed initially for clinical use by topical administration in the treatment of herpes simplex keratitis, and systemic use, except in severe, generalized infections, was usually restricted by the cytoxicity of several compounds. Acyclovir, however, is the safest antiherpes agent to date, with a chemotherapeutic index up to 3000, and the drug has recently been licensed for oral administration so that it can be prescribed for other clinical conditions. An obvious area for extensive use of acyclovir is in the treatment of genital herpes, an increasingly common infection for which no effective treatment has previously been available. If drug-resistant strains are selected through improper use of acyclovir, viruses as pathogenic as the parental virus, which are also resistant to other available drugs, may become prevalent. This is a powerful argument for the continued development of antiviral compounds, but an obvious corollary is the necessity to develop alternative strategies rather than pursue the synthesis of yet more nucleoside analogues. The options are few, but polyamine metabolism could prove a suitable target even though the polyamine inhibitors currently available are relatively inefficient as antiherpes agents. Such a deficiency may be due to their action against anabolic rather than catabolic routes of spermidine and putrescine biosynthesis, as argued earlier. This emphasises the need for further development of polyamine inhibitors.

In conclusion, it is possible to envisage a number of different approaches to the therapeutic use of polyamine inhibitors in the treatment of infectious diseases. Firstly, specific antagonists of enzymes in the polyamine biosynthetic pathway may be used. In several instances such enzymes are peculiar to the pathogen with consequent selective action in the infected host, but qualitative differences in analogous enzyme activities can be exploited where such absolute distinctions do not exist. The exquisite discrimination between virus-specific and host-specific thymidine kinase exhibited by acyclovir is explained more prosaically in terms of substrate affinity. The various halogenated analogues of either substrate or product of ornithine decarboxylase also have significant differences in their inhibitor action against prokaryotic enzymes. In the absence of such qualitative distinctions, quantitative differences may be exploited, since enhanced polyamine biosynthesis is characteristic of active growth, whereas there is minimal activity in quiescent cells. A further stratagem directed against the physiology of the pathogen could be based on structural analogues that perturb the normal functions of polyamines. Enzyme inhibitors alone can prevent the further formation of polyamines, but cell growth is unaffected until their intracellular concentrations fall below optimal levels, and this could result in a consequent delay in any therapeutic effect. Such depletion, however, also results in enhanced uptake of exogenous polyamines, so that the most rapid therapeutic effect should be achieved by a combination of enzyme inhibitor and polyamine analogue. Finally, polyamines as prosthetic groups could direct cytotoxic agents to specific intracellular targets, and the synergistic action between α-difluoromethylornithine and bleomycin may be a reflection of such mechanisms. In order to obtain the best therapeutic effect it is apparent that these different strategies should be matched to particular polyamine requirements of the pathogen. Such demands for clinical efficacy are dependent, in turn, on continued research into the nature and functions of polyamines in both prokaryotic and eukaryotic cells.

ADDENDUM

The efficacy of α-difluoromethylornithine in the chemotherapeutic treatment of human trypanosomiasis has been demonstrated in a recent pilot study (Sjoerdsma and Schechter, 1984). This clinical trial comprised 9 cases, including 6 cases with diagnosis of CNS involvement. The drug was given either orally at up to 20 g/day or intravenously at 20–30 g/day, according to the severity of the disease. Such treatment resulted in clearing of peripheral and CSF parasites within a few days. A rapid reversal of the symptoms of disease was observed in all cases, and there were no indications of toxic side effects. Two patients relapsed after several months: one responded to a further course of treatment, and the other was treated with melarsoprol. Another patient treated successfully with α-difluoromethylornithine had an infection which had not responded to melarsoprol.

ACKNOWLEDGMENTS

We are grateful to Dr. D. J. Jeffries and Dr. P. P. McCann for their helpful comments and to Helen J. Brown for the preparation of the manuscript.

REFERENCES

Abdel-Monem, M. M., Newton, N. E., and Weeks, C. E. (1974). *J. Med. Chem.* **17,** 447–450.
Akamatsu, N., Oguchi, M., Yajima, Y., and Ohno, M. (1978). *J. Bacteriol.* **133,** 409–410.
Alhonen-Hongisto, L. (1980). *Biochem. J.* **190,** 747–754.
Alhonen-Hongisto, L., Veijalainen, P., Ek-Kommonen, C., and Jänne, J. (1982). *Biochem. J.* **202,** 267–270.
Ames, B. N., and Dubin, D. T. (1960). *J. Biol. Chem.* **235,** 769–775.
Ames, B. N., Dubin, D. T., and Rosenthal, S. M. (1958). *Science* **127,** 814–816.
Applebaum, D. M., Dunlap, J. C., and Morris, D. R. (1977). *Biochemistry* **16,** 1580–1584.
Archard, L. C., and Williamson, J. D. (1971). *J. Gen. Virol.* **12,** 249–258.
Archard, L. C., and Williamson, J. D. (1974). *J. Gen. Virol.* **24,** 493–501.
Bacchi, C. J., Lipschik, G. Y., and Nathan, H. C. (1977). *J. Bacteriol.* **131,** 657–661.
Bacchi, C. J., Nathan, H. C., Hutner, S. H., McCann, P. P., and Sjoerdsma, A. (1980). *Science* **210,** 332–334.
Bacchi, C. J., Nathan, H. C., Hutner, S. H., Duch, D. S., and Nichol, C. A. (1981). *Biochem. Pharmacol.* **30,** 883–886.

Bacchi, C. J., Nathan, H. C., Hutner, S. H., McCann, P. P., and Sjoerdsma, A. (1982). *Biochem. Pharmacol.* **31,** 2833–2836.

Bacchi, C. J., Garofalo, J., Mockenhaupt, D., McCann, P. P., Diekema, K. A., Pegg, A. E., Nathan, H. C., Mullaney, E. A., Chunosoff, L., Sjoerdsma, A., and Hutner, S. H. (1983). *Mol. Biochem. Parasitol.* **7,** 209–225.

Bachrach, U. (1970). *Annu. Rev. Microbiol.* **24,** 109–134.

Bachrach, U., Don, S., and Weiner, H. (1974). *J. Gen. Virol.* **22,** 451–454.

Bachrach, U., Brem, S., Wertman, S., Schnur, L. F., and Greenblatt, C. L. (1979a). *Exp. Parasitol.* **48,** 457–463.

Bachrach, U., Brem, S., Wertman, S., Schnur, L. F., and Greenblatt, C. L. (1979b). *Exp. Parasitol.* **48,** 464–470.

Bachrach, U., Abu-Elheiga, L., Talmi, M., Schnur, L. F., El-On, J., and Greenblatt, C. L. (1981). *Med. Biol.* **59,** 441–447.

Balfour, H. H., Bean, B., Mitchell, C. D., Sachs, G. W., Boen, J. R., and Edelman, C. K. (1982). *Am. J. Med.* **73**(No. 1A), 241–248.

Bauer, D. J. (1977). "The Specific Treatment of Virus Disease." MTP Press Ltd., Lancaster, England.

Betts, R. F. (1982). *Prog. Med. Virol.* **28,** 44–64.

Bitonti, A. J., and Couri, D. (1981). *Biochem. Biophys. Res. Commun.* **99,** 1040–1044.

Bitonti, A. J., McCann, P. P., and Sjoerdsma, A. (1982). *Biochem. J.* **208,** 435–441.

Bowman, W. H., Tabor, C. W., and Tabor, H. (1973). *J. Biol. Chem.* **248,** 2480–2486.

Caldarera, C. M., Barbiroli, B., and Moruzzi, G. (1965). *Biochem. J.* **97,** 84–88.

Cheetham, B. F., and Bellett, A. J. D. (1982). *J. Cell. Physiol.* **110,** 114–122.

Cheetham, B. F., Shaw, D. C., and Bellett, A. J. D. (1982). *Mol. Cell. Biol.* **2,** 1295–1298.

Clarkson, A. B., Bacchi, C. J., Mellow, G. H., Nathan, H. C., McCann, P. P., and Sjoerdsma, A. (1983). *Proc. Natl. Acad. Sci. U.S.A.* **80,** 5729–5733.

Coen, D. M., Schaffer, P. A., Furman, P. A., Keller, P. M., and St. Clair, M. H. (1982). *Am. J. Med.* **73**(No. 1A), 351–360.

Cohen, S. S. (1979). *Science* **205,** 964–971.

Cohen, S. S., and Lichtenstein, J. (1960). *J. Biol. Chem.* **235,** 2112–2116.

Cohen, S. S., and McCormick, F. P. (1979). *Adv. Virus Res.* **24,** 331–387.

Cohen, S. S., Hoffner, M., Jansen, M., Moore, M., and Raina, A. (1967). *Proc. Natl. Acad. Sci. U.S.A.* **57,** 721–728.

Collins, P., and Bauer, D. J. (1977). *Ann. N.Y. Acad. Sci.* **284,** 49–59.

Cooke, B. C., and Williamson, J. D. (1973). *J. Gen. Virol.* **21,** 339–348.

Cowan, S. T., and Steele, K. J. (1981). "Manual for the Identification of Medical Bacteria." Cambridge Univ. Press, London and New York.

Cunningham-Rundles, S., and Maas, W. K. (1975). *J. Bacteriol.* **124,** 791–799.

Dion, A. S., and Cohen, S. S. (1972). *J. Virol.* **9,** 423–430.

Dubin, D. T., and Rosenthal, S. M. (1960). *J. Biol. Chem.* **235,** 776–782.

Dykstra, W. G., and Herbst, E. J. (1965). *Science* **149,** 428–429.

Emanuelsson, H., and Heby, O. (1982). *Cell Biol. Int. Rep.* **6,** 951–954.

Ferrari, W., Loddo, B., Gessa, G. L., Spaneda, A., and Brotzu, G. (1964). *Life Sci.* **3,** 755–758.

Ferro, A. J., Barrett, A., and Shapiro, S. K. (1978). *J. Biol. Chem.* **253,** 6021–6025.

Field, H. J., Larder, B. A., and Darby, G. (1982). *Am. J. Med.* **73**(No. 1A), 369–371.

Fillingame, R. H., Jorstad, C. M., and Morris, D. R. (1975). *Proc. Natl. Acad. Sci. U.S.A.* **72,** 4042–4045.

Fox, C. F., and Weiss, S. B. (1964). *J. Biol. Chem.* **239,** 175–185.

Fozard, J. R., and Koch-Weser, J. (1982). *TIPS* pp. 107–110.

Francke, B. (1978). *Biochemistry* **17,** 5494–5499.
Friedrich, B., and Magasanik, B. (1979). *J. Bacteriol.* **137,** 1127–1133.
Fujita, K., Murakami, Y., Kameji, T., Matsufuji, S., Utsunomiya, K., Kanamoto, R., and Hayashi, S. (1983). *Adv. Polyamine Res.* **4,** 683–691.
Furukawa, T., Jean, J.-H., and Plotkin, S. A. (1978). *Virology* **85,** 622–625.
Gale, E. F. (1940). *Biochem. J.* **34,** 392–413.
Gibson, W., and Roizman, B. (1971). *Proc. Natl. Acad. Sci. U.S.A.* **68,** 2818–2821.
Gibson, W., and Roizman, B. (1973). *In* "Polyamines in Normal and Neoplastic Growth" (D. H. Russell, ed.), pp. 123–135. Raven Press, New York.
Gillet, J. M., Boné, G., and Herman, F. (1982). *Trans. R. Soc. Trop. Med. Hyg.* **76,** 776–777.
Goldstein, D. A., Heby, O., and Marton, L. J. (1976). *Proc. Natl. Acad. Sci. U.S.A.* **73,** 4022–4026.
Greene, R. C. (1957). *J. Am. Chem. Soc.* **79,** 3929.
Guirard, B. M., and Snell, E. E. (1964). *J. Bacteriol.* **88,** 72–80.
Guirard, B. M., and Snell, E. E. (1980). *J. Biol. Chem.* **255,** 5960–5964.
Hafner, E. W., Tabor, C. W., and Tabor, H. (1979). *J. Biol. Chem.* **254,** 419–426.
Ham, R. G. (1965). *Proc. Natl. Acad. Sci. U.S.A.* **53,** 288–293.
Hannonen, P., Jänne, J., and Raina, A. (1972). *Biochem. Biophys. Res. Commun.* **46,** 341–348
Hanson, W. L., Bradford, M. M., Chapman, W. L., Waits, V. B., McCann, P. P., and Sjoerdsma, A. (1982). *Am. J. Vet. Res.* **43,** 1651–1653.
Heller, J. S., Kyriakidis, D. A., Fong, W. F., and Canellakis, E. S. (1976). *Proc. Natl. Acad. Sci. U.S.A.* **73,** 1858–1862.
Herbst, E. J., and Snell, E. E. (1948). *J. Biol. Chem.* **176,** 989–990.
Hershey, A. D. (1957). *Virology* **4,** 237–264.
Hibasami, H., and Pegg, A. E. (1978). *Biochem. Biophys. Res. Commun.* **81,** 1398–1405.
Hibasami, H., Tanaka, M., Nagai, J., and Ikeda, T. (1980). *FEBS Lett.* **116,** 99–101.
Hochman, J., Katz, A., and Bachrach, U. (1978). *Life Sci.* **22,** 1481–1484.
Hodgson, J. (1976). Ph.D. Thesis, London University.
Hodgson, J., and Williamson, J. D. (1975). *Biochem. Biophys. Res. Commun.* **63,** 308–312.
Hoffman, P. J., and Cheng, Y.-C. (1979). *J. Virol.* **32,** 449–457.
Hudson, J. B. (1979). *Arch. Virol.* **62,** 1–29.
Isom, H. C. (1979). *J. Gen. Virol.* **42,** 265–278.
Isom, H. C., and Backström, J. T. (1979). *Cancer Res.* **39,** 864–869.
Isom, H. C., and Pegg, A. E. (1979). *Biochim. Biophys. Acta* **564,** 402–413.
Jaffe, J. J. (1965). *Biochem. Pharmacol.* **14,** 1867–1881.
Jänne, J., Pösö, H., and Raina, A. (1978). *Biochim. Biophys. Acta* **473,** 241–293.
Jorstad, C. M., Harada, J. J., and Morris, D. R. (1980). *J. Bacteriol.* **141,** 456–463.
Kallio, A., and McCann, P. P. (1981). *Biochem. J.* **200,** 69–75.
Kallio, A., McCann, P. P., and Bey, P. (1981). *Biochemistry* **20,** 3163–3168.
Kallio, A., McCann, P. P., and Bey, P. (1982). *Biochem. J.* **204,** 771–775.
Kihara, H., and Snell, E. E. (1957). *Proc. Natl. Acad. Sci. U.S.A.* **43,** 867–871.
Kollonitsch, J., Patchett, A. A., Marburg, S., Maycock, A. L., Perkins, L. M., Doldouras, G. A., Duggan, D. E., and Aster, S. D. (1978). *Nature (London)* **274,** 906–908.
Küchler, C., Küchler, W., and Schulze, W. (1968). *Acta Virol. (Engl. Ed.)* **12,** 441–445.
Kyriakidis, D. A., Heller, J. S., and Canellakis, E. S. (1978). *Proc. Natl. Acad. Sci. U.S.A.* **75,** 4699–4703.

Lambros, C., and Bacchi, C. J. (1976). *Biochem. Biophys. Res. Commun.* **68,** 658–667.
Lambros, C., Bacchi, C. J., Marcus, S. L., and Hutner, S. H. (1977). *Biochem. Biophys. Res. Commun.* **74,** 1227–1234.
Lanzer, W., and Holowczak, J. A. (1975). *J. Virol.* **16,** 1254–1264.
Liquori, A. M., Costantino, L., Crescenzi, V., Elia, V., Giglio, E., Puliti, R., Savino, M. de S., and Vitagliano, V. (1967). *J. Mol. Biol.* **24,** 113–122.
Luk, G. D., Civin, C. I., Weismann, R. M., and Baylin, S. B. (1982). *Science* **216,** 75–77.
McCann, P. P. (1980). *In* "Polyamines and Biomedical Research" (J. M. Gaugas, ed.), pp. 109–124. Wiley, New York.
McCann, P. P., Tardif, C., Mamont, P. S., and Schuber, F. (1975). *Biochem. Biophys. Res. Commun.* **64,** 336–341.
McCann, P. P., Tardif, C., Hornsperger, J. M., and Bohlen, P. (1979). *J. Cell. Physiol.* **99,** 183–190.
McCann, P. P., Tardif, C., Pegg, A. E., and Diekema, K. (1980). *Life Sci.* **26,** 2003–2010.
McCann, P. P., Bacchi, C. J., Clarkson, A. B., Seed, J. R., Nathan, H. C., Amole, B. O., Hutner, S. H., and Sjoerdsma, A. (1981a). *Med. Biol.* **59,** 434–440.
McCann, P. P., Bacchi, C. J., Hanson, W. L., Cain, G. D., Nathan, H. C., Hutner, S. H., and Sjoerdsma, A. (1981b). *Adv. Polyamine Res.* **3,** 97–110.
McCormick, F. (1977). *J. Cell. Physiol.* **93,** 285–292.
McCormick, F. (1978). *Virology* **91,** 496–503.
McCormick, F. P., and Newton, A. A. (1975). *J. Gen. Virol.* **27,** 25–33.
Mach, M., Ebert, P., Popp, R., and Ogilvie, A. (1982). *Biochem. Biophys. Res. Commun.* **104,** 1327–1334.
Mamont, P. S., Böhlen, P., McCann, P. P., Bey, P., Schuber, F., and Tardif, C. (1976). *Proc. Natl. Acad. Sci. U.S.A.* **73,** 1626–1630.
Mamont, P. S., Duchesne, M. C., Grove, J., and Bey, P. (1978). *Biochem. Biophys. Res. Commun.* **81,** 58–66.
Mamont, P. S., Danzin, C., Wagner, J., Siat, M., Joder-Ohlenbusch, A. M., and Claverie, N. (1982). *Eur. J. Biochem.* **123,** 499–504.
Mandel, M. (1962). *J. Mol. Biol.* **5,** 435–441.
Marcus, S. L., Lipschik, G. Y., Treuba, G., and Bacchi, C. J. (1980). *Biochem. Biophys. Res. Commun.* **93,** 1027–1035.
Martin, R. G., and Ames, B. N. (1962). *Proc. Natl. Acad. Sci. U.S.A.* **48,** 2171–2178.
Martin, W. H., Pelczar, M. J., and Hanson, P. A. (1952). *Science* **116,** 483–484.
Marton, L. J., Levin, V. A., Hervatin, S. J., Koch-Weser, J., McCann, P. P., and Sjoerdsma, A. (1981). *Cancer Res.* **41,** 4426–4431.
Matsui, I., Kamei, M., Otani, S., Morisawa, S., and Pegg, A. E. (1982). *Biochem. Biophys. Res. Commun.* **106,** 1155–1160.
Metcalf, B. W., Bey, P., Danzin, C., Jung, M. J., Casara, P., and Vevert, J. P. (1978). *J. Am. Chem. Soc.* **100,** 2551–2553.
Mitchell, J. L. A., and Mitchell, G. (1982). *Biochem. Biophys. Res. Commun.* **105,** 1189–1197.
Mitchell, J. L. A., and Rusch, H. P. (1973). *Biochim. Biophys. Acta* **297,** 503–506.
Mitchell, J. L. A., Carter, D. D., and Rybski, J. A. (1978). *Eur. J. Biochem.* **92,** 325–331.
Morris, D. R., and Fillingame, R. H. (1974). *Annu. Rev. Biochem.* **43,** 303–325.
Morris, D. R., and Pardee, A. B. (1966). *J. Biol. Chem.* **241,** 3129–3135.
Murphy, B. J., and Brosnan, M. E. (1976). *Biochem. J.* **157,** 33–39.

Nathan, H. C., Soto, K. V. M., Moreira, R., Chunosoff, L., Hutner, S. H., and Bacchi, C. J. (1979). *J. Protozool.* **26,** 657–660.

Nathan, H. C., Bacchi, C. J., Hutner, S. H., Resigno, D., McCann, P. P., and Sjoerdsma, A. (1981). *Biochem. Pharmacol.* **30,** 3010–3013.

Nickerson, K. W., Dunkle, L. D., and van Etten, J. L. (1977). *J. Bacteriol.* **129,** 173–176.

Niskanen, E., Kallio, A., McCann, P. P., and Baker, D. G. (1983). *Blood* **61,** 740–745.

Noon, R. J., and Barker, H. A. (1972). *J. Bacteriol.* **109,** 44–50.

Obenrader, M. F., and Prouty, W. F. (1977). *J. Biol. Chem.* **252,** 2860–2865.

Obert, G., Tripier, F., Nonnenmacher, H., and Kirn, A. (1980). *Ann. Virol. (Inst. Pasteur)* **131,** 13–24.

Oka, T. (1974). *Science* **184,** 78–80.

Oka, T., Perry, J. W., Takemoto, T., Sakai, T., Terada, N., and Inoue, H. (1981). *Adv. Polyamine Res.* **3,** 309–320.

O'Leary, M. H., and Herreid, R. M. (1978). *Biochemistry* **17,** 1010–1014.

Oredsson, S. M., Deen, D. F., and Marton, L. J. (1982). *Cancer Res.* **42,** 1296–1299.

Ostrander, M., and Cheng, Y.-C. (1980). *Biochim. Biophys. Acta* **609,** 232–245.

Pegg, A. E. (1977). *FEBS Lett.* **84,** 33–36.

Pegg, A. E. (1979). *J. Biol. Chem.* **254,** 3249–3253.

Pegg, A. E., and McCann, P. P. (1982). *Am. J. Physiol.* **243,** C212–C221.

Pegg, A. E., and McGill, S. (1979). *Biochim. Biophys. Acta* **568,** 416–427.

Pegg, A. E., Tang, K.-C., and Coward, J. K. (1982). *Biochemistry* **21,** 5082–5089.

Pegg, A. E., Bitonti, A. J., McCann, P. P., and Coward, J. K. (1983). *FEBS Lett.* **155,** 192–196.

Pett, D. M., and Ginsberg, H. S. (1968). *Fed. Proc., Fed. Am. Soc. Exp. Biol.* **27,** 615.

Pett, D. M., and Ginsberg, H. S. (1975). *J. Virol.* **15,** 1289–1292.

Pösö, H., and Jänne, J. (1976). *Biochem. J.* **158,** 485–488.

Rahiala, A. E.-L., Kekomaki, M., Jänne, J., Raina, A., and Raiha, N. C. (1971). *Biochim. Biophys. Acta* **227,** 337–343.

Raina, A. (1963). *Acta Physiol. Scand.* **60,** Suppl. 218.

Raina, A., and Cohen, S. S. (1966). *Proc. Natl. Acad. Sci. U.S.A.* **55,** 1587–1593.

Raina, A., Eloranta, T., Hyvönen, T., and Pajula, R.-L. (1983). *Adv. Polyamine Res.* **4,** 245–253.

Ramakrisha, S., Guarino, L., and Cohen, S. S. (1978). *J. Bacteriol.* **134,** 744–750.

Rodwell, A. W. (1967). *Ann. N.Y. Acad. Sci.* **143,** 88–109.

Rogasa, M., and Bishop, F. S. (1964). *J. Bacteriol.* **87,** 574–580.

Roizman, B. (1978). *In* "The Molecular Biology of Animal Viruses" (D. B. Nayak, ed.), pp. 769–848. Dekker, New York.

Russell, D. H., and Snyder, S. H. (1968). *Proc. Natl. Acad. Sci. U.S.A.* **60,** 1420–1427.

Schnipper, L. E., Crumpacker, C. S., Marlowe, S. I., Kowalsky, P., Hershey, B. J., and Levin, M. J. (1982). *Am. J. Med.* **73** (No. 1A), 387–392.

Seiler, N., Danzin, C., Prakash, N. J., and Koch-Weser, J. (1978). *In* "Enzyme-Activated Irreversible Inhibitors" (N. Seiler, M. J. Jung, and J. Koch-Weser, eds.), pp. 55–72. Elsevier, Amsterdam.

Seiler, N., Knödgen, B., Bink, G., Sarhan, S., and Bolkenius, F. (1983). *Adv. Polyamine Res.* **4,** 135–154.

Seyfried, C. E., Oleinik, O. E., Degen, J. L., Resing, K., and Morris, D. R. (1982). *Biochim. Biophys. Acta* **716,** 169–177.

Sharkis, S. J., Luck, G. D., Collector, M. J., McCann, P. P., Baylin, S. B., and Sensenbrenner, L. L. (1983). *Blood* **61,** 604–607.

Shortridge, K. F., and Stevens, L. (1973). *Microbios* **7**, 61–68.

Siimes, M., Seppänen, P., Alhonen-Hongisto, L., and Jänne, J. (1981). *Int. J. Cancer* **28**, 567–570.

Sjoerdsma, A. (1981). *Clin. Pharmacol. Ther.* **30**, 3–22.

Sjoerdsma, A., and Schechter, P. J. (1984). *Clin. Pharmacol. Ther.* **35**, 287–300.

Sneath, P. H. A. (1955). *Nature (London)* **175**, 818.

Stevens, L., McKinnon, I. M., Turner, R. M., and North, M. J. (1978). *Biochem. Soc. Trans.* **6**, 407–409.

Sunkara, P. S., and Rao, P. N. (1981). *Adv. Polyamine Res.* **3**, 347–356.

Tabor, C. W., and Kellogg, P. D. (1970). *J. Biol. Chem.* **245**, 5424–5433.

Tabor, C. W., and Tabor, H. (1976). *Annu. Rev. Biochem.* **45**, 285–306.

Tabor, C. W., Tabor, H., and Hafner, E. W. (1978). *J. Biol. Chem.* **253**, 3671–3676.

Tabor, H., and Tabor, C. W. (1964). *Pharmacol. Rev.* **16**, 245–300.

Tabor, H., Rosenthal, S. M., and Tabor, C. W. (1958). *J. Biol. Chem.* **233**, 907–914.

Tabor, H., Hafner, E. W., and Tabor, C. W. (1980). *J. Bacteriol.* **144**, 952–956.

Tabor, H., Tabor, C. W., Cohn, M. S., and Hafner, E. W. (1981). *J. Bacteriol.* **147**, 702–704.

Tait, G. H. (1976). *Biochem. Soc. Trans.* **4**, 610–612.

Tait, G. H. (1979). *Biochem. Soc. Trans.* **7**, 199–201.

Tang, K. C., Pegg, A. E., and Coward, J. K. (1980). *Biochem. Biophys. Res. Commun.* **96**, 1371–1377.

Traub, A., Mager, J., and Grossowicz, N. (1955). *J. Bacteriol.* **70**, 60–69.

Tuomi, K., Mäntyjärvi, R., and Raina, A. (1980). *FEBS Lett.* **121**, 292–294.

Tyms, A. S. (1982). *Med. Lab. Sci.* **39**, 275–286.

Tyms, A. S., and Williamson, J. D. (1980). *J. Gen. Virol.* **48**, 183–191.

Tyms, A. S., and Williamson, J. D. (1982). *Nature (London)* **297**, 690–691.

Tyms, A. S., Scamans, E. M., and Williamson, J. D. (1979). *Biochem. Biophys. Res. Commun.* **86**, 312–318.

Tyms, A. S., Scamans, E. M., and Naim, H. M. (1981). *J. Antimicrob. Chemother.* **8**, 65–72.

Tyms, A. S., Rawal, B. K., Naim, H. M., and Williamson, J. D. (1983). *Adv. Polyamine Res.* **4**, 507–517.

Umezawa, H. (1983). *Adv. Polyamine Res.* **4**, 1–15.

Wade, J. C., Hintz, M., McGuffin, R. W., Springmeyer, S. C., Connor, J. D., and Meyers, J. D. (1982). *Am. J. Med.* **73**(No. 1A), 249–256.

Wallace, H. M., and Keir, H. M. (1981). *J. Gen. Virol.* **56**, 251–258.

Wallace, H. M., Baybutt, H. N., Pearson, C. K., and Keir, H. M. (1980). *J. Gen. Virol.* **49**, 397–400.

Wickner, R. B., Tabor, C. W., and Tabor, H. (1970). *J. Biol. Chem.* **245**, 2132–2139.

Williams-Ashman, H. G., and Schenone, A. (1972). *Biochem. Biophys. Res. Commun.* **46**, 288–295.

Williams-Ashman, H. G., Seidenfeld, J., and Galletti, P. (1982). *Biochem. Pharmacol.* **31**, 277–288.

Williamson, J. D. (1976). *Biochem. Biophys. Res. Commun.* **73**, 120–126.

Williamson, J. D. (1984). To be published.

Williamson, J. D., and Archard, L. C. (1974). *Life Sci.* **14**, 2481–2490.

Williamson, J. D., and Archard, L. C. (1976). *J. Gen. Virol.* **30**, 81–89.

Williamson, J. D., and Cooke, B. C. (1973). *J. Gen. Virol.* **21**, 349–357.

11   Bacterial surface lectins

T. WADSTRÖM and T. J. TRUST

I.   INTRODUCTION

In 1888, Stillmark first reported that castor bean extracts were able to agglutinate erythrocytes from different animal species. The seed extracts were found to contain haemagglutinating proteins, defined as agglutinins, haemagglutinins, or more recently lectins. The term lectin (Latin *legere,* to select or pick out) was based on the observation that some seed extracts could discriminate among human blood groups (Boyd and Reguera, 1949; Boyd and Shapleigh, 1954a,b). As an example, extracts from the lima bean (*Phaseolus lunatus*) were found to selectively agglutinate type A erythrocytes. This ability of seed extracts to selectively agglutinate different human blood groups was confirmed in an extensive survey of 51 plant species encompassing 28 different genera (Renkonen, 1948). These early reports prompted many studies in the 1950s that provided the first evidence that the specificity of major blood groups in humans are determined by sugars (Watkins 1966). These discoveries also came into practical use for the detection, isolation, and characterization of carbohydrate-containing polymers, such as glycoproteins, glycolipids (glycoconjugates) and other polysaccharides.

Despite the many studies on plant lectins and their wide use in many fields of biological research (Nicolson, 1974; Lis and Sharon, 1977, 1981), it has not been widely realized that bacteria also produce lectin-like proteins (Table 1). Some of these proteins have important roles in microbial pathogenicity and include exotoxins and surface proteins that are involved in adhesion of the bacterial cell to the eukaryotic cell. This review focuses on these adhesive proteins and proposes that these carbohydrate-recognizing bacterial proteins are lectins.

Because of the importance of attachment in the pathogenesis of infectious disease, the molecular interactions involving bacterial surface lectins are receiving considerable attention in laboratories around the world. In many cases it is

Medical Microbiology, 4
ISBN 0-12-228004-0

Table 1 Plant and bacterial haemagglutinins (lectins): some landmarks

Castor bean haemagglutinin	Stillmark, 1888, 1889
Escherichia coli haemagglutinin	Guyot, 1908
Escherichia coli D-mannose lectin	de Miranda and Collier, 1955[c]
Escherichia coli (K88)	Gibbons *et al.,* 1975[a]
Vibrio cholerae (L-fucose lectin)	Jones and Freter, 1976[b]

[a] First report indicating specific glycoconjugate receptors involving more than one carbohydrate residue.
[b] First report indicating that carbohydrates coupled to gel bead surface are potent lectin inhibitors compared to corresponding soluble saccharide.
[c] In Duguid and Old (1980).

hoped that a better understanding of these attachment processes will be useful in the rational development of vaccines against organisms where immunoprophylaxis is either not available or inadequate. In other cases, it is hoped that the development of other therapeutic or preventative measures will be facilitated. Because of the breadth of this rapidly expanding topic, this review does not attempt to provide the reader with a detailed consideration of the whole field. Rather, the chapter deals with topics selected to illustrate the nature and importance of bacterial surface lectins.

II. DEFINITION OF BACTERIAL SURFACE LECTINS

In order to define bacterial surface lectins, we first need to consider the status of the classical definition of a plant lectin in the light of recent findings from a variety of disciplines. Plant lectins have classically been defined as proteins that recognize and bind to specific monomeric carbohydrate moieties and exhibit agglutinating or precipitating activity. These plant lectins vary in composition, molecular weight, subunit structure, and sugar-binding specificities (Lis and Sharon, 1977, 1981), and are usually known by their trivial names, concanavalin A (con A), phytohaemagglutinin (PHA), etc., or by a botanical one (e.g., *Dolichos biflorus* lectin) (Goldstein and Hayes, 1978).

It is becoming apparent, however, that this definition of a lectin is too confining. Allowance needs to be made for those sugar-binding proteins that do not agglutinate, and for other proteins that recognize and bind more complex carbohydrates. A broader definition of lectins as sugar-binding proteins permits inclusion of nonagglutinating plant toxins such as abrin and ricin, which are closely related to the agglutinins of *Ricinus communis* and *Abrus precatorius* (Olsnes *et al.,* 1980, 1981), and permits inclusion of several proteins found in connective tissues, such as fibronectin. These proteins show preferential binding to certain complex carbohydrates, such as heparin and some gangliosides (Hart, 1980;

Barondes, 1981), and have recently been proposed as important regulators in normal tissue growth.

There are also good examples of proteins in the microbial world that clearly fit into a broader definition of lectin. For example, in the case of Sendai virus, it is well established that the haemagglutinating protein of this virus recognizes and binds to complex carbohydrates such as gangliosides (Haywood, 1974). In fact, Holmgren *et al.* (1980) have demonstrated that the protein actually recognizes an oligosaccharide with the sequence Neu-Acα2,8NeuAcα2,3βGalNac. Several bacterial toxins are also known to recognize complex sugars and must be considered as lectins. Cholera toxin is a protein that has five or six binding subunits that recognize a carbohydrate moiety on GM_1 gangliosides and similar carbohydrate structures on cell-surface glycoproteins (Cole *et al.*, 1977; Kohn *et al.*, 1978, 1981). The minimal requirement for the binding of cholera toxin is probably several D-galactose residues (Clements and Finkelstein, 1979; Hart, 1980; Ronnberg and T. Wadström, unpublished). Furthermore, cholera toxin has recently been shown to aggregate liposomes bearing GM_1 on the surface (Richards *et al.*, 1979). A second bacterial toxin that must be considered as a lectin is *Shigella* toxin (Olsnes *et al.*, 1981). This toxin recognizes oligosaccharides derived from chitin (i.e., *N*-acetylglucosamine oligomers) and was in fact purified by chitin chromatography (Olsnes *et al.*, 1980). The ability of this toxin to agglutinate

Table 2 Experimental approaches to identify cell-surface receptors for microbial lectins

Inhibition studies with	Example	References
Monosaccharides	Type 1 fimbriae of *Escherichia coli* (D-mannose)	Duguid, 1957
Oligosaccharides	Salivary glycoproteins and peptides (*Streptococcus mutans, Actinomyces viscosus*)	Gibbons *et al.,* 1975 Ellen *et al.,* 1980
Monosaccharide coupled to a solid phase	Adhesin(s) of *Vibrio cholerae* (L-fucose to agar beads)	Jones and Freter, 1976
Glycoconjugates	CFA/I and K99 adhesins of ETEC	Faris *et al.,* 1980
Erythrocytes with different blood group antigens	F7 fimbriae *Escherichia coli* isolated from urinary-tract infections	Källenius *et al.,* 1980a
Blocking experiments with plant lectins	Type 1 fimbriae of *Escherichia coli*	Salit and Gotschlich, 1977
	K88 adhesin of porcine ETEC	Sellwood, 1980
	Gonococcal fimbriae	Buchanan *et al.,* 1978
	Schistosoma haemoparasites	Peireira *et al.,* 1980

Table 3 Some properties of fimbriae of Gram-negative bacteria

Fimbriae	Diameter (nm)	Haemagglutination	Cell adhesin
Type 1	7	MSHA[a]	?[a]
2	7	HA negative	
3	4.8	HA negative	Fungal and plant cells
4	4.0	MRHA	*Proteus mirabilis* adhesin (Silverblatt, 1974)
Escherichia coli F73	7.0	MRHA	p[k] cell receptors (erythrocytes and urinary-tract cells (Källenius *et al.,* 1980a)
Escherichia coli CFA/I	7.0	MRHA	GM$_2$-like glycoconjugate (Faris *et al.,* 1980)
Proteus mirabilis (second type)	7.0	MSHA?	

[a] MSHA, mannose-sensitive haemagglutination; MRHA, mannose-resistant haemagglutination.
[b] Not proven to be an adhesin in *Escherichia coli* mucosal infections by promoting adhesion to epithelial cells. Proposed to cause binding to mucus (Ørskov *et al.,* 1980a).
[c] F7 according to the recently proposed nomenclature for bacterial fimbriae (Ørskov *et al.,* 1980b), after a modified scheme originally proposed by Duguid (1955, 1957).

cells or model membrane systems containing appropriate carbohydrates has yet to be determined.

These examples allow us to arrive at a definition of bacterial surface lectins. These are carbohydrate-binding proteins, involved in cellular adhesion, that may or may not exhibit cell-aggregating activity, and that may or may not be inhibited

Table 4 "Fuzzy layers," fimbriae, or fibrillae on Gram-positive bacteria proposed as surface structures recognizing receptors on eukaryotic cells

Organism	Possible nature	Reference
Streptococcus pyogenes	M-protein + /LT[a]	Gibbons *et al.,* 1972 Beachey *et al.,* 1980
Corynebacterium renale	Fibriae	Honda and Yanagawa, 1974, 1978
Staphylococcus aureus	Unknown	
Lactobacilli	Capsular material[b]	Fuller and Brooker, 1980
Oral streptococci	Unknown	
Actinomyces viscosus	Fimbriae	Ellen *et al.,* 1981

[a] Proposed as the major adhesin of strains isolated from urinary tract infections in cattle. (Similar fimbriae also reported in other species of *Corynebacteria*.)
[b] Staining by ruthenium red carbohydrate stain.

Table 5 Monosaccharide specificities for some bacterial lectins

Source	Organism	Reference
D-Mannose	*Escherichia coli*	Duguid *et al.*, 1955
	Vibrio cholerae	Jones, 1977, 1980
	Klebsiella pneumoniae	Fader *et al.*, 1979
	Salmonella typhimurium	Korhonen, 1980
	Aeromonas hydrophila	Atkinson and Trust, 1980
D-Galactose	*Pseudomonas aeruginosa*	Gilboa-Garber, 1972
	Fusobacterium nucleatum	Mongielo and Falker, 1979
	Actinomyces viscosus	Ellen *et al.*, 1980
	Streptococcus pyogenes	Wadström and Tylewska, 1982
L-Fucose	*Vibrio cholerae*	Jones and Freter, 1976
	Aeromonas hydrophilia	Atkinson and Trust, 1980
Sialic acid	*Mycoplasma pneumoniae*	Gabridge and Taylor-Robinson, 1979

by monosaccharides (Table 2). Indeed, the majority of these surface lectins (adhesins or colonization factors) probably recognize quite complex oligomers on cell surfaces, most of which have yet to be identified. These bacterial surface lectins include both fimbriae (pili) and outer-membrane proteins of Gram-negatives, and the fimbria-like appendages (fibrillae, or fuzzy layers) of Gram positives (Tables 3 and 4). When inhibited by monosaccharides, the concentration of sugar required is usually higher than that required with plant lectins. For instance, inhibition of the binding of Type 1 fimbriae of enteric bacteria requires 0.5–1.0% (w/v D-mannose. This concentration difference is probably a reflection of the lectin multivalence on the bacterial cell surface (Tables 5 and 6).

Table 6 Microbial lectins recognizing terminal *N*-acetylgalactosamine residues

Lectin	Reference
Pseudomonas aeruginosa "broad-spectrum haemagglutinin"	Gilboa-Garber, 1972
K99 adhesin of calf ETEC[a]	Gibbons *et al.*, 1975
Actinomyces viscosus agglutinin	Ellen *et al.*, 1980
Aeromonas hydrophila haemagglutinin	Atkinson and Trust, 1980
Outer bacterial fimbriae[b]	

[a] Nonconclusive studies with colostrum oligosaccharides inhibiting the haemagglutination of this surface fibrillar antigen.
[b] Terminal *N*-acetylgalactosamine residues of gangliosides were proposed as receptor structure for gonococcal fimbriae (Buchanan *et al.*, 1978) and fimbriae of human (CFA/I) and animal (K99) enterotoxigenic *Escherichia coli* (ETEC) (Faris *et al.*, 1980). (Note: Terminal *N*-acetylgalactosamine was also proposed as the natural receptor on glycoproteins and glycolipids for heat-labile LT.)

III.   ASSAYS FOR BACTERIAL SURFACE LECTINS

A.   Haemagglutination

The haemagglutination assay has classically been used to demonstrate bacterial adherence (Table 7). In this assay, the simultaneous adhesion of bacteria to the surfaces of two or more erythrocytes causes red blood cell aggregation via a bridging mechanism. This aggregation is detected visually on a slide, in a tube, or in a microtitre plate. Demonstration of lectin participation in this adherence requires that the haemagglutination be sensitive to inhibition or reversal by monosaccharides. Ineed, this ability of a sugar to interfere with haemagglutination is generally taken to indicate the involvement of this sugar (or a relative) in the receptor structure on the surface of the erythrocyte. The agglutination is often reported as sugar-sensitive or sugar-resistant. For example, D-mannose inhibits the haemagglutination (HA) produced by type 1 fimbriae of enterobacteria, and this is commonly referred to as mannose-sensitive haemagglutination (MSHA) (Duguid *et al.*, 1955; Duguid, 1959). If mannose fails to inhibit, then the haemagglutination may be referred to as mannose-resistant (MRHA). However, care should be taken when evaluating such classifications, since in many cases the workers do not report having tested any other monosaccharides. This means that the true sugar sensitivity is not known. In other cases a whole battery of simple sugars does not inhibit. This often reflects the recognition on the eukaryotic surface of a much more complex carbohydrate. For example, it has recently been shown that while the haemagglutinating activity of a *Myxococcus xanthus*

Table 7   Inhibition of binding of ^{125}I-labelled K88 antigens to intestinal brush borders by carbohydrates and lectins[a]

Substrate	Binding (%)
Control	100
Monosaccharides (except those listed below)	100
D-Glucosamine	81.1
D-Galactosamine	59.9
D-Mannosamine	86.6
Stachyose (α-D-galactosyl-α-D-galactosyl-α-D-glucosyl-β-D-fructose)	69.2
Galactan (polymer of D- and L-galactose)	50.3
Lectins	
Concanavalin A	96.8
Ricinus communis 120	92.8
Soybean agglutinin	82.1
Fucose-binding protein	27.8

[a] From Sellwood (1980).

haemagglutinin could not be inhibited by simple sugars or amino sugars, it could be inhibited with fetuin, a fetal calf serum glycoprotein (Cumsky and Zusman, 1979). The *O*-glycosidically linked trisaccharide of fetuin was shown to be inhibitory by itself, and the penultimate galactose of this glycopeptide was directly implicated in the inhibitory activity. Unfortunately, many of the other complex oligosaccharides present on cell surfaces are not readily available for screening tests.

Many workers have also screened organisms against a battery of erythrocytes from different animal species. Regrettably, the information derived from such an exercise is limited, since the carbohydrate composition on the membranes of the erythrocytes from various animal species is not well defined. Even in the case of human erythrocytes, there are minor glycoconjugates that could serve as lectin receptors and that have only recently been reported, and it is probable that others await identification. In the majority of cases the identity of the receptor on the human erythrocytes is still unknown.

An additional complication that needs to be recognized when attempting to assess complex haemagglutination and sugar inhibition patterns of various bacterial strains is the ability of many bacteria to produce more than one lectin. Indeed, different culture conditions can even be used to advantage when attempting to demonstrate the presence of different lectins on a single strain. For example, the optimal temperature for all plasmid-mediated haemagglutinins (K88, K99, CFA/I, CFA/II) of enterotoxigenic *Escherichia coli* (ETEC) is 37°C, with complete suppression of synthesis at 18°C (Wadström *et al.*, 1978). In contrast, type 1 fimbriae are synthesized at both temperatures. Also, L-alanine can be used to selectively suppress expression of K99 antigen by catebolite repression (de Graaf *et al.*, 1980b).

Recently, an assay of haemagglutination that provides quantitative information on the kinetics, reversibility and adhesive strength of the attachment process has been developed (Brooks and Trust, 1983). The technique is an adaptation of a viscometric assay that has also been applied to the study of lectin-induced agglutination (Brooks *et al.*, 1974; Greig and Brooks, 1979, 1981). It is based on the fact that aggregated suspensions exhibit a higher apparent viscosity than otherwise equivalent but nonaggregated samples. Application of this technique will undoubtedly provide valuable information on the adhesive event. The technique has already been used to demonstrate that the agglutination reaction can proceed in two phases, the second of which is induced by shear forces (Brooks and Trust, 1983). This shear-induced bacterial haemagglutination produced by an MSHA strain of *Aeromonas salmonicida,* and its incomplete reversal by α-methyl mannoside closely parallels the behaviour of the tetravalent lectin concanavalin A in the viscometric assay (Greig and Brooks, 1981) (Fig. 1). These findings provide the strongest evidence that a major mechanism by which bacteria can adhere to cell surfaces is via a lectin interaction. In this haemagglutination assay, the bacterial cell clearly acts as a multivalent lectin.

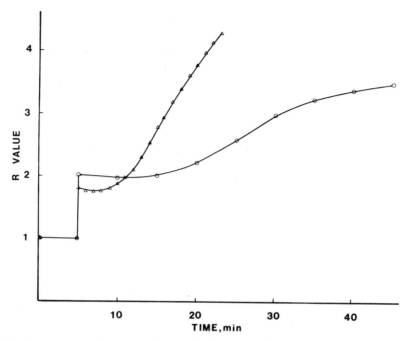

Fig. 1 Aggregation of erythrocytes studied by a viscosimetric method (Brooks *et al.,* 1974; Brooks and Trust, 1983). A plant lectin (concanavalin A, △) or bacterium (*Aeromonas salmonicida,* ○) is added to the erythrocyte suspension at 5 min, and cell aggregation (*R* value) is recorded as a change in higher apparent viscosity compared to controls without addition of a plant or a bacterial lectin, i.e., in this case whole bacterial cells with a surface lectin.

B. Adhesion to other eukaryotic cells

Not all adhesive appendages are haemagglutinating. This is illustrated by the 987p fimbriae of porcine ETEC. This means that other cells may need to be used in defining bacterial lectins. A variety of other cell types have in fact been used in attachment studies. In addition, a variety of assay techniques have been used to examine the bacterial attachment to these various cell types. One problem that is immediately apparent in many of these studies is the poorly defined quality of the cells used. Cells are often obtained by mucosal scrapings in the oral cavity (bucca and pharynx), and in other cases desquamated urine sediment cells have been used. While some studies show that the viability of these single-cell preparations may not be important, at least in some test systems the day-to-day variation in cell preparations from the same and from different individuals often does produce variable results (Svanborg-Eden and Hansson, 1978). The various assay problems have recently encouraged studies to find organ- or tissue-culture systems that allow more standardized test conditions (Jones, 1980). The problem

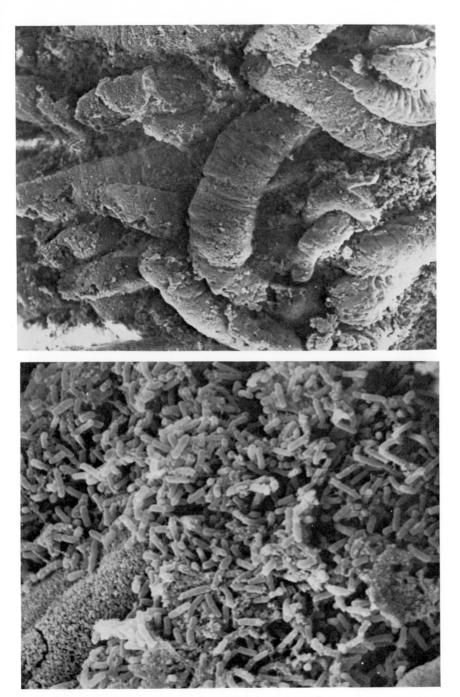

Fig. 2 Scanning electron micrographs of K88 porcine ETEC organisms attaching to the gut epithelial surface. (Kindly supplied by Dr. L. Nagy and P. Walker, Wellcome Research Laboratories, Beckenham, Kent, England.)

of obtaining a continuous supply of biopsy material from different mucosae of animals and humans has in turn focused attention on the development of suitable tissue-culture systems, such as the human intestinal cell line 407. This cell line has recently been used for measuring adhesion of *E. coli* carrying various fimbrial antigens (Jann *et al.*, 1981; Wadstrom *et al.*, 1984) and for studies on the attachment properties of *Vibrio parahaemolyticus* (Gingras and Howard, 1980).

Preparations of mucosal brush borders that can be stored at low temperatures ($-70°C$ in a glycerol medium) (Girardeau, 1980) appear to be a most useful alternative. Rabbit brush borders have recently been used with human entero-pathogenic *E. coli*, while porcine brush borders have been used with porcine K88 ETEC organisms (Sellwood, 1980) (Fig. 2).

C. Other assays

An early observation by Brinton (1965) that fimbriated *E. coli* stick to plastic surfaces has been extended for adherence test systems. Several nonbiological systems have been especially useful for studies on receptor–ligand interactions. Buchanan (1976) showed that gonococcal fimbriae bind latex particles and also bind to tissue-culture cells. Later we found that haemagglutinating *E. coli* display hydrophobic interactions, and this allowed us to develop a rapid simple test for the detection of nonhaemagglutinating adhesions (lectins) such as the 987p of porcine ETEC (Smyth *et al.*, 1978; Wadström *et al.*, 1980a; Faris *et al.*, 1981; Moon *et al.*, 1980). More recently, the development of an autoagglutination test in salt solutions of different molarities (the "salting out principle," Lindahl *et al.*, 1981) has produced a simple test to rapidly screen enterobacteria for the presence of surface protein adhesions (lectins) and to quantitate their relative surface hydrophobicities.

IV. THE PROTOTYPE BACTERIAL SURFACE LECTIN: TYPE 1 D-MANNOSE-SPECIFIC FIMBRIAE

The best-described bacterial surface lectin is the D-mannose-specific type 1 fimbriae of *E. coli*. The first evidence for the presence of adhesive appendages on the surface of *E. coli* was provided by Gyot (1908) (Table 1), who reported that many strains rapidly agglutinated erythrocytes of many animal species. Each bacterial strain was found to react differently with erythrocytes from individual animals of one species, and different strains also reacted differently with red blood cells of different species. This was interpreted as the possession of differ-ent kinds of haemagglutinins. Nearly four decades later, haemagglutinating *E. coli* cultures were shown to also agglutinate other cells such as leukocytes, sperms, yeast cells, fungal spores, and plant pollens (for references, see Duguid and Old, 1980). Haemagglutinins were formed by the majority of the 112 strains of tested *E. coli*. Other enterobacteria were also able to agglutinate human red blood cells.

In 1955, as a rule of an extensive systematic study, Duguid *et al.* divided the haemagglutinating *E. coli* into three groups (I, II and III) on the basis of HA patterns. A fourth group (IV) failed to haemagglutinate erythrocytes from a large number of different animal species (Table 3). Electron-microscopic examination of strains from these HA groups revealed that groups I and II carried numerous filamentous appendages on the cell surface. These were estimated to be about 10 nm in width and up to about 1 μm in length. They were arranged continuously around the whole cell (i.e., peritrichously), and there were between 100 and 250 per cell. Each culture was also found to contain some nonfimbriated bacteria. Group III strains, although able to haemagglutinate, were devoid of surface fimbriae, as were group IV strains. The elegant studies by Duguid and colleagues and by Brinton (1965) also revealed that different culture conditions favored or suppressed production of these fimbriae. Importantly, this variation between a fimbriate and a nonfimbriate phase usually correlated with expression or suppression of haemagglutinating activity. In the case of group I strains of *E. coli* and other species of enterobacteria, the haemagglutinating activity was usually optimal at 37°C in static liquid cultures serially transferred every 24–48 hours. Haemagglutinating activity was also expressed when the same strains were grown at 20°C on agar (Duguid *et al.*, 1955; Duguid and Old, 1980).

The first report of sugar inhibition of haemagglutination was by Collier and Miranda (1955). These workers demonstrated that of many monosaccharides tested, only D-mannose strongly inhibited the haemagglutinating activity of strains of *E. coli*. These strains were later shown to belong to group I of the Duguid scheme. Similar haemagglutinins were also discovered on *Shigella flexneri*, *Klebsiella*, and *Salmonella*. These were all inhibited by low concentrations of D-mannose (0.1–0.5% w/v), α-D-methyl-mannoside, yeast mannan, and related chemical structures (Old, 1972). The mannose-sensitive haemagglutinin in such enterobacterial strains was named the "MS adhesin" by Duguid (1959) and thus became the first defined bacterial protein fulfilling the criteria of a bacterial surface lectin.

Preparations of detached and isolated fimbriae were then shown to produce mannose-sensitive agglutination of red blood cells (Brinton, 1959; Old, 1963; Salit and Gotschlich, 1977), conclusively identifying the fimbriae as the adhesive appendage carrying the lectin activity. Salit and Gotschlich (1977) also found that when type 1 fimbriate cells of *E. coli* were attached to the surface of monkey kidney cells, the fimbriae were in contact with the kidney cell surface over considerable lengths, suggesting that fimbriae possess multiple binding sites.

Recent studies by Sweeney and Freer (1979) have provided further evidence for the presence of multiple binding sites on these haemagglutinating fimbriae. Fimbriae were progressively shortened by treatment with ultrasound. As the fimbriae were shortened, their haemagglutinating capacity was decreased, but their ability to bind to erythrocytes did not decrease to the same extent. The results provide strong evidence that binding sites are located along the length of the fimbriae, rather than being a single terminal binding site. Furthermore, isolated fimbriae did not agglutinate inside-out vesicles prepared from horse erythrocytes, or liposomes, suggesting that the binding mechanism was not based on nonspecific hydrophobic interactions. However, Sweeney and Freer did not test the mannose sensitivity of this fimbrial binding.

While many bacterial species are now known to produce mannose-sensitive haemagglutinating fimbriae, the structural relationships between these fimbriae are still not clear. Although the adhesive activities of the various type 1 fimbriae are similar, antigenic differences between these type 1 fimbriae suggest chemical and structural differences (Duguid and Campbell, 1969). Some of the differences have recently been demonstrated by Korhonen *et al.* (1980). These workers purified type 1 fimbriae from *Salmonella typhimurium* and compared the pilin structure with pilin from *E. coli* type 1 fimbriae. *Salmonella typhimurium* pilin had an apparent molecular weight of 21,000, and the *E. coli* type 1 pilin was 17,000. The *S. typhimurium* pilin contained more proline, serine, and lysine than reported for type 1 pilin of *E. coli*. Despite these differences, the two fimbriae were shown to be similar in their morphology and isoelectric point. Using enzyme-linked immunosorbent assay, the type 1 fimbriae purified from two *E. coli* strains and *S. typhimurium* were shown to be not cross-reactive immunologically. These findings, together with the recent interest in *E. coli* fimbrial vaccines (Levine *et al.*, 1982), suggest that further studies might be warranted on the type 1 fimbriae to reveal the extent of antigenic similarity or diversity.

The sugar inhibition patterns of the various type 1 fimbriae are similar. Old (1972) studied the carbohydrate inhibition of haemagglutination by pilated *S. typhimurium* and *Shigella flexneri* cells and showed that the α-configuration at the C-1 position in the mannopyranoside molecule and unmodified hydroxyl groups at C-2, C-3, C-4, and C-6 of the D-mannose molecule were required for maximum binding to the bacterial fimbrial lectin sites. Similar results have since been reported with purified type 1 *E. coli* fimbriae (Salit and Gotschlich, 1977) and purified *S. typhimurium* type 1 fimbriae (Korhonen *et al.*, 1980). Old (1972) was in fact the first worker to notice and comment on the remarkable similarity in the sugar inhibition pattern of the type 1 fimbriae and the plant lectin concanavalin A.

A. Other mannose-specific surface lectins

A mannose-specific "lectin" has been isolated from the surface of *E. coli* (Eshdat *et al.*, 1978). This lectin is a high-molecular-weight protein aggregate and has a different amino acid composition from that of type 1 pili, the K99 antigen, and the major outer-membrane protein of *E. coli*. A mannose-specific lectin has also been isolated from a *Pseudomonas aeruginosa* strain grown in the presence of acetylcholine or choline (Gilboa-Garber *et al.*, 1977). These workers have also isolated a galactose-specific haemagglutinin from the same strain of *P. aeruginosa*. Both haemagglutinins are proteins with estimated subunit molecular weights of 13,000–13,700 (Gilboa-Garber, 1972) and 11,000 (Gilboa-Garber *et al.*, 1977), respectively. The morphological characteristics of these molecules have not been determined, but Pearce and Buchanan (1980) have suggested that they may be fimbrial precursors.

Mannose-specific surface lectins are not restricted to Gram-negatives. For example, Bagg *et al.* (1980) have recently isolated a mannose-specific surface lectin from the immunologically active *Corynebacterium parvum*. These workers suggest that this lectin may play a role in the adjuvant and antitumour activity of this organism.

V. GLYCOCONJUGATES AS LECTIN RECEPTORS

It has been known for many years that certain pathogens display a predilection for specific tissues. This is illustrated by the colonization of lung tissue by pneumonococci, the colonization of the intestine by *V. cholerae*, and the predilection of the malaria parasite for the erythrocyte. However, it was a long time until the concept of *receptor sites* on cell surfaces, already well defined in pharmacology and hormone chemistry, became recognized in microbiology (Keusch, 1979). Specific surface receptors for microorganisms were first demonstrated in studies on the virulence of influenza virus (Poste and Nicolson, 1977; Lonberg-Holm and Philipsson, 1981). Early studies on the so-called receptor-destroying enzyme (RDE) showed that it abolished the binding of virus to the erythrocyte surface, and so prevented haemagglutination (HA). The enzyme was subsequently recognized as neuraminidase, and its activity shown to remove the terminal sialic acid residues of sialoglycoproteins on the cell surface. Three such sialoglycopeptides (PAS 1, PAS 2 and PAS 3) were identified on human red blood cell membranes, and at least one protein involved in binding influenza virus, glycophorin A, is present in transmembrane configuration. Many other studies on other haemagglutinating viruses lead to the defining of a number of the virus receptors of erythrocytes. It was subsequently proposed that similar glycoconjugates are exposed on the mucosal epithelial cell surfaces of the organ preferentially recognized and infected by each virus.

The presence of sugar sequences of glycoconjugates at the external cell surface places them in a key position to function in receptor phenomena (Keusch, 1979; Hart, 1980; Barondes, 1981). In fact, carbohydrates are especially good candidates for participation in such recognition functions as receptors. A simple glucose disaccharide can exist in 11 distinct forms, and a glucose trisaccharide can yield 176 anomeric configurations. A mixed trisaccharide obviously allows many more structural variants. Typically, oligosaccharides of mammalian cell membranes are composed of between 4 and 20 monosaccharide residues, most commonly of glucose, galactose, mannose, fucose, N-acetylglucosamine, N-acetylgalactosamine, and N-acetylneuraminic acid (Keusch, 1979). This allows for a multitude of different possible receptors.

The first substantial evidence for the key role of bacterial lectin–glycoconjugate receptor interactions in the pathogenesis of bacterial infections was provided by studies on the pathogenicity of intestinal infections in the young piglet. Gibbons *et al.* (1975) discovered that specific glycoproteins in sow colostrum and saliva inhibited the haemagglutination of sheep erythrocytes by K88 ETEC (Tables 8 and 9). These workers proposed a role for specific β-galactosyl residues of glycoproteins and glycolipids as possible natural cell receptors in the gut. Rutter *et al.* (1975) subsequently noticed that some litters of piglets were uniformly susceptible to K88 ETEC infections, while different parents produced piglets that were uniformly resistant. These observations led to the discovery that

Table 8 Haemagglutination of sheep erythrocytes by K88 antigen in the presence of colostrum, components of colostrum, and various glycoconjuates

Inhibitor	Lowest concentration (μg/ml) to inhibit MRHA at 4°C
Colostrum fractionation on Sephadex G200	
Immunoglobulin fraction	200
Neuramine lactose fraction	2,500
Deproteinized whey glycopeptide fraction (a)	1,000
Deproteinized whey glycopeptide fraction (b)	1,000
Glycoproteins	
Porcine submaxillary mucin (PSM)	50
Porcine submaxillary mucin (desialylated)	100
PSM (periodate oxidated/borohydride reduced)	375
Bovine submaxillary mucin (BSM)	375
BSM (desialylated)	100
Ovine submaxillary mucin (OSM)	75
OSM (desialylated)	200
Human A substance	375
Human A substance (periodate oxidized/ borohydride reduced)	200
Fetuin	50,000
Fetuin (desialylated)	250
Fetuin (desialylated, periodate oxidized/ borohydride reduced)	375

Table 9   Inhibition of haemagglutination reactions of CFA/I strains by glycopeptides isolated from human milk[a,c]

	MRHA$_{hum}$2		
Lectin origin[b]	1049a-13	1058a-2	54e-14
Vicia sativa	HA	HA	HAI
Tritium vulgaris	HA	HA	HA
Crotalaria junsea	HA	HAI	HAI

[a] Milk samples were fractionated on lectin–Sepharose columns (B. Lönnerdal, B. Erson, M. Lindahl, A. Faris, and T. Wadström, unpublished). MRHA$_{hum}$, Mannose-resistant haemagglutination of human erythrocytes. HA, Haemagglutination positive. HAI, Haemagglutination reaction inhibited.

[b] Carbohydrate specificity of lectins: *Vicia sativa,* α-methyl mannoside; *Tritium vulgaris,* glucosamine; *Crotalaria juncea,* lactose.

[c] From Lindahl *et al.* (1984).

specific intestinal receptors for K88 were inherited as a Mendelian dominant, and breeding experiments confirmed that it was possible to obtain litters that do not possess the receptor and are resistant to natural and experimental infection with K88+ ETEC organisms (Rutter, 1981). Glycolipid analysis of brush border preparations from susceptible and resistant piglets implicated a specific minor glycolipid as the receptor for the K88 adhesin (Kearns and Gibbons, 1979). This glycolipid is missing in resistant animals (H. Leffler, personal communication). While the demonstration that animals can be bred to have resistance to K88 ETEC infections could have revolutionized piglet production, field studies have unfortunately shown that such litters are highly susceptible to other natural infections. This is illustrated by the recent isolation of porcine ETEC with K99 and 987p surface antigens, indicating that breeding for resistance to a single bacterial adhesin is probably not a simple solution for prevention of neonatal and weaning diarrhoea in young piglets (Rutter, 1981).

There is now evidence for involvement of glycoconjugates in the receptors for K99 and CRA/I adhesins (Table 10). We have systematically investigated inhibition of haemagglutination by K99 and CFA/I ETEC strains with crude and purified ganglioside preparations. The observation that only monosialogangliosides (Type II, Sigma) gave inhibition of K99 and CFA/I ETEC, with no inhibition at concentrations much above the critical micellar concentration (cmc) prompted inhibition studies with highly purified specific gangliosides, with results summarized in Table 11. These results suggest that both K99 and CFA/I recognize terminal galactosyl residues on glycoconjugates in the erythrocyte

Table 10 Haemagglutination activity of CFA/I, K99, and CFA/II strains in the presence of glycoconjugates[e]

Strain type (number)	Poly-α-2-8-NANA[a]	Submaxillary mucin[b]	Fetuin[c]	Control[d]
CFA/I	−	+	+	+
K99	+	−	+	+
CFA/II (24)	−	−	−	+
CFA/II (32)	+	−	+	+
CFA/II (55)	−	−	+	+
CFA/II (5)	+	+	+	+

[a] Purified *Escherichia coli* K1 capsule (0.3 mg/ml), kindly supplied by Dr. K. Jann.
[b] Purified bovine submaxillary mucin (0.3 mg/ml), contains 10% NANA (Boehringer).
[c] Purified fetuin from fetal calf serum (0.3 mg/ml), contains 6.2% NANA (Sigma).
[d] PBS, ph 6.8, was used in control experiments. All experiments performed at pH 6.8.
[e] From Lindahl *et al.* (1984).

membrane. This binding may well involve both glycoprotins and glycolipids. More recent studies by others have confirmed these observations with CFA/I ETEC and show that the inhibition is reversed by lowering the incubation temperature from 37 to 4°C (Bartus *et al.*, 1980).

A glycolipid has also been implicated as a receptor for fimbriated urinary tract (uti) *E. coli*. The attachment of these organisms to human urinary-tract epithelial cells was inhibited by a glycolipid preparation from the same cell source. Subsequent studies suggest that the receptor for this MRHA adhesin of uti *E. coli* is ceramide globoside (Leffler and Svanborg-Eden, 1981). Certainly human erythrocytes devoid of the ceramide globoside pK blood group antigen did not haemagglutinate with the majority of uti *E. coli* tested (Källenius *et al.*, 1980a;

Table 11 Inhibition by glycolipids on haemagglutination with ETEC strains[a]

Strain	K88[b]	K99	CFA/I	CFA/II
Glycolipid Monosialogangliosides	−	Inhibition	Inhibition	−
Disialogangliosides	−	−	−	−
GM$_1$	−	−	−	−
GM$_2$	−	Inhibition	Inhibition	−
GM$_3$	−	−	−	−

[a] All experiments performed at pH 6.8 with a glycolipid concentration of 3.3 mg/ml (~2 mM).
[b] Minus sign indicates no inhibition.

Källenius, 1981). The adhesin of these uti *E. coli* will be termed F7 in a new nomenclature recently proposed by Ørskov *et al.* (1980b).

The glycoconjugate recognized by the bacterial surface lectin does not always have to be of host origin. Some bacteria may in fact only bind to virus-infected cells. This has been demonstrated in the case of group B streptococci. These organisms bind to kidney epithelial cells, but only after these kidney cells have been infected with influenza virus (Pan *et al.*, 1979). Indeed, the adherence of the streptococci appears to involve recognition of viral haemagglutinin, a glycoprotein that is inserted into the mammalian cell membrane before exit of mature virus. It is likely that more examples of this phenomenon will be found.

VI.   ATTACHMENT TO BODY SURFACES

A.   The oral cavity

The concept that specific adherence to surfaces might allow bacteria to avoid rapid eradication due to shear forces imposed by fluid flow was first investigated by oral microbiologists. These studies revealed that the dynamics in the colonization of the oral cavity are similar to an *in vitro* continuous culture with a high dilution rate, resulting in a rapid wash-out of nonadherent organisms (Gibbons and van Houte, 1980). Lectin-like interactions have been identified in the oral cavity. For example, there are specific interactions between the surface of *Streptococcus mutans* and other oral streptococci, and salivary glycoproteins and mucus components (Gibbons and Quareshi, 1978, 1979). This recognition and interaction of bacterial surface lectins with different glycoconjugate receptors in different parts of the oral cavity probably accounts for the differential colonization seen in this cavity. For example, *Actinomyces viscosus* produces a fuzzy layer very similar to the structure of K88 and K99 when viewed electron microscopically, and β-galactosyl residues appear to be involved in the colonization by this organism (Ellen *et al.*, 1980, 1981) (Fig. 3).

The oral microorganisms also produce surface carbohydrate polymers such as dextrans and levans, as well as surface enzymes such as glycosyl transferase. These undoubtedly participate in the colonization of the various surfaces in the oral cavity (Fig. 4). Other nonspecific interactions are also involved in this complex ecosystem. Pioneer studies on the binding of *S. mutans* and other oral streptococci to different artificial surfaces (hydroxyapatite, glass, ion exchangers, etc.) point to a role for charge interactions, while more recent studies on *S. mutans* and *S. salivarius* suggest that hydrophobic interactions also participate (Linder *et al.*, 1984).

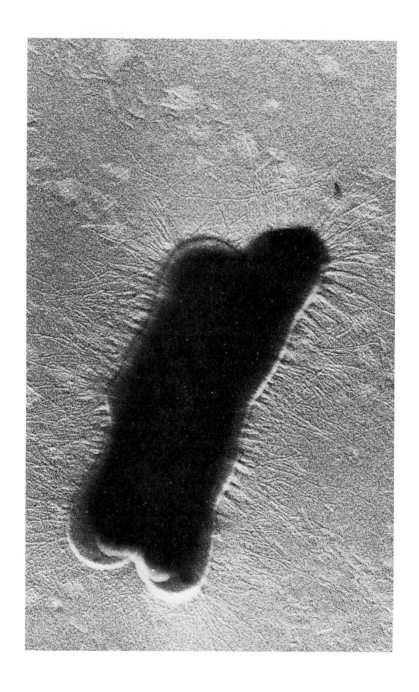

304

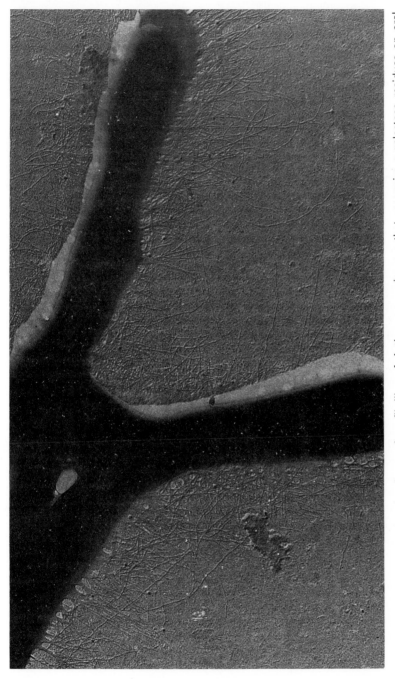

Fig. 3 Electron micrographs showing surface fibrillae of *Actinomyces viscosus* that recognize ᴅ-galactose residues on oral mucosal surfaces (Ellen *et al.*, 1980, 1981). These structures are filaments much thinner than fimbriae on Gram-negative bacteria (see Table 3).

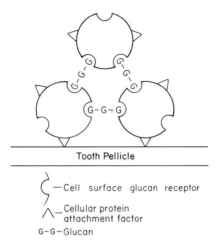

Tooth Pellicle

ζ —Cell surface glucan receptor

$\wedge$ —Cellular protein
            attachment factor

G–G–Glucan

Fig. 4 A proposed model of *Streptococcus mutans* adherence, illustrating the cell surface protein–salivary pellicle attachment phase and a glucan-mediated cell–cell accumulation phase (Staaf *et al.,* 1980).

B. Gastrointestinal tract

1. Vibrio cholerae

Adhesion of *Vibrio cholerae* to the intestinal mucosa is essential to the pathogenesis of cholera. The first recognition that haemagglutinating activity of *V. cholerae* might correlate with an ability to colonize the human gut was by Lankford and Legsomburana (1965). Indeed, *V. cholerae* was shown to agglutinate red blood cells from chicken, sheep, rabbit and humans, and this characteristic was initially exploited to differentiate the classical and El Tor biotypes (Barua and Mukherjee, 1963; Finkelstein and Mukherjee, 1963; Lankford and Legsomburana, 1965). Sugar inhibition studies further revealed that the haemagglutination produced by some strains of *V. cholerae* was inhibited by D-mannose, while other strains were inhibited by L-fucose (Barua and Mukerjee, 1963; Jones and Freter, 1976; Bhathacharjee and Srivastava, 1978). In addition, the attachment of classical *V. cholerae* 01 strains to rabbit brush border membranes was also shown to be inhibited by L-fucose (Jones and Freter, 1976). These studies also revealed for the first time that a bacterial haemagglutinin that was inhibited only at a relatively high concentration of monosaccharide was much more efficiently inhibited when the sugar was coupled to a polymer like Sepharose. This clearly suggested that oligosaccharides or other higher-molecular-weight glycoconjugate compounds could be involved in the binding site of the haemagglutinin receptor. The adhesion of non-01 *V. cholerae* to rabbit brush borders has subsequently been shown to be inhibited by L-fucose, but unlike the classic 01 strains, this mechanism is independent of calcium ion concentration (Levett and Daniel, 1981; Jones *et al.*, 1976).

Recently, Hanne and Finkelstein (1981) have demonstrated the existence of three different haemagglutinins produced by *V. cholerae*. A cell-associated mannose-sensitive haemagglutinin appears to be produced only by the El Tor biotype. This HA is responsible for the haemagglutination biotyping differentiation of El Tor from the classical biotype and has no apparent divalent ion requirement. An L-fucose-sensitive haemagglutinin was detected transiently in early log-phase growth with two of four classical strains and with several MSHA⁻ mutants of El Tor strains. In addition, a "soluble" HA was detected in late log-phase cultures of all strains tested. This HA was not inhibitable by any of the sugars tested, required Ca^{2+} for maximum activity, and had a restricted spectrum of erythrocytes on which it was active. Importantly, pretreatment of the infant rabbit with purified "cholera lectin" prevented intestinal colonization in this model (Finkelstein *et al.*, 1978), giving one of the first indications that receptor blockade may be an efficient way to prevent mucosal colonization with certain microbial pathogens (Keusch, 1979).

It would appear then that multiple adhesive mechanisms occur in *V. cholerae* (Jones, 1980). However, the nature of these various adhesins is still rather unclear. Some *Vibrio* species do bear fimbriae that mediate mannose-sensitive haemagglutination (Tweedy *et al.*, 1968); however, Nelson *et al.* (1976) could not demonstrate such fimbriae in *V. cholerae* 01. The best-characterized HA is clearly the soluble haemagglutinin, "cholera lectin." This has recently been purified to apparent homogeneity, and there appear to be three distinct pH isotypes, which, in the native state, exist as noncovalently associated polymers of 32,000-MW subunits. Electron microscopy revealed long filamentous polymers. The soluble HA does appear to be a bifunctional molecule, since it also displays significant protease activity. Importantly, Fab fragments against the purified HA inhibited attachment of heterologous serotype/biotype *V. cholerae* to infant rabbit small bowel (Finkelstein and Hanne, 1981).

2. Lectin variety of Aeromonas hydrophila

Aeromonas hydrophila was recently convincingly shown to be a human intestinal pathogen inducing diarrhoea by a cytotonic enterotoxin (Wadström *et al.*, 1976; Ljungh *et al.*, 1982). The organism has also been implicated in a wide variety of clinical conditions (Trust and Chipman, 1979). *A. hydrophila* serves as a valuable model for studies on bacterial lectins, since the haemagglutination produced by different strains is inhibited by either D-mannose, L-fucose or D-galactose (Atkinson and Trust, 1980) (Table 12). This inhibition is highly specific and requires only millimolar amounts of the various sugars. The haemagglutinins exhibit acute specificity, recognizing quite subtle structural differences in the positioning of single hydroxyl groups on the sugars. Strains are also available

Table 12 Sugar inhibition of haemagglutination by *Aeromonas hydrophila*

Strain	Sugar inhibiting haemagglutination
A6[a]	D-Mannose or L-fucose
A10[b]	D-Mannose or L-fucose
A46	D-Galactose plus D-mannose
A69	D-Mannose
Ah412	D-Galactose
Ah434	L-Fucose

[a] Strain is fimbriated and agglutinates yeast.
[b] Strain lacks fimbriae and fails to agglutinate yeast.

that are inhibited by both D-mannose and L-fucose. This ability to recognize either sugar is clearly dependent on the similar spatial arrangements of hydroxyl groups when the sugars are in different linkages on the receptor molecule. Recent evidence suggests that, in these strains, the fucose–mannose lectin is not fimbriae-borne, but some other form of surface protein is implicated. Another strain of *A. hydrophila* carries two lectins, and both D-galactose and D-mannose are required to inhibit haemagglutination. The two lectin activities on this strain appear to be involved in attachment of this strain to buccal epithelial cells, and they have quite different pH optima (Trust and Atkinson, unpublished observations).

3. Amoeba lectins

Another lectin interaction probably important in gastrointestinal disease has recently been recognized. This involves the association of amoebae with human cells. These interactions of amoebae may well become more important to microbiologists working on diarrhoeal diseases. Although the microbes involved are not bacteria, in at least one case they appear to recognize a similar receptor to *Shigella* toxin and deserve comment (Kobiler and Mirelman, 1980; Kobiler *et al.*, 1981).

The development of *in vitro* cultivation methods for mammalian parasites now makes it possible to obtain isolated organisms for cell–cell interaction studies. Studies on isolated *E. histolytica* trophozoites demonstrated that isolated organisms and sonicated membrane fragments produced haemagglutination of different red blood cells. The HA profile was similar to that obtained with wheat germ agglutinin (WGA). Subsequent studies demonstrated that this membrane-associated agglutinin was released upon repeated freezing and thawing. Inhibition studies with various carbohydrates and released agglutinin showed that hydroly-sates of purified chitin caused drastic inhibition of the haemagglutination. The trimer and tetramer of *N*-acetylglucosamine gave optimal inhibition on the molar basis. In addition, a variety of *N*-acetylglucosamine-containing compounds, such as bacterial peptidoglycan, rabbit colonic mucus, bovine and human sera, and an IgA fraction isolated from human colostrum, were also found to inhibit the haemagglutination. Attempts were made to purify the agglutinin by affinity chromatography on Sepharose *N*-acetylglucosamine. This technique had pre-viously been successfully used for purification of plant lectins such as wheat germ agglutinin (WGA). Gel electrophoresis of the separated amoeba lectins showed that the preparation was heterogeneous (Kobiler *et al.*, 1981). The recent demonstration that *E. histolytica* also produces a mitogenic protein with lectin-like properties inhibitable by fetuin and *N*-acetylglucosamine (Diamantstein *et al.*, 1980), and the production of a cytotonic enterotoxin with an unknown cell membrane receptor (Ravdin *et al.*, 1980) further point to the importance of complex lectin-like interaction in the pathogenesis of amoeba infections.

C. The respiratory tract

1. Bordetella pertussis

An organism whose haemagglutinating activity has been correlated with vir-ulence is the respiratory pathogen *Bordetella pertussis*. As yet there is little evidence that the haemagglutinins are acting as lectins; however, the question has not been adequately addressed. Keogh and co-workers (1947) were first to report that *B. pertussis* agglutinated erythrocytes and that this ability was associ-ated with mouse virulence. These workers also reported that haemagglutinin (HA) vaccines protected mice against intranasal challenge. Later field trials showed that such an HA vaccine afforded humans significant protection (Rankin and Fischer, 1956). Despite these early observations on the pathogenic signifi-cance of the *B. pertussis* haemagglutinin, it was not until the early 1970s that the structures that allow *B. pertussis* cells to attach onto erythrocytes began to be defined and separated.

Electron microscopic (EM) studies on *B. pertussis* showed that the organism produces hairlike structures of 2–2.5 nm in diameter and 60–100 nm in length. These are found attached to the cells in high numbers in early stages of growth both in liquid and on solid media. These fimbriae seem to detach from cells after 24 hours of growth and are found in increasingly higher concentration in the culture medium (Morse, 1976). Subsequent studies by Morse and co-workers and by Arai and Sato (1976) revealed production of two haemagglutinins. These are known as leucocytosis-promoting-factor haemagglutinin (LPFHA) and fila-

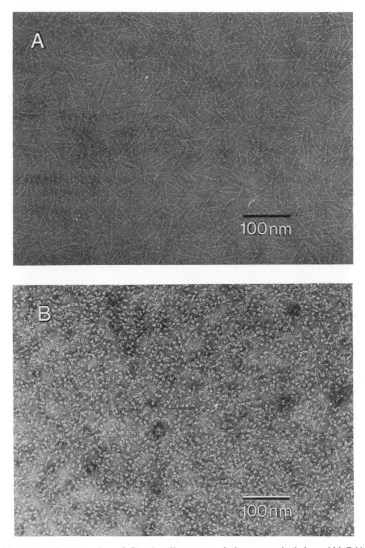

Fig. 5 Electron micrographs of *Bordetella pertussis* haemagglutinins: (A) F-HA; (B)
LPF-HA. Uranyl acetate (1%) was used for negative staining.

mentous haemagglutinin (FHA) (Fig. 5). LPFHA is presumed to be an outer-
membrane protein that exhibits low haemagglutinating activity. LPFHA displays
a single band on electrophoresis at a molecular weight of 108,000. Electron
micrographs showed spherical molecules about 6 nm in diameter (Arai and Sato,
1976; Morse, 1976). FHA exhibits high haemagglutinating activity and is anti-

genically distinct from LPFHA. Predictably, electron micrographs of FHA revealed filamentous structures about 2 × 40 nm in size, presumably derived from the fimbriae.

Mouse protective activity was examined with these two distinct HAs. Sato *et al.* (1978), and Irons and MacLennon (1978) reported that active immunization with FHA protected mice from intracerebral challenge with *B. pertussis.* Formalin-treated LPFHA was a poor protective antigen in mice (Sato *et al.*, 1978), and active LPFHA was also nonprotective (Irons and MacLennon, 1978). In contrast, Munoz and Bergman (1977) found that preparation of LPFHA protected mice from intracerebral *B. pertussis* infection. Sato *et al.* (1981) have recently reexamined this question of mouse protection using HA vaccines. Using an aerosol-induced respiratory infection of mice as a laboratory model for pertussis, they have shown that passive immunization with antibody to either FHA or to LPFHA protects mice from disease. Moreover, anti-FHA but not anti-LPFHA prevented the attachment of *B. pertussis* to mammalian cells (HeLa and Vero) in culture. This latter finding is good evidence that antibodies that are directed against an adhesion can confer protective immunity.

2. Mycoplasma

Mycoplasma are extracellular parasites when they grow *in vivo.* In order to derive nutrients essential for growth, they attach to the surface of animal cells. They are excellent model organisms for studies on bacterial lectins because they must adhere to cells and because they recognize carbohydrate moieties in this attachment process. The close association of mycoplasma organisms with eukaryotic host cells has been well described using electron microscopy, and specialized electron-dense structures at the tips of many mycoplasma cells appear to function as attachment organelles (Bredt *et al.,* 1980; Collier, 1980). This gives rise to polar or "end-on" attachment. Recent scanning electron microscopy evidence suggests that the polar attachment to ciliated respiratory epithelium is a result of the organism's gliding mobility. Thus, the tip is perhaps the part of the organism that leads along the cilia to reach and adhere to the epithelial cell surface. Furthermore, the densely packed cilia may permit the thin and flexible filamentous mycoplasma organisms to progress while preventing spherical organisms from reaching the epithelial cell surface. The mycoplasma's perpendicular orientation in tracheal organ cultures is probably supported by the cilia.

Scanning electron microscopy studies have also shown that some forms of *Mycoplasma pneumoniae* can also adhere to erythrocytes via membrane sites other than the tip structure. These adherent cells are rounded, pear-shaped, or irregular organisms that lack tip structure (Brunner *et al.,* 1979; Razin *et al.,* 1981).

There is strong evidence that sialic acid residues of cell membrane glycoconjugates act as specific receptor sites for *M. pneumoniae* and *M. gallisepticum*

(Banai *et al.*, 1980). Indeed, the predominant sialoglycoprotein of human erythrocytes, glycophorin, has been shown to be a major receptor for *M. gallinarum* and for *M. pneumoniae*. In the case of *M. pneumoniae*, there also appear to be additional receptors on human erythrocytes. These as yet unidentified receptors are destroyed by trypsin. In the case of *M. gallisepticum*, it was demonstrated that neuraminidase-treated glycophorin did not bind. The best inhibitors had a mucin-like structure, with high molecular weights and high sialic acid contents. *N*-Acetylneuraminic acid appeared to be the favoured sialic acid structure for binding, but there was no strict specificity for its anomeric linkage.

This lectin-mediated attachment may have important autoimmune consequences for the host. Certainly *Mycoplasma* infections are often accompanied by autoimmune sequelae (Stanbridge, 1976). Stanbridge and Weiss (1978) have shown that when cells of *M. hyorhinis* infect murine lymphocytes they behave as multivalent ligands and cap on the lymphoid cell surface. Mycoplasma caps are shed from the surface of cells as an aggregate containing host cell-membrane vesicles. If the capped mycoplasmas actually carry the host membrane receptor sites with them and present them to the host in a conformationally altered state, Stanbridge and Weiss (1978) suggest that the host might mount an immune response against these now altered host antigens. Mycoplasmas have in fact been shown to acquire membrane antigens (e.g., Thy 1.1) from infected lymphoid cells (Wise *et al.*, 1978). It is not yet known whether these interactions of mycoplasmas with cell membranes involve membrane fusion.

Studies have been initiated to determine the nature of the mycoplasma lectin. Mild detergent extraction methods have been used to solubilize *M. pneumoniae* cell membranes, and attempts have been made to isolate the receptor structures by glycophorin–Sepharose chromatography (Banai *et al.*, 1980). Elution was 0.2% sodium dodecylsulfate (SDS) yielded two polypeptides (MW 25,000 and 45,000) showing a high affinity to glycophorin–Sepharose beads, although not to Sepharose beads. The binding of this fraction to red blood cells was relatively low but appeared to be specific, as it was inhibited by glycophorin but not by its hydrophobic moiety. This latter control is pertinent, since both sialic acid residues and the hydrophobic moiety of glycophorin are exposed on the Sepharose beads, whereas in red blood cell membranes the hydrophobic portion of glycophorin is immersed in the lipid bilayer.

3. Chlamydia

Another good model for defining the role of lectins in bacterial attachment is the genus *Chlamydia*. These organisms can only multiply within host cells, and to do this they must first attach to these cells. Studies by Levy (1979) have suggested that the attachment of *C. psittaci* and *C. trachomatis* to host cells of diverse origin appears to involve lectin recognition of an *N*-acetyl-D-glucosamine-containing entity that also binds wheat germ agglutinin with high affinity. Studies on surface properties of *C. psittaci* by isoelectric focussing, hydrophobic interaction chromatography, and two-phase systems also indicate that hydrophobic interactions may be important in adhesion to eukaryotic cells (Vance and Hatch, 1980).

D. The urogenital tract

1. Neisseria gonorrhoeae

The attachment of this organism to a variety of cell types has received much attention. However, although we know quite a bit at the molecular level about the attachment mechanisms of this pathogen and some studies suggest that carbohydrates can be involved in the recognition mechanism, it is still too early to conclusively implicate lectin activity in the adhesion of certain strains of gonococcus.

On primary isolation from infected patients, gonococci are invariably fimbriated (Jephcott *et al.*, 1971; Swanson *et al.*, 1971). Some strains of fimbriated gonococci show haemagglutinating activity with erythrocytes of several species (rabbit, guinea pig, sheep, chicken, and human groups O Rh+) and bind to human buccal cells (Punsalanang and Sawyer, 1973). Nonfimbriated strains do not haemagglutinate or bind to buccal cells. These authors reported that antiserum to partially purified fimbriae inhibited both haemagglutination and epithelial cell adherence. Furthermore, the adherence of fimbriated gonococci to erythrocytes and to buccal cells was not inhibited by any of the 12 different monosaccharides tested. Similarly, Watt (1980a,b) reports that the constituent sugars of host-cell glycolipids and glycoproteins, including D-galactose, α-methyl-D-galactoside, α-methyl-D-galactoside, lactose, melibiose, mannose, α-methyl-D-mannoside, L-fucose, *N*-acetyl-D-galactosamine and *N*-acetyl-D-glucosamine at concentrations up to 0.2 *M* did not inhibit binding of either fimbriated or nonfimbriated gonococci to human epithelial cells. Watt (1980a) also reports that when surface carbohydrates of buccal cells were blocked with lectins, the attachment of radiolabelled purified fimbriae was not affected. Taken together, these experimental results imply that gonococcal fimbriae do not function as classical plant lectins binding to single sugars on the host membrane.

There is other evidence, however, suggesting that gonococcal fimbriae do indeed bind to carbohydrate residues on host cell surfaces. Buchanan *et al.* (1978) showed that fimbriae treated with GM_1, GD_{1a}, GD_{1b} or GT gangliosides at a concentration of 10 to 20 μM showed reduced binding at only 70–80% of the control value. Significant binding (40%) remained even at 74 μM concentrations. That is, the effect of the gangliosides on the fimbriae adhesion might be nonspecific, resulting from a hydrophobic detergentlike action of ganglioside micelles. This is further supported by the finding that gangliosides incorporated into ^{3}H-labelled cholesterol/lecithin liposomes do not bind to piliated gonococci (Trust *et al.,* 1980).

Enzymatic and chemical modification of host-cell surfaces provides better evidence for carbohydrate involvement in the receptors on some cells. Buchanan *et al.* (1978) demonstrated that treatment of buccal cells with exoglycosidases reduced the binding of radiolabelled purified fimbriae. Treatment of buccal cells with an exoglycosidase mixture and neuraminidase also decreased the ability of fimbriated gonococci to adhere (Trust *et al.,* 1980). Lamden *et al.* (1980) demonstrated the existence of isogenic variants that produce one of two distinct fimbriae types. The first two fimbriae types were designated α and β. The binding of these two types to host cells differ. Removal of sialic acid residues from buccal cell surface carbohydrates by treatment with neuraminidase markedly affected the binding of α-fimbriae but had minimal effect on β-fimbrial adhesion. Subsequently, treatment of neuraminidase-modified buccal cells with mixed exoglycosidases further drastically reduced the binding of α-fimbriae but not the binding of β-fimbriae. These findings suggest that α-fimbriae bind specifically to a receptor on buccal cells and that this receptor contains both sialic acid and other sugars. The binding of β-fimbriae to buccal and blood cells and of α-fimbriae to blood cells appears not to involve carbohydrates and may result from hydrophobic interactions.

The outer membrane of *N. gonorrhoeae* also contains a protein, Protein II, which appears to mediate attachment. Protein II comprises a family of proteins with molecular weights ranging from 27,500 to 29,000 (Lambden *et al.,* 1979). The presence in the outer membrane of any one of the Protein II family increases attachment to buccal cells, Protein II* giving the best increase in specific attachment. As was the case with purified fimbriae, a variety of simple sugars do not inhibit the attachment mediated by Protein II (Watt, 1980a), but further studies are required to show whether a more complex carbohydrate may be involved in membrane receptor recognition.

2. Urinary-tract pathogens

The recent characterization of a specific glycoconjugate receptor (the p[k] antigen) for the fimbriae antigen (F7) of a strain of *E. coli* isolated from a urinary-tract infection will certainly encourage further studies in this area. The F7 strains were recently shown to dominate in a Swedish survey (G. Källenius, personal communication), but the relative importance of other fimbriated *E. coli* (F8 through F12), as well as related Gram-negative species, has yet to be defined (F. Ørskov and I. Ørskov, personal communication; D. Old, personal communication). In the case of Gram-positive organisms, the common human urinary-tract pathogen *Staphylococcus saprophyticus* has been shown to haemagglutinate (Gunnarsson *et al.,* 1983), and the possibility that the haemagglutinins of this organism possess lectin properties needs to be explored.

VII.   OTHER INTERACTIONS AFFECTING ADHERENCE

All mucosal surfaces are covered to a greater or lesser extent by a layer of mucus. Studies in the gastrointestinal tract indicate that this mucus layer is in a constant state of turnover. The layer has been regarded as having a protective role by serving to prevent adhesion. In fact, bladder mucin has been termed anti-adherence factor (Parsons and Mulholland, 1978). However, there is little quantitative experimental evidence to support such a role for the mucus glycoconjugates. Indeed, Ørskov *et al.* (1980b) have recently suggested that urinary mucus, and perhaps mucus material elsewhere, may function as a trap for Enterobacteriaceae due to the interaction of type 1 fimbriae with glycoconjugates of the mucus, such as Tamm Horsfall protein (Ørskov *et al.,* 1980a; Chick *et al.,* 1981).

In certain cases the bacterial degradation of mucus constituents may be required to allow access to underlying receptors. Early work on germ-free and conventional animals suggested that enteric bacteria utilize mucus glycoproteins and that such compounds may be of considerable nutritional value to microorganisms growing on mucosal surfaces (Hoskins, 1978; Hoskins and Boulding, 1981). Certainly the intestinal anaerobes are rich sources of glycosidases and proteases and may very well be active degraders of surface mucins, thus influencing the degree of exposure of underlying receptors. Degradation of blood-group substances by intestinal bacteria and the relation between certain blood groups and HLA antigens to gut colonization with, for instance, *Klebsiella* strains in ankylosing spondylitis indicate that more work has to be done in this area. Other observations—that glycosidases in human fecal extracts degrade the O antigen of *E. coli* 086 (a structure closely resembling the human blood group B substance), and that mucin oligosaccharides are excreted in urine of germ-free but not in conventional animals—also need to be followed up (Hoskins, 1978; Hoskins and Boulding, 1981).

Bacterial enzymes that degrade components of the eukaryotic cell surface may also influence receptor exposure and availability. Cholera vibrios produce neuraminidase, which leads to the speculation that this enzyme may unmask natural cell receptors for cholera toxin, but no experimental work with intestinal tissue has been performed to support this hypothesis (Jones, 1977, 1980; Freter, 1980a,b). However, treating tissue-culture cells and erythrocytes with neuraminidase has in several cases shown enhancement of cholera toxin activity, as well as binding of bacteria with surface lectins such as mycoplasmas and *N. gonorrhoeae.*

The immune response to organisms is obviously important in determining the range of microorganisms that can colonize and infect. Secretory IgA appears to prevent adherence of some bacterial species to epithelial cells, at least under *in vitro* experimental conditions (Reed and Williams, 1978). In turn, the bacteria may counter this IgA by producing IgA1 protease. This is produced by *Haemophilus influenzae* (Kilian *et al.*, 1979), *N. meningitidis* and *N. gonorrhoeae* (Plaut, 1978). Many other successful adherers appear to be negative for IgA-protease production, at least under the culture conditions used. These include enteric pathogens such as *V. cholerae,* some shigellae, and salmonellae.

Other host factors may play a role in the success or otherwise of the attachment. One example comes from the work of Selinger *et al.* (1978). These workers found that the pharyngeal cells of rheumatic heart disease patients had an increased avidity for adherence for a rheumatic-fever-associated strain of streptococcus. Other studies have suggested that *E. coli* adhere more readily to the vaginal cells of women with a history of recurrent urinary infections than to similar cells from controls with no history of bacteriuria (Fowler and Stamey, 1977; Källenius and Winberg, 1978). In this regard, Schaeffer *et al.* (1979) have also shown that the ability of epithelial cells from a single individual to bind *E. coli* varies in a cyclical and repetitive pattern. Adherence tends to be higher during the early phase of the menstrual cycle and diminishes shortly after the time of expected ovulation.

Tissue damage may also be important. Certainly *P. aeruginosa* exhibits greater adherence to damaged heart valves than to normal heart valves (Ramirez-Ronda, 1978). Indeed, Ramphal *et al.* (1980) have shown that this species adheres to desquamated or desquamating cells of the respiratory tract after influenza virus infections or endotracheal invasion, but does not adhere to normal trachea, the undamaged basal cell layer, or to the regenerating layer of cells. After endotracheal intubation, *P. aeruginosa* also adhered to the basement membrane when this was exposed. Ramphal *et al.* (1980) have also suggested that this species adheres better to a damaged cornea and use the term "opportunistic adherence" to describe the phenomenon.

VIII. MULTIPLICITY OF FIMBRIATION

Many bacterial fimbriae have been purified to homogeneity and extensively characterized (Pearce and Buchanan, 1980). While some species and strains probably produce only a single fimbriated type, there is increasing evidence that a single bacterial strain can produce a variety of fimbriae types. This is well illustrated by *N. gonorrhoeae* strain P9. This organism can exist in at least one of four fimbriated states (Lambden *et al.*, 1980, 1981). Isogenic variants of P9 have been shown to produce fimbriae with subunit molecular weights of 19,500, 20,500, 21,000, and 18,500. These fimbriae are designated α, β, δ, and γ, respectively. The δ- and γ-fimbriae were isolated from α- and β-fimbriated gonococci surviving after 7 days in guinea pig subcutaneous chambers. Despite the differences in molecular weight, γ- and δ-fimbriae show antigenic cross-reactivity with α- and β-fimbriae. Studies utilizing peptide mapping have shown that α- and β-subunits have regions of considerable structural homology and differ only in a small region of the molecule (Lambden *et al.*, 1981). It is likely that γ- and δ-fimbriae represent further modifications to a basic common structural component.

A similar multifimbriated state has been reported by Ørskov *et al.* (1980a,b) with *E. coli* C1212. Using crossed immunoelectrophoresis and immunoelectron microscopy of the same strain, these authors found that the bacteria exhibited three types of fimbriae. Jann *et al.* (1981) have recently reported on an SDS–PAGE and serological analysis of pili from *E. coli* of different pathogenic patterns, and there was always more than one SDS–PAGE band, again suggesting that *E. coli* strains were mixtures of bacteria having different fimbriae.

These findings indicate that considerable care must be taken when attempting to assess experimental findings, and many earlier studies need to be reevaluated. Much more work needs to be done to determine how widespread the phenomenon is, and workers certainly need to devote more attention to clonal selection.

IX. ROLE OF LECTIN SURFACE HYDROPHOBICITY

Studies with a number of plant lectins have shown that they can exhibit hydrophobic surface characteristics. If we take the case of concanavalin A (con A), this lectin binds specifically to sugars with the mannosyl configuration (Cuatrecasas, 1973; Zanetta and Gombos, 1976). When immobilized on agarose, this lectin was found to be a useful adsorbent for the purification of glycoproteins (Zanetta and Gombos, 1976). However, early work on con A also showed that this lectin could adsorb nonspecifically to cell surfaces, glycoproteins and hydrophobic substances. Moreover, only part of adsorbed glycoproteins were elutable with sugar. It was also found that ethylene glycol in combination with mannosides increased the recovery from con A–agarose (Davey *et al.*, 1976). Other authors similarly reported that detergents greatly affected the total adsorptive capacity of immobilized con A, without changing its ability to recognize preferentially mannosyl and/or glycosyl residues of glycoconjugates (Zanetta and Gombos, 1976; Lotan *et al.*, 1977). More recently, con A has been shown to adsorb to alkylagaroses by hydrophobic interactions (Ochoa *et al.*, 1979). This adsorption increases with temperature, salt concentration, and hydrophobicity of the adsorbent, according to the rules for hydrophobic interactions between proteins and hydrophobic ligands (Hjertén, 1981).

Similarly, studies on other plant lectins such as wheat germ agglutinin (WGA) and lectins from *Phaseolus vulgaris* have shown that hydrophobic interactions are important in binding of lectins to adsorbents (Ochoa and Kristiansen, 1978). The polymeric state of the lectin (e.g., tetramer or dimer of con A) also appears to influence the binding of the lectin to hydrophobic adsorbents and to liposomes (Ochoa *et al.*, 1979; Ochoa, 1980).

In the case of Gram-negative bacteria, hydrophobic surface properties were until recently solely attributed to the rough surface character caused by deficient synthesis of complete lipopolysaccharide (LPS) (van Oss, 1978). Studies on separation of virulent (smooth) bacteria and low-virulence rough bacteria in two-phase partition systems or by hydrophobic interaction chromatography (HIC) confirmed the pronounced hydrophobic surface properties of rough *Salmonella* and *E. coli* strains (Magnusson and Johanssson, 1977; Edebo, *et al.* 1980) (Table 13).

However, early work by Brinton (1965) had suggested the importance of hydrophobic interactions in the association of fimbriated bacteria with surfaces. Fimbriated bacteria displayed a lower electrophoretic mobility and a tendency to bind nonspecifically to plastic surfaces such as latex and polystyrene. In fact, these nonspecific interactions disguised for some time the possibility that biospecific interactions might be involved in binding to cell surfaces (Duguid and Old, 1980).

This ability of fimbriated bacteria to adhere to plastic surfaces and to autoaggregate prompted us to systematically investigate the hydrophobic interactions of enterotoxigenic *E. coli* (ETEC) with various surface adhesins (CFA/I, CFA/II, K88, K99) (see Fig. 2). We first found that K88$^+$ strains bound to hydrophobic gels such as octyl and phenyl Sepharose, while K88$^+$ variants failed to bind (Smyth *et al.*, 1978). Subsequent studies with F$^+$ wild type strains and F$^-$ variants of all four adhesin types have convincingly shown that each gives the

Table 13 Methods to measure surface hydrophobicity of cells

Method	Applications by
Phase partition chromatography	Magnusson and Johansson, 1977
Hydrophobic interaction chromatography (HIC)	Wadström *et al.,* 1978
Wide-angle diffraction	van Oss, 1978
Binding to hydrocarbons	Rosenberg *et al.,* 1980
Hydrophobic probes ([^{14}C]dodecanoic acid)	Kjellberg *et al.,* 1980
"The salt aggregation test"	Lindahl *et al.,* 1981

ETEC cell surface a pronounced hydrophobic character (Wadström *et al.*, 1978; Faris *et al.*, 1981; Lindahl *et al.*, 1981). Growth at 18°C suppresses the F^- character of all four types, as shown by haemagglutination and electron microscopy (EM), and also alters the hydrophobic surface to one with a hydrophilic character. More recent studies have shown that fimbriated *E. coli* strains isolated from urinary tract infections and septicemia show hydrophobic interaction with octyl and phenyl Sepharose (Faris *et al.*, 1981). The standard HIC method and the more recently developed autoaggregation test (Lindahl *et al.*, 1981) for quantitative estimation of bacterial hydrophobicity have revealed the following decreasing order of relative surface hydrophobicity: CFA/I > CFA/II ≫ K88 > K99 > type 1. The development of this simple test for quantitative estimations of surface hydrophobicity will allow workers to rapidly screen large numbers of bacterial strains for fimbriae or other hydrophobic surface proteins such as the M-protein in *Streptococcus pyogenes* (Tylewska *et al.*, 1979; Tylewska and Wadström, 1981), and will facilitate studies on the effect of growth conditions on the expression of these hydrophobic surface characters. A study of K99-ETEC organisms has already shown the practical benefit of HIC for such purposes, HIC being almost as sensitive as enzyme-linked immunosorbent assay (ELISA) for the detection of this fibrillar surface antigen (de Graaf *et al.*, 1980a,b).

The hydrophobicity of these various adhesive appendages is due to their nonpolar amino acid content (40–60%) (Tables 14 and 15). These hydrophobic amino acids have a role in the polymerization of the proteins into long hairlike structures, and many are probably exposed on the surface of the appendage, perhaps as hydrophobic surface patches (Tanford, 1980). This is further sug-

Table 14 Hydrophobic content of bacterial fimbriae amino acid compositions[a]

Fimbriae type	% Nonpolar residues (Pro, Gly, Ala, Val, Met, Ile, Leu, Phe, Trp)
Escherichia coli ($B_{am}P^+$, type 1)	54.0
Escherichia coli (K12, type 1)	56.3
Escherichia coli (1474, K99)	54.7
Escherichia coli (D520, K88)	47.8
Neisseria gonorrhoeae (33)	45.8
Neisseria gonorrhoeae (P9 and 201)	43.8–45.8
Pseudomonas aeruginosa (K/2PfS)	53.7
Moraxella nonliquefaciens (NCTC 7784 SC-c)	50.2
Corynebacterium renale (46)	44.7

[a] Modified and abbreviated after Pearce and Buchanan (1980).

Table 15 Chemical and physical properties of fimbriae[a]

Fimbriae source	Subunit molecular weight	Isoelectric point	% Carbohydrate
Escherichia coli (type 1)	16,600–17,500	4.5–5.1 (3 bands)	None
Escherichia coli (K99)	2 Subunits Major: 22,500 Minor: 29,500	10.1	0.6
Escherichia coli (K88)	25,000	—	1.0
Neisseria gonorrhoeae	19,000 ± 2,500 (varies slightly for different strains)	5.3 (minor band at 4.9)	1.3–2.0 (1–2 Hexoses subunit)
Pseudomonas aeruginosa K (PAK)	17,800 ± 300	3.9	None
Moraxella nonliquefaciens	17,000	—	—
Corynebacterium renale (strain type II)	19,000–19,400	4.35	None

[a] Modified and abbreviated after Pearce and Buchanan (1980).

gested by the HIC studies (Wadström *et al.*, 1978; Faris *et al.*, 1981) and would account for the tendency of closely adjacent fimbriae to clump or aggregate together to form bundles.

It is not clear how these hydrophobic bacterial surface lectins interact with the hydrophilic surface carbohydrates on cell membranes. It is tempting to speculate that the first interaction involves the recognition by the lectin of the appropriate sugar residues of the surface glycoconjugate. The next step in the binding process might be the multiple recognition and attachment of many surface lectins to adjacent cell receptors. In the case of fimbrial lectins, this second step could be followed by penetration of the tip of the appendage to give hydrophobic interactions with phospholipids in the cell membrane. Such a penetration and "double receptor" hypothesis has recently been proposed for cholera toxin and for the binding of interferon and hormones (TSH) to glycoproteins and glycolipids in cell membranes (Kohn *et al.*, 1978, 1981). The biospecificity of the binding would clearly reside in the first step. Analogy with the preferential binding of plant lectins to different epithelial cell populations on the surface of the gut mucosa (Etzler, 1979) suggests that this carbohydrate recognition step could determine the type of cell the bacterium recognizes and attaches to.

X. BACTERIAL LECTINS FOR IMMUNOPROPHYLAXIS

Although the studies by H. W. Smith (1977) had demonstrated the importance of K88 and K99 antigens in the colonization of the small intestine of piglets, calves and lambs with ETEC, it was not until nearly a decade later that this finding provoked the first successful experimental immunizations with K88 and K99 antigens (Nagy *et al.*, 1978). These pioneer studies and others in American, Canadian, British and Dutch experimental stations clearly demonstrated the high protective efficacy of vaccinations with adhesins by the subcutaneous route (Brinton *et al.*, 1978; Nagy *et al.*, 1978). In these cases the adult female animal is immunized and transfers protective antibody to the suckling neonates via colostrum. Commercial products have now been developed at VIDO (Veterinary Infectious Disease Organization, University of Saskatchewan, Saskatoon, Saskatchewan, Canada) and at Wellcome Research Laboratories (Beckenham, Kent, England).

One problem that arises during use of these adhesin vaccines has recently been revealed. Epidemiological studies on porcine and calf diarrhoea show that while immunizations of cows and sows with K88 and K99 vaccines clearly lead to protection of newborn against scours caused by K88 and K99 organisms, they may select for infections by organisms with "new" adhesins such as 987p in the young piglets (H. Moon and S. Acres, personal communications).

Attempts to develop a type 1 *E. coli* fimbriae vaccine to protect against urinary tract and intestinal ETEC infections (Brinton *et al.*, 1978) have not been very successful. Human volunteers show a very poor local antibody response to subcutaneous immunizations (Levine, 1981), and it may be that the exposure in early life to type 1 fimbriated *E. coli* induces a state of tolerance to this antigen. However, the recent finding that the type 1 fimbriae in *Salmonella* are not antigenically related to type 1 fimbriae of reference strains of *E. coli* (Korhonen *et al.*, 1980) suggests that it is too early to speculate on this topic.

Although preliminary studies on fimbrial vaccines to protect against gonorrhea gave promising results (Brinton *et al.*, 1978), subsequent studies have not been as hopeful. Not only does the gonococcus produce at least four types of fimbriae, but Buchanan and Hildebrandt (1981) have reported that gonococcal fimbriae are significantly less protective than an outer-membrane complex consisting primarily of LPS and the principle OMP (Protein 1).

XI. PROSPECTS

It is now apparent that there is a very large number of different bacterial surface lectins. Quite a bit of descriptive information has been accumulated on a small number of these. The best studied are those carried by fimbriae, and in many cases there is information available on the amino acid composition of these fimbriae and the amino acid sequence of the pilin subunits. But even with this basic structural information, in no case has the actual lectin portion of the molecule been identified. This gap in our knowledge concerning the bacterial surface lectin (adhesin) needs to be filled. Studies are urgently needed to elucidate the composition, structure and arrangement of those portions of the adhesive molecule that participate in the lectin interaction. We need to know how many lectin sites are present per molecule and per bacterial cell.

Attention also needs to be focused on the lectin multiplicity of a single strain. Greater care needs to be taken in the future in evaluating the lectin status of a given strain, and appropriate measures should be taken to ensure that the mechanism being examined is indeed due to a single lectin. It is also clear that more attention needs to be directed at nonfilamentous lectins, such as the adhesive outer-membrane proteins of Gram-negative cells.

A wider range of techniques will probably be used for the purification of lectin-bearing molecules. So far, conventional protein purification techniques have been employed. However, the hydrophobic properties of the bacterial lectins suggest that methods such as hydrophobic interaction chromatography and phase-partition systems might be powerful for simple large-scale purification (Ochoa et al., 1979; Ochoa, 1980; Faris et al., 1981). Also, once the sugar specificities have been defined for a bacterial surface lectin, bioaffinity chromatography might similarly facilitate large-scale purification. In a number of cases, sugars bound to agarose or acrylamide beads are already commercially available. In other cases it should not be too difficult to couple more complex oligosaccharides or glycoproteins to appropriate carriers. These carbohydrate-coupled gels may also be quite useful for screening bacterial strains for surface lectins.

In view of the wide applications of commercially available plant lectins, the prospects for similar wide-ranging applications for bacterial surface lectins are bright. One key application must be in the identification and purification of glycoconjugate receptors involved in bacterial colonization processes. As already discussed, very little is known about the identity of most of the lectin receptors. However, the great diversity of bacterial lectins suggests that a great diversity of receptors will also be found. The availability of purified lectins should lead to their use in bioaffinity chromatography for isolation and purification of these various receptors. Once we have a variety of purified lectins and purified receptors, we will be in an ideal position to fully detail the adhesive event at a truly molecular level.

The question of disease prophylaxis and therapy will obviously command a great deal of attention. Immunization with critical virulence lectins has met with limited success. These vaccines have generally been monovalent, and greater success might be expected in future when multivalent vaccines can be developed. Considerable care will need to be paid to the design of such multivalent vaccines, in order to overcome the problems posed by the complexity of antigenic types of fimbriae on gastrointestinal pathogens, for example, or on the gonococcus. Route of administration of vaccines in order to obtain effective antibody response at the level of the mucosal surface will also need to be examined. To date the most effective antilectin (antiadhesin) vaccines have been dependent on passive transfer of colostral antibody. Parenterally introduced vaccines have been markedly less effective. In the case of gastrointestinal pathogens, oral vaccines are obviously most likely to induce a protective mucosal immunity. However, methods allowing penetration of mucus layers to the mucosal surface probably have to be considered to permit development of effective vaccines. Mucosal administration of vaccines on surfaces such as those of the urogenital and respiratory tracts will be more difficult, although an aerosol method may be effective in the latter case.

The possibility that purified bacterial surface lectins can be used for blocking receptors on target surfaces also must be explored. One of the few examples of this to date is the protection afforded to mice by oral administration of "cholera lectin" when the animals were subjected to oral challenge with *V. cholereae* (Finkelstein *et al.*, 1978). However, given the diversity of bacterial surface lectins and the probable complexity of their carbohydrate receptor structures, it may be more profitable to attempt to prevent mucosal surface colonization by nonspecific interactions (such as charge and hydrophobic interactions), instead of biospecific interactions based on lectin carbohydrate-binding characteristics. There is already one good example of this line of thought. Based on the concept that bacterial surface lectins of fimbrial nature show pronounced surface hydrophobic properties, hydrophobic gels were used quite successfully to prevent intestinal infections in an infant rabbit model with human ETEC (Wadström *et al.*, 1981a,b).

Another approach might be to use receptor megatherapy for therapy (Keusch, 1978). This may be most appropriate for gastrointestinal infections. Here it may be possible for oral administration of compounds with sufficiently great affinity for a bacterial adherence factor to compete with the natural epithelial cell receptor for binding to the organism. Keusch (1978) has suggested that, placed on a suitably large, indigestible, nonabsorbable carrier such as cellulose, this facsimile receptor would leave the normal flora undisturbed but would bind to pathogens and carry them out of the body. It could be driven in the desired direction by an excess of reactant and removal of the product: hence megatherapy, and use of a large particle which can be efficiently removed by peristalsis to elimination. The early discovery by Gibbons and co-workers (1975) that milk and saliva contain antiadhesive substances, presumably glycoconjugates, may also be important in this regard, and the possible presence of antiadhesive substances in foodstuffs deserves attention.

Receptor megatherapy has been used experimentally in the prevention of colonization of the urinary tract of mice with *E. coli*. In the case of simple sugars, it may even be reasonable to attempt to displace an organism from its binding site by using the appropriate sugar for elution. Aronson *et al.* (1979) have reported that the injection of mannose-sensitive *E. coli* in the presence of methyl-α-D-mannopyranoside resulted in a considerable reduction in the number of bacteriuric mice. A simple variation of receptor megatherapy might also be useful as a prophylactic measure in some cases (Keusch, 1978). Here an excess of some nontoxic molecule capable of binding to the eukaryotic receptor. By occupying the site it would block attachment.

The recent demonstration of the antiadhesive properties of certain antibiotics may also be of considerable therapeutic value. Roland and Heelan (1979) demonstrated that antibiotics such as tetracycline, chloramphenicol and nafcillin inhibited the haemagglutination of ETEC strains. These antibiotics have heterocyclic ring skeletons which give the molecule hydrophobic properties, and it is tempting to speculate that these compounds interact with hydrophobic patches on fimbriae adjacent to the sugar recognition sites and essentially prevent binding by steric blockade. Further studies will reveal if these or other compounds may be useful in inhibiting the colonization of mucosal surfaces by virulent bacteria.

XII.   SUMMARY

The successful colonization of an animal host by a variety of pathogenic bacteria requires an ability to attach to the epithelial surfaces of that host, especially those of the respiratory, alimentary and urogenital tracts. This specific adherence to the surface of epithelial cells is generally the first of a series of events which may include elaboration of toxins and invasion of the host. Successful parasites appear to have evolved special macromolecules that enhance their ability to adhere to epithelial cells. Such protein molecules have been referred to as adhesins (Duguid, 1959) and are expressed on the surface of the bacterium. The most readily recognized and best-studied adhesive proteins are the filamentous appendages known as fimbriae or colonization factors. In other cases, outer-membrane proteins of Gram-negative species have been implicated. The adhesive event involved specific recognition and interaction with carbohydrate moieties carried by glycoconjugate macromolecules on the surface of the eukaryotic cell. These recognition and interaction processes are analogous to plant lectin–polysaccharide interactions. Those bacterial adhesins that recognize and bind to carbohydrates have therefore been defined as bacterial surface lectins.

ADDENDUM

Recent studies on the binding of oral streptococci of different species to hydroxyapatite coated with salivary glycoproteins have confirmed that lectin-like surface components are involved in binding in this teeth-colonization model (Gibbons *et al.*, 1983). Recent studies on *Actinomyces viscosus* (Masuda *et al.*, 1983) have confirmed earlier studies on surface fibrils recognizing galactose residues of salivary glycoproteins and other glycoconjugates. Studies in progress on the ability of *Pseudomonas aeruginosa* to colonize mucus membranes of the respiratory tract indicate that this pathogen, as well as *Mycoplasma pneumoniae*, may recognize terminal sialic acid residues of different glycoconjugates, in addition to galactose and mannose. Most recently, Loomes *et al.* (1984) have reported that the interaction of *M. pneumoniae* with human erythrocytes is mediated by long-chain oligosaccharides of sialic acid joined by α-2,3 linkage to the terminal galactose residues of poly-*N*-acetyllactosamine sequences of the Ii antigen type. Interestingly, such diverse pathogens as *Chlamydia trachomatis* (Bose *et al.*, 1983) and enterotoxigenic *E. coli* with K99 fimbrial antigen may recognize a specific cell-membrane protein, glycophorin (Lindahl and Wadström, 1984). A Dutch group has also recently been able to isolate a glycolipid (haemotoside) with terminal *N*-acetylgalactosamine and sialic acid, which bind the K99 haemagglutinin, thus confirming the observation by Lindahl and Wadström (1983) that both *N*-acetylneuraminic acid (NANA) and terminal *N*-acetylgalactosamine are recognized by this lectin. Recent experiments also indicate that enterotoxigenic *E. coli* with other fimbrial proteins such as CFAI and CFAII may be classified as sialic acid-specific lectins, since neuraminidase treatment of erythrocytes and other cells prevents binding. Sialic acid polymers such as colominic acid (poly-α-2,8-NANA) and sialic-acid-rich glycoconjugates also inhibit binding of CFAI to human erythrocytes. In the case of the K88 lectin, Nilsson and Svensson, at a glycoconjugate symposium (1983), suggested that a specific glycolipid with α-Gal-Gal residues are recognized by this lectin, thus confirming reports already discussed in this review. In addition, Staley and Wilson (1983) have described the isolation of a specific glycoprotein from the porcine small-bowel brush borders that binds the K88 adhesin.

The fimbrial surface proteins of *E. coli* strains causing urinary tract infections have been extensively studied by two Swedish groups, and several review articles have been published on this topic. In brief, it now seems generally accepted that uropathogenic *E. coli* strains may bind to glycolipids containing the sequence Gal-α-1 → 4-Gal in an internal or terminal position (Källenius *et al.*, 1980b; Leffler and Svanborg-Edén, 1980). The name P-fimbriae has been proposed for this class of lectin, and their presence may be assayed by a particle agglutination test or by glycolipid-coated erythrocytes (Källenius *et al.*, 1981; Leffler and Svanborg-Edén, 1981). Subsequent studies have shown that saccharide structures containing Gal-α-1 → 4-Gal will protect young mice and monkeys against experimental ascending urinary tract infections with P-fimbriated *E. coli* strains (Roberts *et al.*, 1983). Recent research with the monkey model and P-fimbriated pyelonephritogenic *E. coli* indicate that α-Gal-1→3-Gal sugar compounds also inhibit colonization of the upper urinary tract (S. Svensson, personal communication). Besides P-fimbriae, uropathogenic *E. coli* carry other surface lectins (adhesins) specific for mannose residues (common type I fimbriae), *N*-

acetyl-D-glucosamine (Väisänen-Rhen *et al.*, 1983), sialic acid (Parkkinen and Finne, 1983), and other unknown receptors. These different adhesins may be carried simultaneously with each other. Since pyelonephritogenic *E. coli* often produce haemolysins and perhaps other cytolytic toxins (Berger *et al.*, 1983), it has been proposed that in the later stages of severe kidney infections, binding to subepithelial basal membrane components such as laminin may be important (Speziale *et al.*, 1982). Haemagglutinating strains of *Staphylococcus saprophyticus* and group A streptococci show lectin-like interactions with galactose residues on cells and carbohydrate polymers (Gunnarsson *et al.*, 1983; Tylewska and Wadström, 1981). In contrast, binding of fibronectin to staphylococci and group A streptococci is a biospecific, non-lectin-like interaction, inhibitable by the N-terminal 29,000-MW peptide fragment. (Binding of immunoglobulin to protein A on the *Staphylococcus aureus* cell surface is another nonlectin protein–protein interaction.) *Pseudomonas aeruginosa* proteases have been implicated in degrading the layer of fibronectin found on the surface of the oral mucosa. This appears to enable epithelial colonization, probably by surface fimbrial lectin(s) (Woods and Iglewski, 1983). Recent studies on *Neisseria gonorrhoeae* fimbrial antigens indicate that fimbrial proteins with different antigenic properties can recognize one specific cell surface ganglioside (GM_3) and probably glycoproteins with a similar terminal sugar sequence (Schoolnik *et al.*, 1982). Structural studies by Schoolnik *et al.* (1982) have also shown that functional and antigenic domains of the gonococcus pilus subunit can be assigned to peptides prepared by chemical cleavage at methionine residues. The receptor-binding function was found to reside in CNBr-2 between Arg-30 and Met-84. This CNBr-2 fimbrial peptide appears to be highly conserved and immunorecessive. The CNBr-3 fimbrial peptide encompasses a variable region of the fimbrial subunit and determines type-specific antigenicity, while the N-terminal CNBr-1 peptide is strongly hydrophobic and may stabilize polymeric structure.

The genetics of bacteria surface lectins has also commanded considerable attention. For example, the genetic determinant for the K88ab fimbriae has been isolated by molecular cloning (Mooi *et al.*, 1983). This study revealed that four genes encoding for polypeptides with apparent molecular weights of 17,000, 26,000 (the fimbrial subunit), 27,000 and 81,000 are implicated in the biosynthesis of the K88ab fimbria. The 81,000-MW polypeptide is probably involved in translocating fimbrial subunits across the outer membrane. Mooi *et al.* (1983) propose that the 27,000-MW polypeptide might be involved in stabilizing a conformation of the fimbrial subunit required to translocate it across the outer membrane, while the 17,000-MW polypeptide might modify the fimbrial subunits to allow assembly into functional fimbriae. A 27,500-MW polypeptide located on a separate operon is also involved in the biosynthesis of K88ab fimbriae, but its role remains to be determined (de Graaf and Gaastra, 1982). The genes coding for K99 fimbria have also been cloned, as have the genes determining production of mannose-resistant fimbriae and P-fimbriae in uropathogenic strains of *E. coli* (Clegg, 1982; Rhen *et al., 1983*). Molecular cloning has also recently provided important information on the expression of fimbriae in *N. gonorrhoeae*. Indeed, Meyer *et al.* (1982) have presented evidence that conversion of the fimbriae-positive to fimbriae-negative state in *N. gonorrhoeae* involves chromosomal rearrangement.

ACKNOWLEDGMENTS

The authors thank all scientists who supplied us with unpublished information. We especially want to thank R. Ellner, R. A. Finkelstein, R. J. Gibbons, and M. Gill.

T. J. Trust is the recipient of a research grant from the Natural Sciences and Engineering Research Council of Canada and NATO Research grant RG126.80. Grants from the Swedish Medical Research Council (16X47023) and the Swedish Board for Technical Development to T. Wadström are also acknowledged.

REFERENCES

Arai, H., and Munoz, J. J. (1981). *Infect. Immun.* **31**, 495–499.
Arai, H., and Sato, Y. (1976). *Biochim. Biophys. Acta* **444**, 765–782.
Ariizumi, K., Oishi, K., and Aida, K. (1980). *J. Gen. Appl. Microbiol.* **26**, 239–244.
Aronson, M., Medalea, O., Schori, L., Mirelman, D., Sharon, N., and Ofek, I. (1979). *J. Infect. Dis.* **139**, 329–332.
Atkinson, H. M., and Trust, T. J. (1980). *Infect. Immun.* **27**, 928–946.
Bagg, J., Paxton, I. R., Doyle, J., Ross, P. W., and Weir, D. M. (1980b). *In* "Microbial Adhesion to Surfaces" (R. C. W. Berkeley, J. M. Lynch, J. Melling, P. R. Rutter, and D. Vincent, eds.), pp. 528–530. Soc. Chem. Ind., Ellis Harwood Ltd., Chichester, England.
Banai, M., Razin, S., Bredt, W., and Kahane, I. (1980). *Infect. Immun.* **32**, 628–634.
Barondes, S. H. (1981). *Annu. Rev. Biochem.* **50**, 207–231.
Bartus, H., Zajac, I., Sedlock, D., and Actor, P. (1980). *Intersci. Conf. Antimicrob. Agents Chemother., 20th.* Abstract 635.
Barua, D., and Mukherjee, A. C. (1963). *Bull. Calcutta Sch. Trop. Med.* **11**, 85–86.
Beachey, E. H., ed. (1980). "Receptors and Recognition," Ser. B, Vol. 6. Chapman & Hall, London.
Beachey, E. H. (1981). *J. Infect. Dis.* **143**, 325–345.
Beachey, E. H., Simpson, W. A., and Ofek, I. (1980). *In* "Microbial Adhesion to Surfaces" (R. C. W. Berkeley, J. M. Lynch, J. Melling, P. R. Rutter, and B. Vincent, eds.), pp. 389–406. Soc. Chem. Ind., Ellis Harwood Ltd., Chichester, England.
Berger, H., Jacker, J., Höf, H., Hughes, C., Juarez, A., Knapp, S., Müller, D., and Goebel, W. (1983). *In* "Experimental Bacterial and Parasitic Infections" (G. Keusch and T. Wadström, eds.), pp. 137–145. Elsevier/North-Holland Biomedical Press, Amsterdam.

Bhattacharjee, J. W., and Srivastava, B. S. (1978). *J. Gen. Microbiol.* **107**, 407–410.

Bose, S. K., Smith, G. B., and Paul, R. G. (1983). *Infect. Immun.* **40**, 1060–1067.

Boyd, W. C., and Reguera, R. M. (1949). *J. Immunol.* **62**, 333.

Boyd, W. C., and Shapleigh, E. (1954a). *J. Lab. Clin. Med.* **44**, 235.

Boyd, W. C., and Shapleigh, E. (1954b). *J. Immunol.* **73**, 226–236.

Bredt, W., Feldner, J., and Hanne, I. (1980). *Ciba Found. Symp.* **80**, 3–16.

Brinton, C. C. (1959). *Nature (London)* **183**, 782–786.

Brinton, C. C. (1965). *Trans. N.Y. Acad. Sci.* [2] **27**, 1003–1054.

Brinton, C. D., Buzzell, A., and Lauffer, M. A. (1954). *Biochim. Biophys. Acta* **15**, 533–542.

Brinton, C. C., Bryan, J., Dillen, J. A., Guerina, N., Jacobson, L. J., Labik, A., Lee, S., Levine, A., Lim, S., McMichael, J., Polen, S., Rigers, K., To, A. C. C., and To, S. C. M. (1978). *In* "Immunobiology of Neisseria Gonorrhoea" (G. F. Brooks, E. C. Gotschlich, K. K. Holmes, W. D. Sawyer, and F. E. Young, eds.), pp. 155–178. Am. Soc. Microbiol. Washington, D. C.

Brooks, D. E., and Trust, T. J. (1983). *J. Gen. Microbiol.* **129**, 3661–3669.

Brooks, D. E., Goodwin, J. W., and Seaman, G. V. F. (1974). *Biorheology* **11**, 69–77.

Brunner, H., Krauss, H., Schaar, H., and Scheifer, H.-G. (1979). *Infect. Immun.* **24**, 906–901.

Buchanan, T. M. (1976). *In* "Microbiology 1976" (D. Schlessinger, ed.), Am. Soc. Microbiol., Washington, D.C.

Buchanan, T. M., and Hildebrandt, J. F. (1981). *Infect. Immun.* **22**, 985–994.

Buchanan, T. M., Pearce, W. A., Schoolnik, G. K., and Arko, R. J. (1977). *J. Infect. Dis.* **136**, 5132–5137.

Buchanan, T. M., Pearce, W. A., and Chen, K. C. S. (1978). *In* "Immunobiology of Neisseria Gonorrhoea" (G. F. Brooks, E. C. Gotschlich, K. K. Holmes, W. D. Sawyer, and F. E. Young, eds.), pp. 242–249. Am. Soc. Microbiol. Washington, D.C.

Chick, S., Harber, M. J., Mackenzie, R., and Asscher, A. W. (1981). *Infect. Immun.* **34**, 256–261.

Clegg, S. (1982). *Infect. Immun.* **38**, 739–744.

Clements, J., and Finkelstein, R. A. (1979). *Infect. Immun.* **24**, 760–766.

Cole, H. D., Staley, T. E., and Whipp, S. C. (1977). *Infect. Immun.* **16**, 374–481.

Collier, A. M. (1980). *Recept. Recognition, Ser. B* **6**, 159–184.

Cuatrecasas, P. (1973). *Biochemistry* **12**, 1312–1323.

Cumsky, M., and Zusman, D. R. (1979). *Proc. Natl. Acad. Sci. U.S.A.* **76**, 5505–5509.

Davey, M. W., Sulkowski, E., and Carter, W. A. (1976). *Biochemistry* **15**, 704–712.

de Graaf, F. K., and Gaastra, W. (1982). *Microbiol. Rev.* **46**, 129–161.

de Graaf, F. K., Wientjes, F. B., and Klaasen-Boor, P. (1980a). *Infect. Immun.* **27**, 216–221.

de Graaf, F. K., Klaasen-Boor, P., and van Hees, J. E. (1980b). *Infect. Immun.* **30**, 125–128.

Diamantstein, T., Trisse, D., Klos, M., Gold, D., and Hahn, H. (1980). *Immunology* **41**, 347–351.

Duguid, J. P. (1959). *J. Gen. Microbiol.* **21**, 271–286.

Duguid, J. P., and Campbell, J. (1969). *J. Med. Microbiol.* **2**, 535–553.

Duguid, J. P., and Old, D. C. (1980). *Recept. Recognition, Ser. B* **6**, 185–218.

Duguid, J. P., Smith, I. W., Dempster, G., and Edmunds, P. N. (1955). *J. Pathol. Bacteriol.* **70**, 335–348.

Edebo, L., Hed, J., Kihlström, E., Magnusson, K. E., and Stendahl, O. (1980). *Scand. J. Infect. Dis., Suppl.* **124**, 93–99.

Ellen, R. P., Loung, W. L. S., Pillery, E. D., and Grove, D. A. (1980). *Infect. Immun.* **26**, 427–434.

Ellen, R. P., Illery, E. D., Chan, K. H., and Grove, D. A. (1981). *Infect. Immun.* **27**, 335–343.

Eshdat, Y., Ofek, I., Yashouv-Gan, Y., Sharon, N., and Mirelman, D. (1978). *Biochem. Biophys. Res. Commun.* **85**, 1557–1559.

Etzler, M. E. (1979). *Am. J. Clin. Nutr.* **32**, 133–139.

Evans, D. G., Evans, D. J., and Selvidge, L. A. (1981). *Abstr. Annu. Meet. Am. Soc. Microbiol.* p. 152.

Fader, R. C., Avots-Avotins, A. E., and Dais, C. P. (1979). *Infect. Immun.* **25**, 729–737.

Falker, W. A., and Hawley, C. E. (1977). *Infect. Immun.* **15**, 230–238.

Faris, A., Lindahl, M., and Wadström, T. (1980). *FEMS Microbiol. Lett.* **7**, 265–269.

Faris, A., Wadström, T., and Freer, J. H. (1981). *Curr. Microbiol.* **5**, 67–72.

Finkelstein, R. A., and Hanne, I. (1982). *Infect. Immun.* **36**, 1199–1208.

Finkelstein, R. A., and Mukherjee, S. (1963). *Proc. Soc. Exp. Biol. Med.* **112**, 355–359.

Finkelstein, R. A., Arita, M., Clements, J. A., and Nelson, E. T. (1978). *In Proc. J. Conf. Cholera (U.S.-Jpn. Coop. Med. Sci. Program), 13th, 1977* pp. 137–151.

Formisano, S., Johnson, M. L., Lee, G., Aloj, S. M., and Edelhoch, H. (1979). *Biochemistry* **18**, 1119–1124.

Fowler, J. E., and Stamey, T. A. (1977). *J. Urol.* **117**, 472–476.

Freter, R. (1980a). *Ciba Found. Symp.* **80**, 47–55.

Freter, R. (1980b). *Recept. Recognition, Ser. B* **6**, 439–458.

Fuller, R., and Brooker, B. E. (1980). *In* "Microbial Adhesion to Surfaces" (R. C. W. Berkeley, J. M. Lynch, J. Melling, R. P. Rutter, and B. Vincent, eds.), pp. 495–507. Soc. Chem. Ind., Ellis Harwood Ltd., Chichester, England.

Gabridge, M. G., and Taylor-Robinson, D. (1979). *Infect. Immun.* **25**, 455–459.

Garber, N., Glick, J., Gilboa-Garber, N., and Heller, A. (1981). *J. Gen. Microbiol.* **123**, 359–363.

Gibbons, R. J., and Quareshi, J. V. (1978). *Infect. Immun.* **22**, 665–671.

Gibbons, R. J., and Quareshi, J. V. (1979). *Infect. Immun.* **26**, 1214–1217.

Gibbons, R. J., and van Houte, J. (1980). *Recept. Recognition, Ser. B* **6**, 61–104.

Gibbons, R. J., van Houte, J., and Liljemark, W. F. (1972). *J. Dent. Res.* **51**, 424–425.

Gibbons, R. J., Etherden, I., and Moreno, E. C. (1983). *Infect. Immun.* **42**, 1006–1012.

Gibbons, T. R. A., Jones, G. W., and Sellwood, R. (1975). *J. Gen. Microbiol.* **186**, 228–240.

Gilboa-Garber, N. (1972). *FEBS Lett.* **20**, 282–284.

Gilboa-Garber, N. (1982). *Meth. Enzym.* **83**, 378–385.

Gilboa-Garber, N., Mizrahi, L., and Garber, N. (1977). *Can. J. Biochem.* **55**, 975–981.

Gingras, S. P., and Howard, L. V. (1980). *Appl. Environm. Microbiol.* **39**, 369–371.

Girardeau, J. P. (1980). *Ann. Microbiol. (Paris)* **131B**, 31–37.

Goldstein, I. J., and Hayes, C. E. (1978). *Adv. Carbohydr. Chem. Biochem.* **35**, 128–340.

Greig, R. G., and Brooks, D. E. (1979). *Nature (London)* **282**, 738.

Greig, R. G., and Brooks, D. E. (1981). *Biochim. Biophys. Acta* **641**, 410–415.

Gunnarsson, A., Mardh, P. A., Lundblad, A., and Svensson, S. (1983). *In* "Glycoconjugates" (M. A. Chester, D. Heinegård, A. Lundblad, and S. Svensson, eds.), pp. 645–646. Rahms, Lund.

Gyot, G. (1908). *Zentralbl. Bakteriol., Parasitenkd. Infektionskr. Hyg., Abt. 1: Orig.* **47**, 640–657.

Hanne, L. F., and Finkelstein, R. A. (1982). *Infect. Immun.* **36**, 209–214.
Hart, D. A. (1980). *Am. J. Clin. Nutr.* **33**, 2416–2439.
Haywood, A. M. (1974). *J. Mol. Biol.* **83**, 427–436.
Hermodsen, M. A., Chen, K. C. S., and Buchanan, T. M. (1978). *Biochemistry* **17**, 442–445.
Hjertén, S. (1981). *Methods Biochem. Anal.* **27**, 89–94.
Holmgren, J. (1978). *In* "Bacterial Toxins and Cell Membranes" (J. Jeljaszewicz and T. Wadström, eds.), pp. 333–366. Academic Press, London.
Holmgren, J., Elwing, H. G., Fredman, P., Strannegård, Ö., and Svennerholm, L. (1980). *Adv. Exp. Med. Biol.* **125**, 453–470.
Honda, E., and Yanagawa, R. (1974). *Infect. Immun.* **10**, 1426–1432.
Honda, E., and Yanagawa, R. (1978). *Am. J. Vet. Res.* **39**, 155–158.
Hoskins, L. C. (1978). *In* "The Glycoconjugates" (M. I. Horowitz and W. Pigman, eds.), Vol. 2, pp. 235–255. Academic Press, New York.
Hoskins, L. C., and Boulding, E. T. (1981). *J. Clin. Invest.* **67**, 163–172.
Howard, R. J., and Miller, L. H. (1981). *Ciba Found. Symp.* **80**, 202–219.
Irons, L. I., and MacLennan, A. P. (1978). *Dev. Biol. Stand.* **40**, 338–349.
Jann, K., Schmidt, G., Blumenstock, E., and Vosbeck, K. (1981). *Infect. Immun.* **32**, 484–489.
Järvinen, A. K., and Sandholm, M. (1980). *Invest. Urol.* **17**, 443–446.
Jephott, A. E., Reyn, A., and Birch-Hansen, A. (1971). *Acta Pathol. Microbiol. Scand., Sect. B: Microbiol. Immunol.* **79B** 437–439.
Jones, G. W. (1977). *Recep. Recognition, Ser. B* **3**, 139–176.
Jones, G. W. (1980). *Recept. Recognition, Ser. B* **6**, 219–250.
Jones, G. W., and Freter, R. (1976). *Infect. Immun.* **14**, 240–245.
Jones, G. W., Abrams, G. D., and Freter, R. (1976). *Infect. Immun.* **14**, 232–239.
Källenius, G. (1981). Dissertation, Reproprint AB, Stockholm.
Källenius, G., and Winberg, J. (1978). *Lancet* **2**, 540–543.
Källenius, G., Möllby, R., Svensson, S. B., Winberg, J., Lundblad, A., Svensson, S., and Cedergren, B. (1980a). *FEMS Microbiol. Lett.* **7**, 297–302.
Källenius, G., Möllby, R., Svensson, S. B., Winberg, J., and Hultberg, H. (1980b). *Infection* **8**, S288–S293.
Källenius, G., Möllby, R., Svensson, S. B., Helin, I., Hultberg, H., Cedergren, B., and Winberg, J. (1981). *Lancet* **2**, 1369–1372.
Kearns, M. J., and Gibbons, R. A. (1979). *FEMS Microbiol. Lett.* **6**, 165–168.
Keogh, E. V., and North, E. A. (1947). *Nature (London)* **160**, 63.
Keogh, E. V., North, E. A., and Warburton, M. F. (1947). *Aust. J. Exp. Biol. Med. Sci.* **26**, 315–322.
Keusch, G. I. (1978). *Am. J. Clin. Nutr.* **31**, 2208–2218.
Keusch, G. T. (1979). *Rev. Infect. Dis.* **1**, 517–529.
Kilian, M., Mestecky, J., and Schrohenloher, R. E. (1979). *Infect. Immun.* **26**, 143–149.
Kjelleberg, S., Lagercrantz, C., and Larsson, T. (1980). *FEMS Microbiol. Lett.* **7**, 41–44.
Kobiler, D., and Mirelman, D. (1980). *Infect. Immun.* **29**, 221–225.
Kobiler, D., Mirelman, D., and Mattern, C. F. T. (1981). *Ciba Found. Symp.* **80**, 17–35.
Kocourec, J., and Horejsic, V. (1981). *Nature (London)* **290**, 188.
Kohn, L. D., Grollman, E. F., Ledley, F. D., Mullin, B. R., Friedman, R. M., Meldolesi, M. F., and Aloj. S. M. (1978). *In* "Cell Surface Carbohydrate Chemistry" (R. E. Harmon, ed.), pp. 103–133. Academic Press, New York.
Kohn, L. D., Consiglio, E., Aloj, S. M., Beguinot, F., De Wolf, M. J. S., Yavin, E.,

Yavin, Z., Meldolesi, M. F., Shifrin, S., Gill, D. L., Vitti, P., Lee, G., Valente, W. A., and Grollman, E. F. I. (1981). *In* "International Cell Biology" (H.-G. Schweiger, ed.), pp. 696–706. Springer-Verlag, Berlin.

Korhonen, T. K. (1980). *FEMS Microbiol. Lett.* **6**, 421–425.

Korhonen, T. K., Eden, S., and Svanborg-Eden, C. (1980). *FEMS Microbiol. Lett.* **7**, 237–240.

Korhonen, T. K., Leffler, H., and Svanborg-Eden, C. (1981). *Infect. Immun.* **32**, 796–804.

Kronvall, G., Björck, L., Myhre, E., and Wannamaker, L. W. (1979). *Pathogen. Streptococci, Proc. Int. Symp., 7th, 1978* pp. 74–76.

Kuusela, P. (1978). *Nature (London)* **276**, 718–720.

Lambden, P. R., Heckels, J. E., James, L. T., and Watt, P. J. (1979). *J. Gen. Microbiol.* **114**, 305–310.

Lambden, P. R., Robertson, J. N., and Watt, P. J. (1980). *J. Bacteriol.* **141**, 393–396.

Lambden, P. R., Heckels, J. E., McBride, H., and Watt, P. J. (1981). *FEMS Microbiol. Lett.* **10**, 339–341.

Lankford, C. E., and Legsomburana, U. (1965). *In* "Proceedings of the Cholera Research Symposium," pp. 109–120. U.S. Govt. Printing Office, Washington, D.C.

Leffler, H., and Svanborg-Eden, C. (1980). *FEMS Microbiol. Lett.* **8**, 127–143.

Leffler, H., and Svanborg-Edén, C. (1981). *Infect. Immun.* **34**, 920–929.

Levett, P. N., and Daniel, R. R. (1981). *J. Gen. Microbiol.* **125**, 167–172.

Levine, M. (1981). *Ciba Found. Symp.* **80**, 142–160.

Levine, M. M., Black, R. E., Brinton, C. C., Jr., and Clements, M. L. (1982). *Scand. J. Infect. Dis. Suppl.* **33**, 83–95.

Levy, N. J. (1979). *Infect. Immun.* **2**, 946–953.

Lindahl, M., and Wadström, T. (1983). *IRCS Med. Sci.: Libr. Compend.* **11**, 790.

Lindahl, M., and Wästrom, T. (1984). *Vet. Microbiol.* (in press).

Lindahl, M., Faris, A., Wadström, T., and Hjertén, S. (1981). *Biochim. Biophys. Acta* **677**, 471–476.

Lindahl, M., Faris, A., Hjertén, S., and Wadström, T. (1984). *In* "Attachment of Microorganisms to Intestinal Mucosa" (E. Boedeker, ed.). CRC Press, Boca Raton, Florida (in press).

Linder, L., Lund, M. L., Hjertén, S., and Wadström, T. (1984). To be published.

Lis, H., and Sharon, N. (1977). *In* "The Antigens", (M. Sela, ed.), Vol. 4, pp. 429–529. Academic Press, New York.

Ljungh, Å., Eneroth, P., and Wadström, T. (1982). *Toxicon* **20**, 787–797.

Lonberg-Holm, K., and Philipsson, L. (1981). *Recept. Recognition, Ser. B* **8**, Part 2, 217 pp.

Loomes, L. M., Vemura, K., Childs, R. A., Paulson, J. C., Rogers, G. N., Scudder, P. R., Michalski, J.-C., Hounsell, E. F., Taylor-Robinson, D., and Feizi, T. (1984). *Nature (London)* **307**, 560–563.

Lotan, R., Beattle, G., Hubell, W., and Nicolson, G. L. (1977). *Biochemistry* **16**, 1787–1794.

MacLagan, R. M., and Old, D. C. (1980). *J. Appl. Bacteriol.* **49**, 353–360.

Magnusson, K. E., and Johansson, G. (1977). *FEMS Microbiol. Lett.* **2**, 225–227.

Masuda, N., Ellen, R. P., Fillery, E. D., and Grove, D. A. (1983). *Infect. Immun.* **39**, 1325–1333.

Meyer, T. F., Mlawer, N., and So, M. (1982). *Cell* **30**, 45–52.

Mongiello, J. R., and Falker, W. A. (1979). *Arch. Oral Biol.* **24**, 539–543.

Mooi, F. R., Wijfjes, A., and de Graaf, F. K. (1983). *J. Bacteriol.* **154**, 41–49.

Moon, H. W., Kohler, E. M., Schneider, R. A., and Whipp, S. C. (1980). *Infect. Immun.* **27**, 222–230.

Morse, S. I. (1976). *Adv. Appl. Microbiol.* **20**, 9–26.

Munoz, J. J. and Bergman, R. K. (1977). "Bordetella Pertussis, Immunological and other Biological Activities," pp. 47–65. Dekker, New York.

Nagy, B., Moon, H. W., Isaacson, R. E., To, C. C., and Brinton, C. C. (1978). *Infect. Immun.* **21**, 269–274.

Nalin, D. R. (1978). *Lancet* **2**, 958.

Nicolson, G. L. (1974). *Int. Rev. Cytol.* **39**, 89–190.

Nilsson, G., and Svensson, S. (1983). *In* "Glycoconjugates" (M. A. Chester, D. Heinegård, A. Lundblad, and S. Svensson, eds.), pp. 637–638. Rahms, Lund.

Nelson, E. T., Clements, J., and Finkelstein, R. A. (1976). *Infect. Immun.* **14**, 527–547.

Ochoa, J. L. (1980). Dissertation, University of Uppsala, Sweden.

Ochoa, J. L., and Kristiansen, T. (1978). *FEBS Lett.* **90**, 145–148.

Ochoa, J. L., Kristiansen, T., and Påhlman, S. (1979). *Biochim. Biophys. Acta* **577**, 102–109.

Old, D. C. (1963). Ph.D. Thesis, University of Edinburgh, Scotland.

Old, D. C. (1972). *J. Gen. Microbiol.* **71**, 149–157.

Old, D. C., and Scott, S. S. (1981). *J. Bacteriol.* **146**, 404–408.

Olsnes, S., Eikleid, K., and Jonsen, J. (1980). *In* "Natural Toxins" (D. Eaker and T. Wadström, eds.), pp. 471–479. Pergamon, Oxford.

Olsnes, S., Resibig, R., and Eiklid, K. (1981). *J. Biol. Chem.* **256**, 8732–8738.

Ørskov, I., Frencz, A., and Ørskov, F. (1980a). *Lancet* **1**, 265–269.

Ørskov, I., Ørskov, F., and Birch-Andersen, A. (1980b). *Infect. Immun.* **27**, 657–666.

Pan, Y. T., Schmitt, J. W., Sanford, B. A., and Elbein, A. D. (1979). *J. Bacteriol.* **139**, 507–514.

Parkkinen, J., and Finne, J. (1983). *Eur. J. Biochem.* **136**, 355–361.

Parsons, C. L., and Mulholland, S. G. (1978). *Am. J. Pathol.* **93**, 423–432.

Pearce, W. A. and Buchanan, T. M. (1980). *Recept. Recognition, Ser. B* **6**, 289–344.

Pereira, M. E., Loures, M. A., Vialta, F., and Andrade, A. F. B. (1980). *J. Exp. Med.* **152**, 1375–1392.

Pittman, M. (1979). *Rev. Infect. Dis.* **1**, 410–412.

Plaut, A. G. (1978). *N. Engl. J. Med.* **298**, 1459–1463.

Poste, G., and Nicolson, G. (1977). *Cell Surf. Rev.* **2**, 5–194.

Punsalang, A. P., and Sawyer, W. D. (1973). *Infect. Immun.* **8**, 255–263.

Ramirez-Ronda, C. H. (1978). *Clin. Res.* **26**, 404A.

Ramphal, R., Small, P. M., Shands, J. W., Fischlschweiger, W., and Small, P. A. (1980). *Infect. Immun.* **27**, 614–619.

Rankin, D. W., and Fischer, S. (1956). *Med. J. Aust.* **1**, 873–875.

Ravdin, J. I., Croft, B. Y., and Guerrant, R. L. (1980). *J. Exp. Med.* **152**, 377–390.

Razin, S., Kahane, I., Banai, M., and Bredt, W. (1981). *Ciba Found. Symp.* **80**, 98–118.

Reed, W. P., and Williams, R. C. (1978). *J. Chronic Dis.* **31**, 67–72.

Renkonen, K. P. (1948). *Ann. Med. Exp. Biol. Fenn.* **26**, 66.

Rhen, M., Knowles, J., Penttilä, M. E., Sarvas, M., and Korhonen, T. K. (1983). *FEMS Microbiol. Lett.* **19**, 119–123.

Richards, R. L., Moss, J., Alving, C. R., Fishman, P. H., and Brady, R. O. (1979). *Proc. Natl. Acad. Sci. U.S.A.* **76**, 1673–1676.

Roberts, J. A., Kaack, B., and Dominque, G. J. (1983). *In* "Experimental Bacterial and Parasitic Infections" (G. Keusch and T. Wadström, eds.), pp. 125–129. Elsevier/North-Holland Biomedical Press, Amsterdam.

Roland, F., and Heelan, J. (1979). *Ann. Microbiol. (Paris)* **130B**, 33–42.

Rosenberg, M., Gutnik, D., and Rosenberg, E. (1980). *FEMS Microbiol. Lett.* **7**, 265–269.

Rutter, J. M. (1981). *In* "Proceedings of the Third International Symposium on Neonatal Diarrhea" (S. C. Acres, A. J. Forman, and H. Fast, eds.), pp. 183–200. Vet. Infect. Dis. Organ. (VIDO) Publications, University of Saskatchewan, Saskatoon, Canada.

Rutter, J. M., Burrows, M. R., Sellwood, R., and Gibbons, R. A. (1975). *Nature (London)* **257**, 135–136.

Rydén, C., Rubin, K., Höök, M., Speziale, P., Lindahl, M., and Wadström, T. (1981). *J. Biol. Chem.* **258**, 3396–3401.

Salit, I. E., and Gotschlich, E. C. (1977). *J. Exp. Med.* **146**, 1182–1193.

Sato, Y., Izumiya, K., Oda, M. S., and Sato, H. (1978). *Dev. Biol. Stand.* **40**, 51–57.

Sato, Y., Izumiya, K., Sato, H., Cowell, J. L., and Manclark, C. R. (1981). *Infect. Immun.* **31**, 1223–1231.

Schaeffer, A. J., Amundsen, S. K., and Schmidt, L. N. (1979). *Infect Immun.* **24**, 753–759.

Schoolnik, G. K., Tai, J. Y., and Gotschlich, E. C. (1982). *In* "Microbiology—1982" (D. Schlessinger, ed.), pp. 312–316. Am. Soc. Microbiol., Washington, D.C.

Selinger, D. S., Julie, N., Reed, W. P., and Williams, R. C. (1978). *Science* **201**, 455–457.

Selinger, D. S., Adler, S. W., Kelly, R. P., and Reed, W. P. (1980). *Curr. Chemother. Infect. Dis., Proc. Int. Congr. Chemother. 11th, 1979* pp. 790–792.

Sellwood, R. (1980). *Biochim. Biophys. Acta* **632**, 326–335.

Sharon, N., Esdat, Y., Silverblatt, F. J., and Ofek, I. (1981). *Ciba Found. Symp.* **80**, 119–141.

Silverblatt, I. J. (1974). *J. Exp. Med.* **140**, 1696–1711.

Smith, H. W. (1976). *Soc. Appl. Bacteriol. Symp.* **4**, 227–242.

Smith, H. W. (1977). *Bacteriol. Rev.* **41**, 475–500.

Smyth, C. J., Jonsson, P., Olsson, E., Söderlind, O., Hjertén, S., and Wadström, T. (1978). *Infect. Immun.* **22**, 462–472.

Speziale, P., Höök, M., Wadström, T., and Timpl, R. (1982). *FEBS Lett.* **146**, 55–58.

Staaf, R. H., Langley, S. D., and Doyle, R. J. (1980). *Infect. Immun.* **27**, 657–681.

Staley, T. E., and Wilson, I. B. (1983). *Mol. Cell. Biochem.* **52**, 177–189.

Stanbridge, E. J. (1976). *Annu. Rev. Microbiol.* **30**, 169–187.

Stanbridge, E. J., and Weiss, R. L. (1978). *Nature (London)* **276**, 583–587.

Stillmark, H. (1888). Inaugural Dissertation, University of Dorpat, Dorpat, Estonia.

Stillmark, H. (1889). "Arbeiten des Pharmakologischen Institutes zu Dorpat," Vol. III, pp. 59–151. Enke, Stuttgart.

Svanborg-Eden, C., and Hansson, L. Å. (1978). *Infect. Immun.* **21**, 229–237.

Swanson, J., Kraus, S. J., and Gotschlich, E. C. (1971). *J. Exp. Med.* **134**, 886–906.

Sweeney, G., and Freer, J. (1979). *J. Gen. Microbiol.* **112**, 321–328.

Switalski, L. (1976). *Zentralbl. Bakteriol., Parasitenkd., Infektionskr. Hyg., Abt. 1, Suppl.* **5**, 413–426.

Takenaka, A., Oishi, K., and Aida, K. (1979). *J. Gen. Appl. Microbiol.* **25**, 297–400.

Tanford, C. (1980). "The Hydrophobic Effect," 2nd ed. Wiley (Interscience), New York.

Trust, T. J., and Chipman, D. C. (1979). *Can. Med. Assoc. J.* **120**, 942–946.

Trust, T. J., Lambden, P. R., and Watt, P. J. (1980). *J. Gen. Microbiol.* **119**, 179–187.

Tweedy, J. M., Park, W. A., and Hodgkiss, W. (1968). *J. Gen. Microbiol.* **51**, 235–244.

Tylewska, S., Hjertén, S., and Wadström, T. (1979). *FEMS Microbiol. Lett.* **6**, 248–253.

Väisänen-Rhen, V., Korhonen, T. K., and Finne, J. (1983). *FEBS Lett.* **159**, 233–236.
Vance, D. W., and Hatch, T. P. (1980). *Infect. Immun.* **29**, 175–180.
van Oss, C. J. (1978). *Annu. Rev. Microbiol.* **32**, 19–39.
Wadström, T., and Tylewska, S. (1982). *Curr. Microbiol.* **7**, 343–348.
Wadström, T., Ljungh, Å., and Wretlind, B. (1976). *Acta Pathol. Microbiol. Scand., Sect. B: Microbiol.* **84B**, 112–114.
Wadström, T., Smyth, C. J., Faris, A., Jonsson, P., and Freer, J. H. (1978). *In* "Proceedings of the Second International Symposium on Neonatal Diarrhea" (S. C. Acres, ed.), pp. 29–55. Stuart Bundle Press, Saskatoon, Canada.
Wadström, T., Faris, A., Hjertén, S., and Lindahl, M. (1980a). *In* "Microbial Adhesion to Surfaces" (R. C. W. Berkeley, J. M. Lynch, J. Melling, P. R. Rutter, and D. Vincent, eds.), pp. 537–540. Soc. Chem. Ind., Ellis Harwood Ltd., Chichester, England.
Wadström, T., Faris, A., Freer, J. H., Habte, D., Hallberg, D., and Ljungh, Å. (1980b). *Scand. J. Infect. Dis., Suppl.* **24**, 148–153.
Wadström, T., Faris, A., Lindahl, M., Hjertén, S., and Ågerup, B. (1981a). *Scand. J. Infect. Dis.* **13**, 129–132.
Wadström, T., Faris, A., Lindahl, M., Lövgren, K., Ågerup, B., and Hjertén, S. (1981b). *In* "Proceedings of the Third International Symposium on Neonatal Diarrhea" (S. C. Acres, A. J. Forman, and H. Fast, eds.), pp. 237–250. Vet. Infect. Dis. Organ. (VIDO) Publications, University of Saskatchewan, Saskatoon, Canada.
Wadström, T. *et al.*, (1984a). In preparation.
Wadström, T. *et al.*, (1984). In preparation.
Watkins, W. M. (1966). *BBA Libr.* **5**, 462–513.
Watt, P. J. (1980a). *In* "Microbial Adhesion to Surfaces" (R. C. W. Berkeley, J. M. Lunch, J. Melling, R. P. Rutter, and B. Vincent, eds.). Soc. Chem. Ind., Ellis Harwood Ltd., Chichester, England.
Watt, P. J. (1980b). *Symp. Br. Soc. Cell Biol.* **3**, 137–170.
Wise, K. S., Cassell, G. H., and Acton, R. T. (1978). *Proc. Natl. Acad. Sci. U.S.A.* **75**, 4479–4483.
Woods, D. E., and Iglewski, B. H. (1983). *Rev. Infect. Dis.* **5**, Suppl. 4S, 715–722.
Zanetta, J. P., and Gombos, G. (1976). *In* "Con A as a Tool" (H. Bittiger and H. P. Schnebli, eds.), pp. 389–398. Wiley, London.

Index